NEPHROLOGY SECRETS

DONALD E. HRICIK, M.D.

Professor of Medicine
Chief, Division of Nephrology
Case Western Reserve University
    School of Medicine
Medical Director, Transplantation Services
Department of Medicine
University Hospitals of Cleveland
Cleveland, Ohio

JOHN R. SEDOR, M.D.

Professor of Medicine, Physiology,
    and Biophysics
Case Western Reserve University
    School of Medicine
Chief, Division of Nephrology
Department of Medicine
MetroHealth Medical Center
Cleveland, Ohio

MICHAEL B. GANZ, M.D.

Associate Professor of Medicine
Case Western Reserve University
    School of Medicine
Chief, Division of Nephrology
Department of Medicine
Veterans Affairs Medical Center
Cleveland, Ohio

HANLEY & BELFUS, INC./ Philadelphia

Publisher: HANLEY & BELFUS, INC.
Medical Publishers
210 South 13th Street
Philadelphia, PA 19107
(215) 546-7293; 800-962-1892
FAX (215) 790-9330
Web site: http://www.hanleyandbelfus.com

Note to the reader: Although the information in this book has been carefully reviewed for correctness of dosage and indications, neither the authors nor the editors nor the publisher can accept any legal responsibility for any errors or omissions that may be made. Neither the publisher nor the editors make any warranty, expressed or implied, with respect to the material contained herein. Before prescribing any drug, the reader must review the manufacturer's current product information (package inserts) for accepted indications, absolute dosage recommendations, and other information pertinent to the safe and effective use of the product described. This is especially important when drugs are given in combination or as an adjunct to other forms of therapy.

Library of Congress Cataloging-in-Publication Data

Nephrology secrets / edited by Donald E. Hricik, John R. Sedor,
  Michael B. Ganz.
      p.   cm. — (The secrets series)
   Includes bibliographical references and index.
   ISBN 1-56053-309-9 (alk. paper)
   1. Kidneys—Diseases Miscellanea. 2. Nephrology Miscellanea.
 I. Hricik, Donald E. II. Sedor, John R. III. Ganz, Michael Bruce.
 IV. Series.
  [DNLM: 1. Kidney Diseases Examination Questions. WJ 18.2 N439
1999]
RC903.N477 1999
616.6'1—dc21
DNLM/DLC
for Library of Congress   99-14494
                                      CIP

£21.00

NEPHROLOGY SECRETS   ISBN 1-56053-309-9

Last digit is the print number: 9 8 7 6 5 4 3 2 1

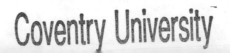

DEDICATION

This book is dedicated to past and present faculty members and fellows in the Division of Nephrology at Case Western Reserve University.

CONTENTS

I. PATIENT ASSESSMENT

III. PRIMARY GLOMERULAR DISEASE

IV. SECONDARY GLOMERULAR DISEASE

V. OTHER PARENCHYMAL RENAL DISEASES

IX. ACID-BASE AND ELECTROLYTE DISORDERS

CONTRIBUTORS

Hany S. Y. Anton, M.D.
Nephrology Fellow, Department of Medicine, Case Western Reserve University School of Medicine, University Hospitals of Cleveland, Cleveland, Ohio

Carolyn P. Cacho, M.D.
Assistant Professor of Medicine, Division of Nephrology, Department of Medicine, Case Western Reserve University School of Medicine; Staff Nephrologist, University Hospitals of Cleveland, Cleveland, Ohio

Chokchai Chareandee, M.D.
Senior Nephrology Fellow, Department of Medicine, Case Western Reserve University School of Medicine, University Hospitals of Cleveland, Cleveland, Ohio

Diane M. Cibrik, M.D.
Nephrology Fellow, Department of Medicine, Case Western Reserve University School of Medicine, University Hospitals of Cleveland, Cleveland, Ohio

Ira D. Davis, M.D.
Associate Professor of Pediatrics, Division of Pediatric Nephrology, Department of Pediatrics, Case Western Reserve University School of Medicine; Medical Director of Pediatric Nephrology, Rainbow Babies and Children's Hospital, Cleveland, Ohio

Ashwin Dixit, M.D.
Nephrology Fellow, Department of Medicine, Case Western Reserve University School of Medicine, University Hospitals of Cleveland, Cleveland, Ohio

Elashi Essam, M.D.
Nephrology Fellow, Department of Medicine, Case Western Reserve University School of Medicine, University Hospitals of Cleveland, Cleveland, Ohio

Michael B. Ganz, M.D.
Associate Professor of Medicine, Department of Medicine, Case Western Reserve University School of Medicine; Chief, Division of Nephrology, Department of Medicine, Veterans Affairs Medical Center, Cleveland, Ohio

Donald E. Hricik, M.D.
Professor of Medicine; Chief, Division of Nephrology, Department of Medicine, Case Western Reserve University School of Medicine; Medical Director, Transplantation Services, Department of Medicine, University Hospitals of Cleveland, Cleveland, Ohio

Thomas C. Knauss, M.D.
Associate Professor, Department of Medicine, Case Western Reserve University School of Medicine; Veterans Affairs Medical Center; University Hospitals of Cleveland, Cleveland, Ohio

Eduardo K. Lacson, Jr., M.D.
Instructor of Medicine, Renal Division, Department of Medicine, Harvard Medical School; Associate Physician, Brigham and Women's Hospital, Boston, Massachusetts

Lavinia A. Negrea, M.D.
Assistant Professor, Department of Medicine, Case Western Reserve University School of Medicine; Veterans Affairs Medical Center; University Hospitals of Cleveland, Cleveland, Ohio

Mahboob Rahman, M.D., M.S.
Assistant Professor of Medicine, Department of Medicine, Case Western Reserve University School of Medicine; Attending Physician, University Hospitals of Cleveland, Cleveland, Ohio

Edmond Ricanati, M.D.
Professor of Medicine, Department of Medicine, Case Western Reserve University School of Medicine; Director of Peritoneal Dialysis, MetroHealth Medical Center, Cleveland, Ohio

Jeffrey R. Schelling, M.D.
Assistant Professor, Department of Medicine, Case Western Reserve University School of Medicine; Staff Physician, MetroHealth Medical Center, Cleveland, Ohio

John R. Sedor, M.D.
Professor of Medicine, Physiology, and Biophysics, Department of Medicine, Case Western Reserve University School of Medicine; Chief, Division of Nephrology, Department of Medicine, MetroHealth Medical Center, Cleveland, Ohio

Ashwini Sehgal, M.D.
Assistant Professor of Medicine, Biomedical Ethics, and Epidemiology and Biostatistics, Case Western Reserve University School of Medicine; Staff Nephrologist, MetroHealth Medical Center, Cleveland, Ohio

Marcia R. Silver, M.D.
Assistant Professor of Medicine, Department of Medicine, Case Western Reserve University School of Medicine; Staff Physician, Director of Hemodialysis Program, MetroHealth Medical Center, Cleveland, Ohio

Michael S. Simonson
Associate Professor of Medicine, Department of Medicine, Case Western Reserve University School of Medicine, Cleveland, Ohio

Michael C. Smith, M.D.
Professor of Medicine, Department of Medicine, Case Western Reserve University School of Medicine; Physician, University Hospitals of Cleveland, Cleveland, Ohio

Beth A. Vogt, M.D.
Assistant Professor, Department of Pediatrics, Case Western Reserve University School of Medicine; Pediatric Nephrologist, Rainbow Babies and Children's Hospital, Cleveland, Ohio

Miriam F. Weiss, M.D.
Associate Professor, Division of Nephrology, Department of Medicine, Case Western Reserve University School of Medicine; University Hospitals of Cleveland, Cleveland, Ohio

Jay B. Wish, M.D.
Professor, Department of Medicine, Case Western Reserve University School of Medicine; Medical Director, Hemodialysis Services, University Hospitals of Cleveland, Cleveland, Ohio

Linda Zarif, M.D.
Nephrology Fellow, Department of Medicine, Case Western Reserve University School of Medicine, University Hospitals of Cleveland, Cleveland, Ohio

PREFACE

The roots of the specialty of nephrology are firmly entrenched in disciplines such as histopathology, immunology, and physiology—the basic sciences that helped to elucidate both the pathogenesis of various renal diseases and the kidney's role in hypertension and common electrolyte and acid-base disturbances. With the availability of hemodialysis, peritoneal dialysis, and effective immunosuppressive therapy for kidney transplant recipients, however, the clinical practice of nephrology has centered increasingly on the management of patients with end-stage renal disease. Technological improvements in renal replacement therapies (i.e., dialysis and kidney transplantation) have resulted in a dramatic increase in the numbers of patients whose lives can be sustained despite end-stage renal disease. In the United States alone, more than 300,000 patients currently are receiving renal replacement therapy. A growth rate of 5–8% per year is anticipated for at least the next 5 years.

To the extent that renal disorders such as hypertension, electrolyte and acid-base disturbances, and various kidney diseases occur in patients cared for by virtually all medical and surgical specialists, students and house officers should regard basic concepts in nephrology as an essential element of training. *Nephrology Secrets* provides information about all aspects of nephrology that should be of value to trainees learning this specialty and to more advanced health care professionals who seek a review of essential topics in the field. Using the informal question-and-answer format of the popular *Secrets Series*®, it is hoped that the material presented here will provide an enjoyable learning experience and a foundation for excellent patient care

Donald E. Hricik, M.D.
John R. Sedor, M.D.
Michael B. Ganz, M.D.

I. Patient Assessment

1. PHYSICAL DIAGNOSIS

Thomas C. *Knauss*, M.D.

1. What is the single most important question to ask a patient suspected of having renal disease?

"Have you had this before?" A prior history of renal disease is important in constructing a differential diagnosis and assessing the acuity or chronicity of disease.

2. What renal diseases should be considered when there is a strong family history of kidney problems?

Polycystic kidney disease
Alport syndrome
Hypertensive nephrosclerosis
Diabetic nephropathy

Fabry's disease
Lupus nephritis
Focal segmental glomerulosclerosis
  (rarely familial)

3. What features of the medical history should be elicited in hospitalized patients who develop acute renal failure?

- Recent episodes of hypotension
- Exposure to intravenous contrast
- Treatment with nephrotoxic drugs
- Recent systemic infection
- Risk factors for volume depletion (e.g., gastrointestinal losses, diuretic therapy)

4. Describe the physical exam findings that may be seen in patients with uremia.

Hypertension
Signs of fluid overload
Pallor of skin and mucous membranes
Asterixis
Peripheral neuropathy
Pericardial friction rub
Uremic frost (in advanced uremia)

5. What are the physical signs of fluid overload?

Hypertension
Elevated jugular venous pressure
Hepatojugular reflux
S_3 heart sound

Pulmonary crackles
Ascites
Edema

6. What are the signs and symptoms of volume depletion?

Postural hypotension
Dizziness
Dry mucous membranes
Skin tenting
Flat neck veins (low jugulovenous pressure)

Dark yellow urine
Decreased urine output

7. Which kidney diseases are frequently associated with skin rashes?

Rash	Associated Kidney Disease
Purpura	Idiopathic thrombocytopenic purpura (ITP) Henoch-Schönlein purpura Other forms of vasculitis
Petechiae	Hemolytic uremic syndrome Focal glomerulonephritis secondary to subacute bacterial endocarditis Acute interstitial nephritis
Hives	Henoch-Schönlein purpura Acute interstitial nephritis
Discoid lupus	Systemic lupus erythematosus
Impetigo	Poststreptococcal glomerulonephritis
Angiokeratoma	Fabry's disease

8. Which kidney diseases are frequently associated with signs and symptoms of arthritis?
Lupus nephritis
Amyloidosis
Henoch-Schönlein purpura
Cryoglobulinemia
Sarcoidosis

9. What physical finding best characterizes the nephrotic syndrome?
Edema.

10. What happens to blood pressure in nephrotic syndrome?
Blood pressure may be normal in patients with nephrotic syndrome, especially if renal function is well preserved. Nephrotic patients with severe hypoalbuminemia (< 2 gm/dl) sometimes exhibit a postural drop in blood pressure due to relative intravascular volume depletion.

11. What physical finding in a patient with nephrotic syndrome and diabetes mellitus best correlates with diabetic nephropathy?
Proliferative diabetic retinopathy. Forty-five percent of patients with biopsy-proven diabetic nephropathy will have retinopathy at the time they present with proteinuria. By the time these patients reach end-stage renal disease, 95% will have retinopathy.

12. Peripheral neuropathy due to uremia can be seen in advanced azotemia. Which diseases can independently cause peripheral neuropathy and renal dysfunction?
1. **Diabetes mellitus** can cause distal polyneuropathy.
2. **Vasculitis** can cause mononeuritis multiplex.
3. **Fabry's disease** can cause distal polyneuropathy.
4. **Amyloidosis** can result in bilateral carpal tunnel and distal neuropathy.

13. Which renal diseases are associated with hemoptysis?
• Pulmonary edema secondary to acute or chronic renal failure
• Goodpasture's syndrome
• Pulmonary embolus or infarct in a patient with glomerulonephritis and renal vein thrombosis
• Bacterial endocarditis

14. What renal disease is associated with deafness?
Alport syndrome.

15. What are some renal causes of flank pain and gross hematuria?
Renal stone disease
Renal neoplasms
Renal vein thrombosis
Papillary necrosis
Pyelonephritis

16. What physical findings can be seen in patients with cholesterol atheroembolic disease?
Cyanosis and microinfarcts in toes
Livedo reticularis in buttocks and thighs
Cholesterol plaques at branch points of retinal arteries

17. List some of the extrarenal physical findings that may be seen in patients with systemic lupus erythematosus.
Alopecia
Nasal or oral ulcerations
Pleural or pericardial effusion or rub
Hepatosplenomegaly
Ascites
Edema
Arthritis, fever

BIBLIOGRAPHY
1. Abuelo JG: Diagnosing vascular causes of renal failure. Ann Intern Med 123:601–614, 1995.
2. Breyer JA: Diabetic nephropathy in insulin-dependent patients. Am J Kidney Dis 6:533–547, 1992.
3. Cameron JS: The nephrotic syndrome and its complications. Am J Kidney Dis 10:157–171, 1987.
4. Fraser CL, Arieff A: Nervous system complications in uremia. Ann Intern Med 109:143–153, 1988.
5. Gleeson MJ: Alport's syndrome: Audiological manifestations and implications. J Laryngol Otol 98:449–465, 1984.
6. Kassirer JP: Atheroembolic renal disease. N Engl J Med 280:812–818, 1969.
7. Liano F, Pascual J: Epidemiology of acute renal failure: A prospective multicenter community-based study. Kidney Int 50:811–818, 1996.
8. Turner AN, Rees AJ: Goodpasture's disease and Alport's syndrome. Annu Rev Med 47:377–386, 1996.
9. Vanholder R: The uremic syndrome. In Greenberg A (ed): Primer on Kidney Diseases, 2nd ed. San Diego, Academic Press, 1998, pp 403–407.

2. URINALYSIS

Michael B. Ganz, M.D.

1. What are the major determinants of urine color?

The color of urine (usually yellow!) is determined predominantly by chemical content and concentration. Urine may be relatively colorless when volume is high and concentration is low. Cloudy urine may be the result of phosphates (usually normal) or white blood cells and bacteria (abnormal). Red urine reflects hemoglobin, while red urine without red blood cells indicates either free hemoglobin or myoglobin. Other colors can be seen. For instance, green urine may reflect exogenous chemicals (e.g., methylene blue) or *Pseudomonas* bacteriuria, while orange color may indicate the presence of bile pigments.

2. What is the importance of the urine specific gravity?

A standard part of the urinalysis, specific gravity reflects the concentration of dissolved solutes in urine. It is best measured using a hygrometer. Specific gravity normally ranges between 1.003 and 1.030. However, this range decreases as one ages, reflecting a decreased ability to dilute and concentrate urine. Urine osmolality, normally ranging between 50 and 1,200 mOsm/L also reflects the concentration of urine but is more cumbersome to measure and is not part of the routine urinalysis. Monitoring specific gravity or urine osmolality may aid in the management of stone-forming patients who should be encouraged to maintain a dilute urine. These measurements also provide a general sense of the patient's state of hydration and may provide clues in the differential diagnosis of patients with hypo- or hypernatremia (see Chapter 65, Hyponatremia and Hypernatremia).

3. What is the significance of urine pH?

Usually measured with a reagent strip, urine pH values in humans range from 4.5 to 7.8. Throughout the course of the day, urine pH is most often closer to the lower limit of this range, reflecting the renal hydrogen ion excretion that is necessary to maintain acid-base balance in the face of endogenous acid production of about 1 mEq/kg/day. The urine is transiently alkaline after meals or the ingestion of bicarbonate loads. Persistently alkaline urine (pH > 7.5) may aid in making a diagnosis of distal renal tubular acidosis (see Chapter 20, Disorders of Tubular Function). Infection with urea-splitting organisms such as *Proteus* also is associated with a high urine pH resulting from bacterial conversion of urea to ammonia.

4. Can urine glucose be used to monitor glycemic control in patients with diabetes mellitus?

Dipstick reagents generally detect concentrations of glucose as low as 50 mg/dl. The renal threshold for tubular reabsorption of glucose is approximately 180 mg/dl (i.e., with plasma glucose concentrations of 180 mg/dl or less, all of the glucose filtered by glomeruli is reabsorbed in the proximal tubules). Thus, detection of glucose in the urine crudely indicates a blood sugar of at least 230 mg/dl. Used as a screening test, this finding suggests the diagnosis of diabetes mellitus. However, glucosuria occasionally occurs when the blood sugar is normal, either as an isolated finding in patients with a defect in tubular glucose transport or in patients with more generalized tubular dysfunction (e.g., Fanconi syndrome) or tubulointerstitial disease. Furthermore, in diabetics, glucose may appear in the urine long after the blood sugar has normalized, rendering urine glucose measurements virtually worthless in the day-to-day management of diabetes.

5. What is the significance of finding ketones in the urine?

Ketones, generally detected with a nitroprusside assay, are detected in the urine of patients with diabetic, alcoholic, or starvation ketoacidosis. In patients with severe ketoacidosis and an altered redox state, urine ketones initially may be negative due to relative overproduction of beta-hydroxybutyrate but later become positive as the redox states return to normal.

6. What is the meaning of a positive dipstick determination for "blood"?

Reagent strips use peroxidase-like activity of hemoglobin to catalyze a reaction wherein both hemoglobin and myoglobin react positively. The major cause of a positive dipstick test for blood is the presence of hemoglobin-containing red blood cells. Free hemoglobin also can be filtered at the glomerulus and appears in the urine when the capacity for plasma protein binding with haptoglobin is exceeded. Some of the hemoglobin is catabolized by proximal tubules. The major cause for increased hemoglobin is hemolysis, while rhabdomyolysis gives rise to myoglobinuria.

7. What is the significance of positive dipstick tests for leukocyte esterase and nitrites?

The esterase assay relies on the fact that esterases are released from lysed white blood cells in the urine. Urinary bacteria convert nitrates to nitrites. Positive tests for leukocyte esterase or nitrites generally indicate leukocyturia and possible urinary tract infection.

8. What urinary proteins are detected by the standard dipstick?

Most dipstick reagents contain a pH-sensitive colorimetric indicator that changes color when bound to negatively charged proteins such as albumin. Positively charged proteins, such as immunoglobulin light chains, are less well detected even when large amounts are present (see Chapter 4, Measurement of Urinary Protein, and Chapter 13, Asymptomatic Proteinuria).

9. Name the cellular elements from urinalysis depicted in the following figure.

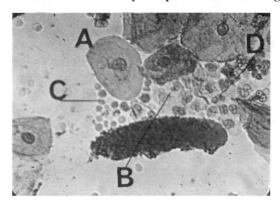

A, Squamous epithelial cell. *B* and *D*, White blood cells (polymorphonuclear cells). *C*, Red blood cells. Also shown in the lower center of the figure is a granular cast.

10. Name the urine crystals depicted in the following figure.

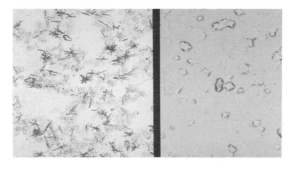

Left, Calcium phosphate crystals. *Right*, Calcium oxalate crystals.

11. What are red blood cell casts?

Red blood cell casts are formed elements that are excreted into the urine when an active glomerular lesion is present (i.e., acute glomerulonephritis) and red blood cells are extravasated through the glomerulus into the tubular lumen. In acute glomerular disease, there is usually urinary stasis. Proteins secreted from the tubules (e.g., Tamm-Horsfall glycoproteins) remain in the tubular lumen for a prolonged period of time, quite often in the presence of an acid urine, thereby forming a "cast" of the lumen. Any cell in the lumen will be trapped in that cast and excreted into the urine.

12. What are white blood cell casts?

Formed in the same manner as red blood cell casts (see question 11), white blood cell casts are indicative of some form of interstitial nephritis including suppurative pyelonephritis. Again, there is often urinary stasis allowing a cast to be formed that traps white blood cells (granulocytes) in the secreted glycoprotein material.

13. What are the causes of eosinophiluria?

Eosinophils are best detected with a Wright stain or Hansel stain. In the proper clinical setting, the presence of eosinophils in the urine suggests drug-induced acute interstitial nephritis. However, eosinophiluria is not specific for that disorder and can also be seen in acute prostatitis, other urinary tract infections, and renal transplant rejection.

14. What is the significance of lipiduria?

The presence of free lipid droplets or lipid droplets within tubular cells (oval fat bodies) is best detected with microscopy, using a polarizing lens. These droplets generally are found in the urine of patients with heavy proteinuria or nephrotic syndrome (see Chapter 17, Nephrotic Syndrome).

BIBLIOGRAPHY

1. Kasiske BL, Keane WF: Laboratory assessment of renal disease: Clearance, urinalysis, and renal biopsy. In Brenner B (ed): The Kidney, 5th ed. Philadelphia, W.B. Saunders, 1996, pp 233–278.
2. McCormack M, Dessureault J, Guitard M: The urine specific gravity dipstick: A useful tool to increase fluid intake in stone forming patients. J Urol 146:1475–1482, 1991.
3. McNagny SE, Parker RM, Zenilman JM, Lewis JS: Urinary leukocyte esterase test: A screening test: A screening method for the detection of symptomatic chlamydial and gonococcal infections in men. J Infect Dis 165:573–577, 1992.
4. Schwab SJ, Dunn FL, Feinglos MN: Screening for microalbuminuria. Diabetes Care 15:1581–1587, 1992.

3. MEASUREMENT OF GLOMERULAR FILTRATION RATE

Michael S. Simonson

1. What is the glomerular filtration rate (GFR)?

GFR is the amount of plasma filtered through glomeruli per unit of time. Although the term can refer to the function of single nephrons, GFR most often refers to the sum filtration rate of all functioning nephrons.

2. What is the clinical significance of the GFR?

Clinical assessment and management of patients with renal disease generally require an estimate of GFR, the single best index of functioning renal mass. Serial measurements of GFR are used to monitor the severity and course of renal disease. Measurement of GFR is also useful for determining appropriate doses of drugs that are excreted by the kidney. Excretion of such drugs (see Chapter 8, Drug Therapy in Renal Disease) falls when GFR declines. Without lowering drug dosage accordingly, plasma drug concentrations can rapidly accumulate to toxic levels.

3. What are normal values for GFR in adults?

The range of normal values for GFR are:
Men: 115–125 ml/min
Women: 90–100 ml/min

4. What is the relationship between GFR and renal function?

GFR varies directly with renal function. A decline in GFR signifies progression of underlying renal disease (i.e., nephron injury) or a condition associated with decreased renal perfusion (e.g., volume depletion). In contrast, an increase in GFR usually indicates improvement of renal function. Stable but subnormal GFR suggests stable renal disease.

5. How is GFR estimated in routine clinical practice?

In most patients, it is unnecessary to determine an exact value for GFR. Instead, it is important to know whether GFR is declining (indicating renal disease), increasing, or stable. The most widely used clinical index of GFR is the serum concentration of creatinine. Creatinine is a by-product of the nonenzymatic conversion of creatine and phosphocreatine in skeletal muscle. Production of creatinine by skeletal muscle is proportional to muscle mass and remains relatively constant. These and other properties make creatinine a convenient, endogenous marker for GFR. Serum creatinine is determined in a routine panel of biochemical blood tests and can, therefore, be serially analyzed in the same patient to monitor renal function. Convenience, reproducibility, and low cost account for the popularity of serum creatinine as an index of GFR. Serum creatinine varies inversely with GFR.

6. Why does serum creatinine correlate inversely with GFR?

The amount of creatinine filtered at the glomerulus (GFR × plasma creatinine) approximates the amount excreted by the kidney, and the amount of creatinine produced by the muscle mass remains relatively constant. In the steady state, creatinine excretion equals creatinine production. Thus, the following relationship holds true:

Creatinine excretion (approximated by filtered creatinine) = Muscle production of creatinine
   or
GFR × Plasma creatinine = Constant
   or
Plasma creatinine = Constant/GFR

It is apparent from this relationship that a decline in GFR increases serum creatinine.

7. What are normal values for serum creatinine in adults?

Men: Serum creatinine = 0.8–1.3 mg/dl (or 70–114 µmol/L)

Women: Serum creatinine = 0.6–1.0 mg/dl (or 53–88 µmol/L)

Reduced muscle mass and correspondingly lower rates of creatinine synthesis account for the slightly lower normal values of serum creatinine in women. To convert serum creatinine from mg/dl to Standard International units (mmol/L), multiply by 0.088.

8. What are normal values for serum creatinine in children?

Because growing children have an increasing muscle mass, serum creatinine increases somewhat with age. The following formulas estimate normal values for serum creatinine in children ages 1–20 years[4]:

Boys: Serum creatinine = 0.35 + age in years/40

Girls: Serum creatinine = 0.35 + age in years/55

9. What are the major limitations of serum creatinine as a clinical index of renal disease?

A low serum creatinine concentration may be misleading in patients with reduced muscle mass. In addition, serum creatinine is a somewhat insensitive index of renal function, especially in early and late stages of renal disease. As shown in the Figure, serum creatinine does not increase (i.e., > 1.0 mg/dl) until major declines in GFR have occurred. Two mechanisms account for the relative insensitivity of serum creatinine as an indicator of renal disease. As part of the adaptation of the kidney to renal injury, uninjured nephrons undergo hypertrophy and hyperfiltration to compensate for the loss of functioning nephrons (i.e., compensatory hyperfiltration). Thus, total GFR and serum creatinine remain relatively normal despite a decrease in functioning nephrons. Another potential problem is that tubular secretion of creatinine, which normally contributes little to overall creatinine clearance, increases progressively as renal disease worsens. Thus, both the serum creatinine concentration and the creatinine clearance (see question 11) become increasingly unreliable as estimates of GFR in patients with advanced renal disease. Finally, certain circumstances are associated with spurious elevations of serum creatinine independent of changes in GFR. Rhabdomyolysis or ingestion of cooked meat can transiently increase creatinine production and elevate serum creatinine, as can certain drugs (e.g., cimetidine, trimethoprim) that decrease tubular secretion of creatinine. High concentrations of certain exogenous compounds (e.g., flucytosine, cefoxitin, and other cephalosporin antibiotics) can be detected as creatinine. In patients with ketoacidosis, acetoacetic acid can be detected as creatinine leading to false elevations.

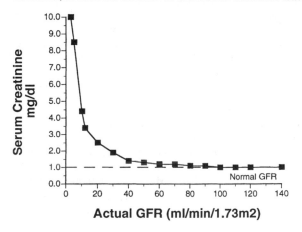

Relationship between serum creatinine and actual values for GFR in patients with renal failure. Normal value of serum creatinine is indicated by the dashed line. (Adapted from Shemesh O, Golbetz H, Kriss JP, Myers BD: Limitations of creatinine as a filtration marker in glomerulopathic patients. Kidney Int 28:830–838, 1985.)

10. Can serum creatinine be used clinically to predict the course of renal disease in patients?

Some nephrologists use plots of the reciprocal of serum creatinine versus time (i.e., 1/serum creatinine versus time) to predict the course of renal failure. Although this technique yields useful information in some patients (i.e., time to end-stage renal failure), in many patients, the decline in renal function is nonlinear and is therefore poorly modeled by such plots. Clinical predictions based on reciprocal plots should be interpreted with great care.

11. What other methods are available to measure GFR?

Effective management of patients with renal disease sometimes requires actual estimates of GFR, as opposed to the index of GFR provided by serum creatinine. To estimate GFR, one must measure the clearance of molecular markers that are (1) freely filtered at the glomerulus, (2) present at a stable plasma concentration, and (3) not reabsorbed, secreted, or metabolized by the kidney. Clearance is defined as the volume of plasma cleared of a specific compound (i.e., creatinine, glucose) per unit time. The clearance (C) of any compound X can be determined from the following formula:

$$C = ([U_X] \times V)/[P_X]$$

where $[U_X]$ is the concentration of X in urine, V is the volume of urine containing X, and $[P_X]$ is the plasma concentration of X.

The most common clinical method for directly estimating GFR consists of measuring the clearance of endogenous creatinine (see question 12). Variable tubular secretion of creatinine makes creatinine clearance an imperfect marker of GFR. Measurements of the clearance of the polysaccharide inulin or the radioisotope ^{125}I-iothalamate are gold standards for estimates of GFR. However, the technical challenges and expense of inulin and ^{125}I-iothalamate clearances render these tests impractical for clinical use except in research or therapeutic trials.

12. How is creatinine clearance measured?

Creatinine clearance is usually determined by using venous blood for serum creatinine and a 24-hour urine collection, using the following formula:

$$\text{Creatinine clearance} = ([U_{Cr}] \times V)/[\text{serum creatinine}]$$

where $[U_{Cr}]$ is the urine concentration of creatinine, and V is the 24-hour urine volume.

Normal values for creatinine clearance are 120 ± 25 ml/min in men and 95 ± 20 ml/min in women. In practice, several problems can severely compromise the utility of creatinine clearance. Because the renal tubules secrete creatinine, measurements of creatinine clearance can significantly overestimate true GFR, particularly in patients with renal disease. Accurate measurements of creatine clearance also require complete and carefully timed urine collections; inadequate urine collections yield spurious results.

13. What is a cimetidine-enhanced creatinine clearance?

One approach for enhancing the accuracy of creatinine clearance measurements is to assess clearance after oral administration of the histamine H_2-receptor antagonist cimetidine, which blocks tubular secretion of creatinine thereby improving its accuracy as a true marker of GFR. Creatinine clearance with cimetidine has been reported to be nearly identical to GFR, even in patients with mild or severe renal failure. A single dose of 1,200 mg of cimetidine given 2 hours before starting the 24-hour urine collection has been proven effective.[7]

14. Can creatinine clearance and GFR be estimated from simple measurements of serum creatinine?

In an attempt to improve the accuracy of serum creatinine as a measure of GFR, variations in sex- and age-dependent differences in muscle mass have been incorporated into formulas that estimate GFR (in ml/min) from serum creatinine. The most widely used estimate is derived from the Cockcroft-Gault formula:

$$\text{Creatinine clearance} = [(140 - \text{age}) \times \text{body weight}]/(72 \times \text{plasma creatinine})$$

where lean body weight is in kg, age is in years, and plasma creatinine is in mg/dl. For women, multiply the result by a factor of 0.85 to compensate for the lower average muscle mass. The utility of this formula is dramatically illustrated when one considers that a serum creatinine of 1.7

mg/dl corresponds to a creatinine clearance of 79 ml/min in an 80-kg, 20-year-old man but only a clearance of 36 ml/min in a 45-kg, 75-year-old woman.

For children older than 2 years, creatinine clearance is estimated as follows:

$$[0.55 \times \text{height (cm)}]/[\text{serum creatinine (mg/dl)}]$$

15. Can measurements of blood urea nitrogen (BUN) serve as an index of GFR?

BUN is not a reliable index of GFR. The renal tubules reabsorb urea in quantities that vary depending on the state of hydration, thus rendering the BUN an inaccurate marker for GFR. BUN concentration is also strongly affected by changes in catabolism and protein intake.

BIBLIOGRAPHY

1. Cockroft DW, Gault MH: Prediction of creatinine clearance from serum creatinine. Nephron 16:31–39, 1976.
2. Kasiske BL, Keane WF: Laboratory assessment of renal disease: Clearance, unianalysis, and renal biopsy. In Brenner BM (ed): The Kidney, 5th ed. Philadelphia, W.B. Saunders, 1996, pp 1137–1174.
3. Levey AS: Measurement of renal function in chronic renal disease. Kidney Int 38:167–184, 1990.
4. Schwartz GJ, Haycock GB, Spitzer A: Plasma creatinine and urea concentration in children: Normal values for age and sex. J Pediatr 88:828–837, 1976.
5. Shemesh O, Golbetz H, Kriss JP, Myers BD: Limitations of creatinine as a filtration marker in glomerulo-pathic patients. Kidney Int 28:830–838, 1985.
6. Vander AJ: Renal clearance. In Vander AJ (ed): Renal Physiology, 5th ed. New York, McGraw-Hill, 1995, pp 51–61.
7. Walser M: Assessing renal function from creatinine measurements in adults with chronic renal failure. Am J Kidney Dis 32:23–31, 1998.

4. MEASUREMENT OF URINARY PROTEIN

Michael S. Simonson

1. How does the kidney normally restrict the excretion of plasma proteins?

The glomerulus functions as a size- and charge-selective ultrafilter that largely prevents filtration of plasma proteins into the tubules. As shown in the Figure, glomerular capillaries comprise three distinct structures: a fenestrated endothelium, a glomerular basement membrane, and a lining of epithelial cells attached to the basement membrane by podocytes ("foot processes").

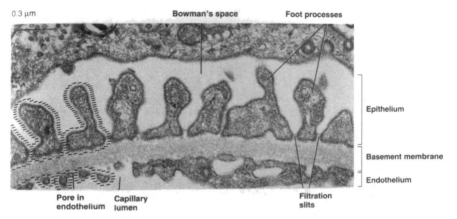

Ultrastructure of the glomerular capillary membrane as depicted by electron microscopy. Note the negative charges illustrated on the fenestrated endothelium, basement membrane, and epithelial foot processes.

Size-selective properties reflect poorly characterized "pores" in the glomerular capillary wall structure that prevent filtration of proteins above a specific molecular radius. Charge-selective properties arise from the presence of negatively charged sialoproteins and proteoglycans in the endothelium, basement membrane, and epithelial podocytes. Because most plasma proteins including albumin are negatively charged, they are electrostatically repelled and fail to filter through the glomerulus. The glomerular capillary membrane is not a perfect filter. However, a large fraction of the plasma protein filtered through glomeruli is subsequently reabsorbed by renal tubular cells.

2. What is the clinical significance of proteinuria?

Urinary protein excretion exceeding 150 mg per day is often associated with renal disease and warrants further evaluation. Unlike measurements of glomerular filtration rate, which indicate the severity of renal dysfunction, proteinuria per se does not always correlate with the severity of renal disease. Some renal diseases cause heavy proteinuria (> 3.5 gm/24 hr) whereas others are associated with normal or only slightly elevated levels of urinary protein excretion. Furthermore, proteinuria is not always associated with renal disease and can result from benign conditions (see Chapter 13, Asymptomatic Proteinuria). The degree of proteinuria can, however, strongly point to specific kinds of renal damage. Heavy proteinuria usually indicates the presence of glomerular disease.

3. What is the pathophysiology of proteinuria?

Glomerular proteinuria results from structural damage to any of the charge- or size-selective properties of the glomerular capillary. Tubular proteinuria results when the tubular absorption of the few normally filtered proteins is disrupted. The pathophysiology of these and other forms of proteinuria is discussed further in Chapter 13, Asymptomatic Proteinuria, and Chapter 17, Nephrotic Syndrome.

4. What proteins are present in normal urine?

The upper limit of total urinary protein excretion in normal individuals is 150 mg/day. A variety of proteins are excreted by the kidneys including small amounts of albumin (< 20 mg/day) and the Tamm-Horsfall mucoprotein (30–50 mg/day), also called uromodulin. Tamm-Horsfall protein, which is secreted by epithelial cells in the loop of Henle, is clinically important because it forms the matrix for most urinary casts (see Chapter 2, Urinalysis).

5. How is proteinuria measured?

Two methods are used clinically to estimate proteinuria semiquantitatively. In the most common procedure, a colorimetric analysis is performed using a dipstick (i.e., Albustix) impregnated with an indicator dye such as tetrabromophenol blue. The indicator color changes according to the amount of protein present; negative protein results in a yellow color while increasing amounts of protein, 1+ to 4+, shift the color from green to blue. The dipstick method is rapid and easy to perform. Dipstick measurements of proteinuria are relatively insensitive (limit of detection of 10–30 mg/dl) and primarily detect albumin.

The second, less common procedure involves adding 5.0% sulfosalicylic acid to a urine sample to denature the urine proteins. Denatured urine proteins cause turbidity, and the amount of urine protein is proportional to the observed turbidity (1+ to 4+). The sulfosalicylic acid method is more sensitive (limit of detection 5–10 mg/dl) than the dipstick technique, and it measures all urine proteins.

6. How are these tests for proteinuria interpreted?

Semiquantitative tests for proteinuria are interpreted as follows:

Dipstick Method	Sulfosalicylic Acid Method
Trace ≅ 10–30 mg/dl	Trace ≅ 20 mg/dl (slight turbidity)
1+ ≅ 30 mg/dl	1+ ≅ 50 mg/dl (print visible through specimen)
2+ ≅ 100 mg/dl	2+ ≅ 200 mg/dl (print invisible)
3+ ≅ 500 mg/dl	3+ ≅ 500 mg/dl (flocculation)
4+ > 2000 mg/dl	4+ > 1000 mg/dl (dense precipitate)

Quantitative measurements of urinary protein excretion are usually obtained using timed urine collections (e.g., a 24-hour collection).

7. Can proteinuria be estimated without performing a 24-hour urine collection?

A newer method for estimating proteinuria involves extrapolation of 24-hour values from a single, randomly collected urine sample. This method is especially valuable for estimating proteinuria when accurate urine collections are inconvenient or impossible (e.g., incontinent patients or small children). Proteinuria is estimated by calculating the ratio of total urine protein to urine creatinine (in mg/mg) in a single urine sample. The ratio approximates 24-hour protein excretion in gm/day per 1.73 m^2 body surface area (see Figure, top of next page).

Using this approximation, normal individuals have a ratio less than 0.2, whereas patients with any type of renal disease can have values between 0.2 and 3.5. Patients with nephrotic syndrome (see Chapter 17, Nephrotic Syndrome) will have ratios greater than 3.5. Consider the following example: A patient with a single random urine specimen has a urine protein of 100 mg/dl (2+ dipstick) and a urine creatinine of 50 mg/dl. The patient's proteinuria would be approximately 2 gm/day per 1.73 m^2 (100/50 = 2).

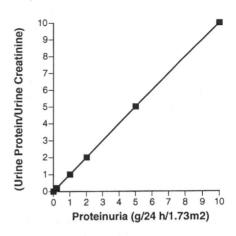

The ratio of urine protein to creatinine in a single urine specimen closely approximates the actual 24-hour protein excretion. Patients with normal protein excretion have a ratio < 0.2. Patients with proteinuria can have ratios between 0.2 and 3.5 or higher. (Adapted from Ginsberg JSM, Chang BS, Maltarese RA, Garella S: Use of single voided urine samples to estimate quantitative proteinuria. N Engl J Med 309:1543–1546, 1983, with permission.)

8. How accurate and specific are clinical tests for proteinuria?

In most patients, the dipstick and sulfosalicylic acid techniques yield similar results that roughly correlate with exact measurements of urine proteins using more sophisticated techniques. Dipstick indicators are more sensitive to albumin whereas sulfosalicylic acid recognizes all proteins. Immunoglobulin light chains are detected by sulfosalicylic acid but not by dipstick. Thus, in patients with multiple myeloma, proteinuria can be missed unless the sulfosalicylic acid test is used. False-positive dipstick results can occur in highly alkaline urine and in highly concentrated or dilute urine. Occasionally, false-positive readings in the sulfosalicylic acid test can occur if large amounts of radiocontrast materials, tolbutamide, penicillin, or cephalosporin antibiotics are present.

9. What is microalbuminuria?

Normal individuals excrete extremely low levels of albumin, usually less than 20 mg/day and well below the limit of detection by dipstick (300–500 mg/day). In diabetics, even small increases in renal albumin excretion (> 30 mg/day) are highly predictive of subsequent overt diabetic nephropathy. By the time elevated albumin excretion is detected by dipstick, significant glomerular damage has already occurred. To improve early diagnosis of diabetic renal disease, sensitive tests (i.e., enzyme-linked immunosorbent assays) have been developed to specifically measure low levels of urine albumin (microalbuminuria). Detection of microalbuminuria can signal the need for therapeutic interventions such as the use of angiotensin-converting enzyme (ACE) inhibitors or strict glycemic control. Note that microalbuminuria can occur even when total protein excretion remains normal (i.e., < 150 mg/day). Many nephrologists and diabetologists recommend that patients with type I and type II diabetes be screened regularly for microalbuminuria.

BIBLIOGRAPHY

1. Anderson S: Proteinuria. In Greenberg A (ed): Primer on Kidney Diseases, 2nd ed. San Diego, Academic Press, 1998, pp 42–46.
2. Bernard DB, Salant DJ: Clinical approach to the patient with proteinuria and the nephrotic syndrome. In Jacobson HR, Striker GE, Klahr S (eds): The Principles and Practice of Nephrology, 2nd ed. St. Louis, Mosby, 1995, pp 110–121.
3. Brenner BM, Hostetter TH, Humes DH: Molecular basis of proteinuria of glomerular origin. N Engl J Med 298:826–833, 1978.
4. Ginsberg JSM, Chang BS, Maltarese RA, Garella S: Use of single voided urine samples to estimate quantitative proteinuria. N Engl J Med 309:1543–1546, 1983.
5. Larson T: Evaluation of proteinuria. Mayo Clin Proc 69:1154–1159, 1994.

5. RENAL IMAGING TECHNIQUES

Elashi Essam, M.D., and Mahboob Rahman, M.D., M.S.

1. List the most commonly used imaging modalities for the kidneys.
- Urographic procedures (plain film, excretory urography, retrograde pyelography, and cystography)
- Ultrasonography
- Computed tomography (CT) scan and spiral CT scan
- Magnetic resonance imaging (MRI) and magnetic resonance angiography (MRA)
- Radionuclide imaging
- Renal angiography

2. What factors determine the choice of imaging procedure?
1. The information needed to guide further management of an individual patient
2. Accuracy and reliability of a given study
3. Invasiveness and the risk of the study
4. Cost of the study

In general, the simplest noninvasive studies are performed first as long as they provide the information needed. If the diagnostic yield is low, more invasive studies may be warranted.

3. Name the different urographic procedures and the information they provide about the urinary tract.

Procedure	Information
Plain abdominal film (kidneys, ureters, bladder [KUB])	Bone: Changes of renal osteodystrophy and either lytic or blastic metastases
	Soft tissue changes: Obliteration of psoas or renal outline may indicate inflammation or tumor
	Air: Air within or adjacent to the kidneys may be due to severe infection, especially in diabetics
	Calcifications: Renal calculus, calcified neoplasm, sloughed papilla, medullary or cortical nephrocalcinosis, ureteric or bladder calculus or tumor
Renal tomography	Renal calcification not observed on plain film especially when bowel gas or stool obscures the renal shadows
Excretory urography (intravenous pyelography)	Evaluation of the collecting structures, ureters, and bladder; provides the greatest spatial resolution of any imaging technique for evaluation of the urinary tract
Retrograde pyelography	Evaluation of possible filling defects not definite on excretory urography
	Selective cytological studies and cultures
	Additional delineation of an obstructed lesion, especially the length of the obstruction and the ureter distal to the obstruction
	Evaluation of ureteral trauma
Cystography	Evaluation of vesicoureteral reflux
	Anatomic delineation of the bladder in patients with reduced renal function
	Evaluation of urethra after pelvic trauma

Table continued on next page

Procedure	Information
Cystography *(cont.)*	Evaluation of vesicovaginal or vesicoenteric fistulas
	Evaluation of urinary incontinence
Voiding cystourethrography	Evaluation of ureteral valve
	Evaluation of ureteral strictures
	Evaluation of incontinence
	Evaluation of vesicoureteral reflux

4. What are the relative contraindications to excretory urography?

1. Previous allergic reaction to contrast media
2. Concern about contrast-induced nephrotoxicity in certain high-risk groups:
   - Preexisting renal insufficiency
   - Diabetic nephropathy
   - Multiple myeloma
   - Volume depletion
3. Cardiac diseases (especially patients with arrhythmias and cardiac irritability)
4. Pregnancy (radiation hazard)

5. List the strengths and weaknesses of ultrasonography in the evaluation of renal disease.

Strengths	Weaknesses
Sensitive detector of intrarenal fluid collections, pelvicalyceal dilatation, and cysts	Does not show fine pelvicalyceal detail
	Does not show the normal ureter
	Shows the retroperitoneum poorly
Differentiates cortex and medulla	Can miss small renal calculi and most ureteric calculi
Differentiates cystic and solid masses	Gives no functional information
Shows the whole renal contour and perinephric space	Operator dependent
Demonstrates renal blood flow by Doppler technique	
Provides good renal imaging irrespective of renal function	
Portable—can be used at bedside in the intensive care unit	
Uses no irradiation or contrast medium	

6. What are the clinical circumstances in which ultrasound may be of value?

Ultrasonography is a good first-line diagnostic method for:
- Estimating kidney size
- Assessing the echogenicity of the kidney. Increased echogenicity may indicate chronic renal disease, but it can also be seen in other pathologic states.
- Diagnosing collecting system dilatation, including possible obstruction in renal failure, pelvic neoplasm, renal transplants, and acute urinary tract infection with suspected pyonephrosis
- Assessing renal blood flow by Doppler technique
- Diagnosing adult polycystic kidney disease and screening involved families
- Guiding interventional procedures such as renal biopsy and cyst aspiration
- Detecting perinephric fluid collections
- Evaluating a renal allograft to assess any suspected fluid collection in the pelvis such as lymphocele, hematoma, or urinoma. Obstruction also can be detected by ultrasound and differentiated from rejection and acute tubular necrosis. Moreover, Doppler ultrasound can be used in evaluating the blood flow to the transplanted kidney without the use of nephrotoxic contrast media.

7. When is a CT scan superior to ultrasound for evaluation of renal disease?
- For evaluation of a solid mass especially if a malignant neoplasm is suspected. CT can define the extent of the neoplasm and lymph node involvement and help in staging.
- For evaluation of perirenal and pararenal spaces and Gerota's fascia
- CT is the imaging method of choice in evaluation of suspected renal trauma. Nonexcretion, contusion, fracture, shattered kidney, and perirenal fluid collection are readily detected on CT. Additional information about other organ injuries can be obtained at the same time.
- CT and MRI are the most efficacious imaging modalities for visualizing retroperitoneal structures including the adrenal glands. CT is particularly helpful in excluding the presence of disease when unusual positions of the kidney or changes in the renal axes have suggested a retroperitoneal mass.

8. What is the role of MRI in evaluating renal disease?
Though most renal diseases can be adequately imaged with other modalities, MRI may be especially helpful in the evaluation of extension of renal cell carcinoma into the renal veins or inferior vena cava when equivocally demonstrated by CT or ultrasound. MRI may play a role in staging of transitional cell carcinoma involving the pelvic floor and evaluation of carcinoma of the prostate. MRI, like CT, is useful in evaluation of the retroperitoneum.

9. What are the indications for radionuclide renal imaging?
The most common uses of nuclear medicine studies are:
- Measurement of renal function including glomerular filtration rate and effective renal plasma flow even in cases of renal impairment
- Measurement of "split" renal function to determine whether nephrectomy is warranted or safe
- Diagnosis of renovascular hypertension by differential blood flow studies using 99m technetium diethylenetetraaminonpentaacetic acid (99m Tc DTPA) or 99m technetium mercaptoacetyltriglycerine (99m Tc MAG3) pre- and postadministration of an angiotensin-converting enzyme (ACE) inhibitor such as captopril in appropriately screened hypertensive patients with intact renal function. The sensitivity and specificity approach 90%.
- Evaluation of renal transplants: Radionuclide imaging can detect impaired blood flow at renal arterial anastomotic site, urinary tract obstruction, and extravasation of the urine.
- Differentiation of obstructive from nonobstructive hydronephrosis

10. How can renal perfusion and excretion be evaluated by radionuclide scan?
After intravenous administration of 99m Tc DTPA, serial nuclear images are displayed pictorially, and corresponding radioactive counts from the kidneys are plotted over time in a graphic form. Early images and counts primarily reflect renal perfusion whereas later images and counts reflect renal excretion.

11. How can a renal scan differentiate between obstructive and nonobstructive distention of the collecting system?
In both obstructive and nonobstructive distention, the excretory phase of the renogram shows initially low but gradually increasing activity over time. Differentiation is possible based on the response to furosemide administration (Lasix renogram). In nonobstructive disease, the intravenous administration of furosemide results in prompt decrease of nuclear activity reflecting the diuresis, whereas, in obstruction, washout of the activity is limited.

12. What is an ACE inhibitor–stimulated radionuclide renal scan?
ACE inhibitor renal scanning is an imaging technique for diagnosis of renovascular hypertension. In the setting of renovascular hypertension, both glomerular filtration rate and renal plasma flow depend on angiotensin II–mediated constriction of the glomerular efferent arteriole. Treatment with ACE inhibitor antagonizes this vasoconstriction and decreases renal uptake and excretion of radioactive tracer. A renogram is considered abnormal if there is evidence of:

- Marked delay in the tracer uptake
- Decrease in the tracer count compared to the normal kidney
- Delay in the excretion of the tracer

Estimates of the sensitivity and specificity of ACE inhibitor–stimulated renography vary widely, but on average probably exceed 80%.

13. What other modalities can be used for evaluation of renovascular hypertension?

Duplex ultrasound: The use of color-flow Doppler in the diagnosis of renovascular hypertension combines anatomic information from ultrasound with hemodynamic information from Doppler. This technique is limited by the fact that the proximal main renal artery is not visualized in 25% of cases. Duplex ultrasound is highly operator-dependent and requires over 1 hour to perform correctly. In experienced hands, the sensitivity and specificity of the duplex ultrasonography are greater than 90%.

MRA: This is a noninvasive modality that can provide information about both anatomy and blood flow. Studies suggest that MRA can detect renal artery stenosis with 70–90% sensitivity and 78–94% specificity.

14. List the indications for renal angiography.

1. Evaluation of renovascular hypertension
2. Interventional angiography:
    - Use of special catheters and embolization technique to control hemorrhage or to occlude arteriovenous fistulas
    - Balloon angioplasty for management of renovascular hypertension and renal artery stenosis due to atherosclerosis
3. Preoperative evaluation of the donor kidney
4. Evaluation of the renal graft for renal artery occlusion or stenosis
5. Establishing the diagnosis of renal vein thrombosis
6. Complex renal masses or complications of polycystic disease or trauma may require angiography.

15. What is a percutaneous nephrostomy?

Percutaneous nephrostomy is the nonoperative placement of a catheter into the renal pelvis under imaging control for drainage of an obstructed kidney. It has largely replaced surgical nephrostomy and can be used for short- and long-term drainage.

16. What is antegrade pyelography?

Antegrade pyelography is a percutaneous injection of an iodinated contrast medium into the renal pelvis under ultrasound guidance of fluoroscopy. It is indicated when evaluation of the anatomy of the upper urinary tract is necessary but cannot be done with excretory urography or retrograde pyelography.

17. What imaging studies should be used to evaluate a renal mass?

The choice of imaging study for evaluation of a renal mass depends on the clinical situation. Although cystic or solid parenchymal masses may first be detected with excretory urography, they require ultrasound or CT for further differentiation, staging, and possible biopsy. Further testing depends on the findings:

- For a probable cystic mass, confirm it by ultrasound.
- For a probable solid mass, do a CT or MRI according to the clinical setting.
- To determine mass versus normal, evaluate by radionuclide renal scan.

18. What are the ultrasonographic features of a simple renal cyst?

Simple renal cysts occur in up to 30% of normal adults and can easily be differentiated from solid masses or tumor. Simple renal cysts:

• Are round and sharply demarcated with smooth borders
• Have no echoes within the mass

19. What imaging studies are needed for evaluating renal failure?
Generally, imaging is needed to define the size and shape of the kidneys and to exclude obstruction as the cause of renal failure. This can be done by:
1. Ultrasound:
   • Evaluates renal size. Generally, small atrophic kidneys are seen in chronic disease.
   • Calculi are shown as echogenic foci with shadowing.
2. CT: Provides additional information about extrinsic causes of ureteral obstruction.
3. Retrograde pyelography:
   • Demonstrates the presence of papillary necrosis and calyceal abnormalities
   • May help to determine the site and cause of obstruction. Bilateral peritoneal narrowing indicates retroperitoneal fibrosis.

20. Describe the radiologic evaluation of patients with suspected urinary tract obstruction.
The radiographic evaluation of suspected urinary tract obstruction should be guided by the results of the history, physical examination, and laboratory data. When an approach is chosen for a patient with renal insufficiency, the risk associated with the use of radiocontrast agents needs to be considered. The following are possible approaches:
Ultrasonography is the preferred screening modality for obstruction because of its high sensitivity for hydronephrosis (sensitivity and specificity about 90%), safety, low cost, and lack of radiation exposure. Moreover, it can be used in patients with elevated serum creatinine. Ultrasonography can determine renal size and reveal dilatation of calyces, the renal pelvis, and occasionally the proximal ureter. In addition, it may show the cortical thickness that may indicate longstanding obstruction.
Abdominal film is used for possible stones or masses.
Excretory urography can be used to identify the site of obstruction and detect associated conditions such as papillary necrosis; however, it is does require the administration of a contrast. It is performed when ultrasound or CT is unable to provide the necessary information, especially when acute calcular obstruction is suspected, because there will be no collecting system dilatation. In obstructive kidneys, the renal density (nephrogram) increases with time after contrast injection. Visualization of the collecting system may be delayed for hours or may not be seen in cases of chronic obstruction. Signs of obstruction are:
• Abrupt termination of the contrast-filled pelvis or ureter
• Dilatation of the collecting system proximally
• Negative pyelogram effect sign, which represents the dilated collecting system seen as branching lucency against the background of density of the nephrogram
• Full-column ureter sign, which is the appearance of the ureter as a full column of contrast rather than the normally interrupted one caused by peristalsis of the normal ureter
Retrograde pyelogram may allow better delineation of the exact point of obstruction and the collecting system distal to the obstruction and may be used to relieve the obstruction
CT is most helpful in obstruction related to a mass and in evaluation of hydronephrosis if simpler methods of evaluation are unsuccessful.
Antegrade studies such as percutaneous antegrade pyelography may be used to delineate the point of obstruction and provide drainage from above. Pressure measurement can be done and may be helpful in separating nonobstructive from obstructive hydronephrosis.
Radionuclide studies are used primarily in the evaluation of the effect of chronic outflow disorders on renal function.

21. What imaging studies are helpful in evaluation of hematuria?
The choice of an imaging study depends on the age of the patient and the suspected cause of hematuria. Infection and calculi are common in young patients, whereas tumors are more common in older patients. The following is usually suggested:

1. **Excretory urography:** This is the primary study in most cases. It may demonstrate:
   - Parenchymal lesions (neoplasm, arteriovenous malformation, non-neoplastic mass, or papillary necrosis)
   - Collecting system tumors, stones, or medullary sponge kidney
2. **Cystoscopy:** This is the procedure of choice for evaluation of suspected mass in the bladder.
3. **CT:** With persistent hematuria and if the above studies are negative, it is reasonable to perform CT. CT is also used to evaluate solid masses and their extent before surgery.
4. **Renal biopsy:** This is used if clinical evidence suggests acute glomerulonephritis or other glomerular problems (proteinuria or red cell casts)
5. **Selective renal arteriography:** This is used for suspected arteriovenous malformation and small renal carcinomas.

BIBLIOGRAPHY

1. Blaufox MD (ed): Radionuclides in Nephro-urology, 2nd ed. Basel, Karger, 1990.
2. Greenberg A (ed): Primer on Kidney Diseases, 2nd ed. San Diego, Academic Press, 1998.
3. Pollack HM (ed): Clinical Urology. Philadelphia, W B. Saunders, 1990.
4. Resnick MI, Rifkin MD: Ultrasonography for the Urinary Tract, 3rd ed. Baltimore, Williams & Wilkins, 1991.

6. RENAL BIOPSY

Jeffrey R. Schelling, M.D.

1. What are some of the indications for renal biopsy?

Persistent hematuria (especially if accompanied by red blood cell casts)
Persistent proteinuria (especially if greater than 3 gm per 24 hr)
Unexplained acute renal failure
Renal transplant allograft dysfunction

2. What are the benefits of a renal biopsy?

A renal biopsy may:
- Help to establish the diagnosis of disease that is either limited to the kidney or part of a systemic disease complex
- Help to provide a prognosis regarding possible renal disease progression and subsequent need for renal replacement therapy
- Help to guide therapeutic options
- Help to limit the pursuit of additional diagnostic studies
- Be used as an investigational tool to better understand the pathophysiology of renal disease

3. What are the risks of renal biopsy?

Up to 80% of renal biopsies are accompanied by a small hematoma within the renal parenchyma. Clinically significant bleeding (persistent gross hematuria, clots within the urinary tract, retroperitoneal bleeding, need for a transfusion) occurs in about 1–2% of renal biopsies. Surgical intervention for intractable bleeding is required in approximately 0.3% of renal biopsies. The risk of introducing infection is very small, particularly when sterile technique is carefully practiced. Arteriovenous fistulas and aneurysms have been described as complications of renal biopsies, although both are rarely clinically significant. Death from a renal biopsy is extremely rare, occurring in approximately 1 in 8,000 procedures.

4. What are the contraindications to renal biopsy?

Coagulation disorders and thrombocytopenia predispose to bleeding complications. Uremic platelet dysfunction is a relative contraindication to renal biopsy, but this can usually be controlled with dialysis or administration of desmopressin (DDAVP), a vasopressin analogue that stimulates platelet coagulation. Uncontrolled hypertension is a relative risk, and it is advisable to maintain blood pressure less than 140/90. Preexisting pyelonephritis may increase the risk of subsequent abscess development. Anatomic abnormalities, particularly the presence of a solitary kidney, are usually considered a contraindication to biopsy. This rationale is based on concerns that (1) uncontrolled bleeding from a solitary kidney may lead to nephrectomy and an anephric state and (2) urinary tract obstruction from a blood clot may result in renal failure. However, there are case series demonstrating the safety of performing biopsy in patients with a solitary kidney. It remains unclear whether a surgical wedge resection ("open biopsy") is associated with a lower morbidity in the setting of a solitary kidney. Patients with impaired mental status may not be candidates for a renal biopsy if they are unable to follow instructions required during the procedure (see question 6).

5. What laboratory studies should be performed prior to a renal biopsy?

It is customary to obtain a baseline hematocrit, platelet count, prothrombin time, and partial thromboplastin time. Some nephrologists will request additional tests to assess the hemostasis adequacy (e.g., bleeding time measurement), but it is unclear whether such studies alter the morbidity and mortality associated with a renal biopsy.

6. How is a renal biopsy performed?

For native kidney biopsies, the patient is generally given a mild general anesthetic or anxiolytic agent (e.g., oral or intravenous benzodiazepine), then placed in a prone position. The kidneys are imaged (see question 7) to identify the lower kidney pole. The skin overlying this area is then prepared with a cleansing solution (e.g., Betadine) and draped with autoclaved towels or sheets to create a sterile field. The region where the biopsy needle will enter the skin is locally anesthetized, typically with 1% lidocaine (Xylocaine). Vital signs, especially pulse and blood pressure, should be obtained immediately prior to the biopsy, to ensure there is no hypotensive effect of the general or local anesthesia and to establish a baseline for postbiopsy comparison. The biopsy needle is advanced only when the patient is holding his or her breath, until it comes in contact with the renal capsule. At this point, the biopsy needle will sway in a superior-inferior direction upon normal respiration. Again while the patient is holding his or her breath, the biopsy needle is quickly advanced to obtain a piece of renal cortex and quickly removed. With these methods, the patient will occasionally describe a sensation of increased pressure on penetration of the renal capsule with the biopsy needle, but there should not be sharp or severe pain.

7. What radiology procedures are used to aid in the renal biopsy?

Renal biopsies are most commonly performed under ultrasound or computed tomography (CT) guidance, at the discretion of the operator. Fluoroscopic guidance is also possible, although this requires administration of a radiocontrast agent, which is relatively contraindicated in patients with preexisting renal insufficiency.

8. What is a biopsy gun?

A biopsy gun is a spring-loaded device that enhances the probability of obtaining kidney tissue by limiting the mechanical manipulation by the operator. In theory, this technique would result in a safer biopsy, because fewer passes with the biopsy gun should be required compared to a standard needle biopsy.

9. What constitutes an adequate biopsy?

Because the most commonly suspected clinical diagnosis is usually a form of glomerular disease, a biopsy core from renal cortex containing a minimum of 6–8 glomeruli is preferable. Two such samples are usually necessary to provide enough tissue for light, immunofluorescence, and electron microscopy studies.

10. How should the patient be monitored following a renal biopsy?

After a native kidney biopsy, the patient should be instructed to lie on his or her back for approximately 6 hours after the biopsy. Following a transplant biopsy, it is also advisable to maintain constant pressure over the biopsy site, for example, with weighted sandbags. Pulse and blood pressure should be checked every 15 minutes for the first 2 hours as an index of hemodynamically significant bleeding. If stable, vital signs can be checked less frequently thereafter. All urine specimens should be saved and observed for gross hematuria. One should not be alarmed at the presence of initial gross hematuria, provided that subsequent specimens reveal resolution of the hematuria. A hematocrit should be measured 4–6 hours after the biopsy to assess change from the baseline value. If there is no evidence of complications at this point, further observation within the hospital is generally not necessary. Therefore, if procedures are performed early in the day, renal biopsies can be done safely on an outpatient basis. Particularly with active children, it is advisable to avoid contact sports for 2–4 weeks postbiopsy, to avoid the possibility of rupturing a renal hematoma.

BIBLIOGRAPHY

1. Falk RJ, Jennette JC: Renal biopsy and treatment of glomerular disease. In Kelley WN (ed): Textbook of Internal Medicine, 3rd ed. Philadelphia, Lippincott-Raven, 1997, pp 1048–1062.
2. Fraser IR, Fairley KF: Renal biopsy as an outpatient procedure. Am J Kidney Dis 25:876–878, 1995.

3. Kasiske BL, Keane WF: Laboratory assessment of renal disease: Clearance, urinalysis and renal biopsy. In Brenner BM (ed): The Kidney, 5th ed. Philadelphia, W.B. Saunders, 1996, pp 1161–1165.
4. Madaio MP: Clinical conference: Renal biopsy. Kidney Int 38:529–543, 1990.
5. Menon SK, Kirchner KA: The role of percutaneous renal biopsy in clinical nephrology. Curr Opin Nephrol Hypertension 2:968–973, 1993.
6. Tisher CC, Croker P: Indications for and interpretations of the renal biopsy: Evaluation by light, electron, and immunofluorescence microscopy. In Schrier RW, Gottschalk CW (eds): Diseases of the Kidney, 6th ed. Boston, Little, Brown, 1997, pp 435–461.

7. INDICATIONS FOR DIALYSIS

Edmond Ricanati, M.D.

1. What is dialysis?

Dialysis is a procedure that removes excess fluid and the toxic end products of metabolism. The two major forms of dialysis are hemodialysis and peritoneal dialysis (see Chapter 44, Technical Aspects of Hemodialysis, and Chapter 47, Technical Aspects of Peritoneal Dialysis). Dialysis is usually prescribed to patients with impaired renal function resulting from acute or chronic renal failure. It is also used occasionally to remove ingested drugs and other toxins in patients who may have normal renal function.

2. What are the common indications for initiating dialysis in patients with acute renal failure?
- Uremic symptoms (e.g., anorexia, nausea, vomiting, encephalopathy)
- Electrolyte or acid-base abnormalities refractory to medical therapy, especially:
    Hyperkalemia
    Metabolic acidosis
    Hyponatremia
- Fluid overload or pulmonary edema refractory to diuretic therapy
- Uremic pericarditis

3. Is there a role for early, prophylactic dialysis in patients with acute renal failure?

There is no evidence that early dialysis improves morbidity or mortality in patients with acute renal failure. Indeed, early dialysis might even delay recovery of renal function. Initiation of dialysis in the setting of acute renal failure is sometimes associated with an abrupt decline in urine output. This phenomenon could be related to dialysis-induced hypotension or to activation of vasoactive compounds as a consequence of blood-dialysis membrane interactions.

4. What are the common indications for initiating dialysis in patients with chronic renal failure?
- Persistent nausea, vomiting, and weight loss. Patients with such symptoms are at increased risk for malnutrition and uremic complications. This is of concern especially when there is a progressive decrease in serum albumin concentration.
- Uremic pericarditis
- Fluid overload and pulmonary edema refractory to diuretic therapy
- Uremic neuropathy, especially when associated with uremic encephalopathy (restlessness, insomnia, anxiety, difficulty with memory, confusion, asterixis)
- Uncontrolled hypertension, especially when associated with fluid overload
- Significant bleeding attributed to uremia
- Glomerular filtration rate of less than 10 ml/min (usually estimated either by creatinine clearance or, more accurately, by the mean of the creatinine and urea clearances)

5. Is there a role for early, prophylactic dialysis in patients with chronic renal failure?

Some studies suggest that long-term patient survival is enhanced when dialysis is initiated "early," that is, before patients have developed significant symptoms of uremia. Other studies indicate better long-term outcomes in patients who are referred to a nephrologist early in the course of their renal disease.

6. How important is the assessment of the nutritional state of the patient as an indicator for early initiation of chronic maintenance dialysis?

According to the Dialysis Outcomes Quality Initiative (DOQI) guidelines, which were based on an extensive and critical review of the literature, dialysis should be initiated when evidence of malnutrition develops in a patient with advanced chronic renal failure. Patients with chronic progressive renal failure develop anorexia, and their protein intake gradually diminishes with progressive drops in creatinine clearance despite efforts to increase nutrition. The long-term survival and the potential for rehabilitation of patients on dialysis are significantly decreased when patients develop malnutrition prior to initiating chronic dialysis.

7. What markers are commonly used in clinical practice for the detection of malnutrition in advanced chronic renal failure?

1. **Anorexia, nausea, vomiting, weight loss**
2. **Low plasma albumin and prealbumin concentrations**. The plasma albumin concentration correlates quite well with body protein stores. Plasma prealbumin has a shorter half-life than albumin and changes rapidly when there are changes in nutritional status. A value below 13 mg/dl is indicative of malnutrition.
3. **Diminished dietary protein intake**. A protein intake of less than 0.8 gm/kg/day or nPNA (protein equivalent of nitrogen appearance normalized using ideal body weight) less than 0.8 gm/kg/day is strongly suggestive of malnutrition.
4. **Abnormal anthropometric measurements**. This is a rapid and reproducible method for evaluating body fat and muscle mass. Values obtained below reference standards for healthy adults are suggestive of malnutrition.
5. **Abnormally low plasma creatinine concentration**. The blood level of plasma creatinine reflects muscle mass. Patients with a plasma creatinine concentration of less than 10 mg/dl at the start of dialysis are considered to be malnourished. This is substantiated by data from the United States Renal Data Systems (USRDS) that revealed that later mortality rate is higher in patients with a plasma creatinine concentration below 10 mg/dl at the time of initiation of dialysis.
6. Other markers of malnutrition are **decreased plasma concentrations of cholesterol, transferrin**, and **somatomedin C**.

BIBLIOGRAPHY

1. CANUSA Peritoneal Dialysis Study Group: Adequacy of dialysis and nutrition in continuous peritoneal dialysis: Association with clinical outcomes. J Am Soc Nephrol 7:198–207, 1995.
2. Chertow GM, Miller SB: Intensity of dialysis in established renal failure. Semin Nephrol 9:476–481, 1996.
3. Conger JD: Does hemodialysis delay the recovery from acute renal failure? Semin Dial 3:146–154, 1990.
4. Hamel MB, Phillip RS, Davis RB, et al: Outcomes and cost-effectiveness of initiating dialysis and continuing aggressive care in seriously ill hospitalized adults. Ann Intern Med 127:195–202, 1997.
5. Lazarus JM, Hakim RM: Timing the initiation of dialysis. J Am Soc Nephrol 6:1319–1326, 1996.
6. US Renal Data System: Patient Mortality and Survival. In USRDS 1996 Annual Report. Bethesda, MD, National Institutes of Health, National Institutes of Diabetes and Digestive and Kidney Diseases, 1996, pp 68–84.

8. DRUG THERAPY IN RENAL DISEASE

Michael B. Ganz, M.D.

1. What are the pharmacokinetic determinants of drug action?
- Absorption or bioavailability of the drug (i.e., the amount of drug that reaches the systemic circulation after administration)
- Degree of protein binding
- Biotransformation in various organs
- Whether biotransformation generates active or inactive metabolites
- Excretion of the parent drug and metabolites (e.g., via the gastrointestinal tract, liver, or kidney)

2. How does plasma protein binding affect drug distribution and action?
Drugs that are easily bound to plasma proteins are confined largely to the vascular space and, therefore, have relatively small volumes of distribution. Protein binding renders the drug pharmacologically inactive by preventing it from getting to its site of action or metabolism. The proportion of free (active) drug will be increased whenever drug protein binding is decreased. Malnutrition and proteinuria lower serum protein levels, effectively reducing proteins available for drug binding. Uremia per se also may alter the protein binding of many drugs (e.g., phenytoin, salicylates, diazepam, methotrexate). It is sometimes necessary to measure both total and free levels of drugs to monitor drug therapy in patients with heavy proteinuria or renal impairment.

3. What mechanisms account for the renal clearance of drugs?
Clearance of drugs by the kidney is dependent on the processes of glomerular filtration and tubular transport. Unbound molecules of appropriate size (including most drugs) can readily pass through the glomerular filtration barrier. Protein-bound molecules usually are not filtered because plasma proteins are restricted by the barrier based on their relatively large size (see Chapter 4, Measurement of Urinary Protein). In patients with glomerular proteinuria, protein-bound drugs may move into the tubular fluid and effectively disappear from plasma at accelerated rates. Many drugs are secreted into tubular lumina from peritubular capillaries via renal tubular cells through active transport mechanisms. When renal disease leads to a reduction in nephrons, the kidney's ability to eliminate drugs declines in proportion to the decline in glomerular filtration rate. As renal failure progresses, drugs filtered or secreted by the kidney can accumulate, potentially resulting in toxicity.

4. Can the kidney metabolize drugs?
The kidney metabolizes a number of endogenous compounds and some drugs. Components of the cytochrome P-450 drug-metabolizing enzymes exist within renal epithelial cells. In patients with renal disease, decreased metabolism may result in increased drug levels. Insulin, for example, is metabolized by the kidney. Plasma insulin levels can increase as renal function decreases, thereby decreasing the need for exogenous insulin or oral hypoglycemic agents.

5. What is the effect of renal disease on drug absorption, distribution, and metabolism?
Absorption of some drugs may be altered in uremia as a consequence of edema of the gastrointestinal tract coupled with uremic nausea, vomiting, or gastroparesis. Alterations in the distribution of drugs vary depending on the agent. Acidic drugs will have a higher free fraction in the plasma of uremic patients as a consequence of decreased protein binding.

Specific metabolites of some pharmacologic agents can accumulate in renal failure. Accumulation of normeperidine, a major metabolite of meperidine (Demerol), in patients with

renal failure can cause seizures. Thiocyanate, a metabolite of nitroprusside, also can cause central
nervous system toxicity. Metabolites of procainamide accumulate in renal failure and may enhance the cardiac toxicities of the parent compound.

6. How is drug dosing altered in patients with renal failure?

Some drugs require a loading dose to generate a therapeutic steady-state drug level within a
short period. In patients with renal failure, the loading dose of a drug is usually not different from
normal. Maintenance doses may be modified in patients with renal failure by interval extension,
that is, lengthening the time interval between doses. This method is more practical for drugs with
long half-lives. Alternatively, the drug dose can be reduced while maintaining the usual dosing
interval. The latter method usually sustains more constant blood levels.

7. How is drug treatment of diabetes mellitus influenced by the presence of renal failure?

As noted in question 4, insulin metabolism declines with deterioration of renal function.
Blood glucose levels should be monitored closely because insulin requirements may change un-
predictably. In the presence of renal failure, oral hypoglycemic agents that are excreted primarily
by the kidney should be avoided or used with caution because prolonged hypoglycemia may
result from drug accumulation. Metformin should not be used in the patient with renal impairment because of an increased risk of lactic acidosis.

8. Which drugs interfere with laboratory tests of renal function?

Cimetidine, trimethoprim, and acetylsalicylic acid increase serum creatinine concentrations
by interfering with tubular secretion of creatinine. Other drugs artifactually elevate serum creatinine levels by interfering with its assay (cefoxitin, methyldopa). Some drugs can change the color
or urine to red-brown (rifampin, phenothiazines) or blue-green (nitrofurantoin, triamterene,
amitriptyline). Finally drugs such as tolbutamide, penicillins, cephalosporins, sulfonamides, and
contrast media can cause a false-positive reaction for protein as measured with a dipstick.

**9. What are special concerns regarding the use of antimicrobial agents in patients with
renal failure?**

The majority of antimicrobial agents are excreted at least partially by the kidney so that dose
reductions often are appropriate in patients with glomerular filtration rates less than 50% of
normal. Gastrointestinal absorption of tetracycline and ciprofloxacin may be decreased if they
are taken with phosphate-binding antacids. Decreased protein binding may contribute to increased neurotoxicity of beta-lactam antibiotics in patients with renal failure.

Nephrotoxicity of antimicrobial agents is a major concern in patients with impaired renal
function and limited renal reserve. The major offenders are the aminoglycosides and amphotericin. Acute allergic interstitial nephritis occurs idiosyncratically with certain antibiotics (especially the beta-lactam agents); however, there are no identifiable risk factors or preventive
measures. The catabolic effects of tetracycline may result in a rise in blood urea nitrogen (BUN),
and, therefore, its use should be avoided in patients with advanced renal insufficiency. Many of
the penicillins are prepared with sodium or potassium. High doses of such agents may be problematic in renal patients with volume overload or hyperkalemia.

10. How does dialysis influence drug therapy?

Dialysis is sometimes employed therapeutically for drug overdoses, even in patients with
normal renal function. On a day-to-day basis, the more important issue is whether dialysis will
eliminate a given drug from the circulation and necessitate an upward adjustment in dose.

11. What drug properties affect dialysis clearance?

Molecule size
Volume of distribution
Degree of protein binding
Water solubility

In general, smaller molecules are more easily dialyzed than large molecules. Drugs that are highly protein-bound or lipophilic (i.e., not water soluble) tend to have large volumes of distribution that render them relatively unavailable for filtration across the dialysis membrane.

BIBLIOGRAPHY

1. Gibson TP: Problems in designing hemodialysis drug studies. Pharmacotherapy 5:23–29, 1985.
2. Golper TA, Bennett WM: Drug usage in dialysis patients. In Nissenson A, Fine R, Gentile D (eds): Clinical Dialysis, 3rd ed. East Norwalk, CT, Appleton & Lange, 1996, pp 608–652.
3. Keller F, Wilms H, Schultze G, et al: Effect of plasma protein binding, volume of distribution, and molecular weight on the fraction of drugs eliminated by hemodialysis. Clin Nephrol 19:201–218, 1993.
4. Madaerazo E, Sun HE, Jay GT: Simplification of antibiotic dose adjustments in renal insufficiency. The DREM system. Lancet 340:767–785, 1992.
5. Reetze-Bonorden P, Bohler J, Keller E: Drug dosage in patients during continuous renal replacement therapy. Clin Pharmacokinetics 18:104–131, 1990.

II. Clinical Syndromes

9. ETIOLOGY, PATHOPHYSIOLOGY, AND DIAGNOSIS OF ACUTE RENAL FAILURE

Miriam F. Weiss, M.D.

1. What is acute renal failure?

Acute renal failure is a sudden decrease in renal function usually manifested by azotemia (increase in blood urea nitrogen [BUN] and serum creatinine concentration) and sometimes associated with oliguria.

2. Define oliguria.

Oliguria refers to urine volumes less than 400 ml/day or 20 ml/hour.

3. What is the difference between acute renal failure and acute tubular necrosis?

Acute renal failure refers to any condition characterized by decreased renal excretory capacity. The differential diagnosis of acute renal failure includes prerenal azotemia (about 70% of cases) and obstructive uropathy (5% of cases) (see Chapter 11, Prerenal Azotemia, and Chapter 12, Obstructive Uropathy). Renal parenchymal disease is the cause of acute renal failure in about 25% of patients. Renal diseases associated with acute renal failure include conditions such as acute glomerulonephritis, acute interstitial nephritis, and rapidly progressive glomerulonephritis. The vast majority of patients with parenchymal renal disease and acute renal failure have acute tubular necrosis. Thus, the two terms often are used synonymously even though patients with acute tubular necrosis represent only a subset of patients with acute renal failure.

4. How common is acute renal failure?

Acute renal failure develops in up to 5% of patients admitted to medical or surgical services.

5. What laboratory parameters help to differentiate prerenal azotemia from acute tubular necrosis?

	Prerenal Azotemia	Acute Tubular Necrosis
Urine specific gravity	> 1.018	~ 1.010
Urine sodium	< 10 mEq/L	> 20 mEq/L
Fractional excretion of sodium	< 1%	> 2%
Urine osmolality	> 500 mOsm/L	~ 280 mOsm/L
Urine sediment	Normal, or clear hyaline casts	Renal tubular cells and "muddy-brown" granular casts

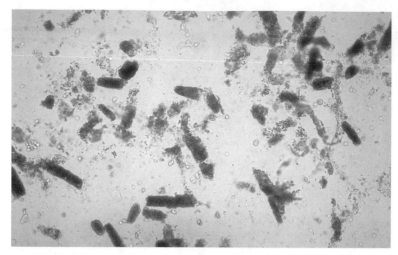

Light microscopic view of unstained urinary sediment from patient with acute tubular necrosis (ATN). Note multiple granular casts, typical of the "dirty brown" urine of ATN. (Original magnification ×40.)

6. Calculate the fractional excretion of sodium (FE Na), %.

$$FENa = \frac{Na^+ \text{ excreted}}{Na^+ \text{ filtered}} \cdot 100 = \frac{U \ Na^+ \cdot V}{P \ Na^+ \cdot \dfrac{U \ creat \cdot V}{P \ Creat}} \cdot 100 = \frac{U/P \ Na^+}{U/P \ creatinine} \cdot 100$$

where U = urine, P = plasma, and V = volume.

7. What are the two major categories of acute tubular necrosis?
1. Ischemic   2. Nephrotoxic

8. What is ischemic acute tubular necrosis?
    Ischemic acute tubular necrosis results from hypoperfusion of the kidneys and can occur in any of the conditions associated with prerenal azotemia (see Chapter 11, Prerenal Azotemia) when the hypoperfusion is sustained and severe.

9. What are the causes of nephrotoxic acute tubular necrosis?
   • Exogenous toxins
      Radiocontrast agents
      Nephrotoxic antibiotics (e.g., aminoglycosides)
      Nephrotoxic anticancer agents
      Heavy metals (lead, mercury)
      Lithium
      Fluorinated anesthetics (methyoxyflurane, halothane)
      Organic solvents (e.g., ethylene glycol)
   • Endogenous toxins
      Rhabdomyolysis (myoglobin)
      Hemolysis (hemoglobin)
      Tumor lysis syndrome
      Myeloma
      Hypercalcemia

10. What is the pathophysiology of acute tubular necrosis?
    Results of animal studies have generated several speculated mechanisms that may account for the decrease in glomerular filtration that characterizes acute tubular necrosis:

- **Intratubular obstruction:** Following an ischemic or nephrotoxic insult, tubular cells, cellular debris (brush border membranes), and crystals (uric acid, etc.) slough into the tubular lumen and occlude the flow of filtrate.
- **Tubular backleak:** Disruption in tubular basement membranes leads to abnormal reabsorption of filtrate.
- **Vasoconstriction:** Damage to tubules evokes neurohumoral mechanisms that secondarily decrease renal blood flow.
- **Changes in glomerular permeability:** The ischemic or nephrotoxic insult directly alters the intrinsic permeability of glomerular capillary membrane.

These mechanisms are not mutually exclusive; some combination of mechanisms is likely involved in humans with acute tubular necrosis. In patients with ischemic acute tubular necrosis, recent interest has focused on the role of **reperfusion injury,** which is characterized by the generation of oxygen radicals, disruption of cell membranes, leak of calcium and other cations into the cell, depletion of high-energy phosphate compounds, and mitochrondrial dysfunction leading to cell death.

11. Which underlying conditions increase the risk of developing acute tubular necrosis after exposure to radiocontrast agents?

Chronic renal insufficiency
Diabetes mellitus
Dehydration

12. Characterize the course of acute tubular necrosis.

The **initiation phase** is the period of time during which exposure to a nephrotoxic agent or ischemia takes place. In clinical practice, it is common for there to be more than one cause of acute tubular necrosis; ischemic and nephrotoxic insults often coexist. The **maintenance phase** may last from days to as long as 6 weeks. This period of time is characterized by persistent oliguria. During the maintenance phase, patients are often dependent on some form of renal replacement therapy (dialysis or continuous hemofiltration). With stabilization of other underlying disease processes and nutritional support, the patient may enter the **recovery phase** of acute tubular necrosis. This period, also called the "diuretic phase," is characterized by increasing urine output and the gradual recovery of renal function. BUN and creatinine levels generally return to normal. However, evidence of tubular dysfunction (e.g., failure to maximally concentrate the urine in response to water deprivation) may persist for months to years after recovery from acute tubular necrosis.

13. How do nephrotoxic and ischemic acute tubular necrosis differ from each other?

Nephrotoxic acute tubular necrosis is more likely to be associated with a nonoliguric presentation. The increase in BUN and creatinine may be relatively gradual. Acute tubular necrosis caused by nephrotoxins also is more likely to fit the criteria for the "intermediate syndrome." Patients with intermediate syndrome show some characteristics of reversible prerenal azotemia, such as a relatively low urine sodium, a partial response to fluid challenge, and a shorter maintenance phase.

14. Describe the pathologic lesion of acute tubular necrosis.

Whether acute tubular necrosis follows ischemia or toxic injury, renal parenchymal changes are patchy and irregular. There is tubular cell necrosis with varying degrees of regeneration. Reflecting the findings on urinalysis, loss of tubular brush border membranes and renal tubular cell casts are frequent findings. Interstitial edema and interstitial inflammation may be present. The findings are relatively nonspecific and may persist even during the recovery phase.

15. What is the mortality rate in patients with acute tubular necrosis?

Overall, mortality rates are between 50% and 70%.

16. What are the common causes of death in patients with acute renal failure?
1. Infections (30–70%)
2. Cardiovascular events (5–30%)
3. Gastrointestinal, pulmonary, or neurologic complications (7–30%)
4. Hyperkalemia or technical issues related to dialytic therapy (1–2%)

BIBLIOGRAPHY

1. Brady HR, Singer GG: Acute renal failure. Lancet 346:1533–1540, 1995.
2. Klahr S, Miller SB: Acute oliguria. N Engl J Med 338:671–675, 1998.
3. Proceedings of the First International Course on Critical Care Nephrology. Kidney Int 64(suppl):S1–S90, 1998.
4. Weisberg LS, Kurnik PB, Kurnik BRC: Risk of radiocontrast nephropathy in patients with and without diabetes mellitus. Kidney Int 45:259–265, 1994.

10. MANAGEMENT OF ACUTE RENAL FAILURE

Miriam F. Weiss, M.D.

1. What are the principles of managing patients with acute tubular necrosis?

There is currently no specific therapy, but there has been some interest in the use of calcium channel blockers, oxygen radical scavengers, nucleotides, and certain growth factors to hasten recovery. Usually, recovery from acute tubular necrosis is spontaneous. Management is supportive and based on the following principles:

- Restrict fluid, sodium, potassium, and phosphate intake.
- Restrict protein intake to reduce the generation of urea.
- Use diuretics to control hypervolemia.
- Administer $NaHCO_3$ to correct acidemia.
- Adjust the dosage of medications that rely on the kidney for clearance or metabolism.
- Dialyze the patient when conservative management is not sufficient to maintain solute and water balance.

2. Can diuretics prevent acute tubular necrosis?

Definitive controlled trials are lacking. However, it has become routine to administer IV fluids and diuretics under certain circumstances. For example, IV fluids and mannitol are administered routinely prior to cross-clamping of the aorta in patients undergoing repair of abdominal aortic aneurysms. Aggressive hydration and forced alkaline-osmotic diuresis using $NaHCO_3$ and mannitol have been used in patients with rhabdomyolysis to maintain a high-output state and minimize the risk of acute renal failure. In patients at high risk for the development of radiocontrast-induced renal failure, administration of IV fluids (0.45% saline) before the imaging procedure has been found to be more effective in preventing acute renal failure than the combination of IV fluids and diuretics (either furosemide or mannitol).

3. Can diuretics convert oliguric to nonoliguric acute tubular necrosis?

Because the etiologies of acute tubular necrosis are diverse, the benefit of diuretics remains undetermined. However, it is widely believed that the prognosis of patients with nonoliguric renal failure is better than those with oliguria. Consequently, high doses of loop diuretics often are administered to patients in the early phase of acute tubular necrosis to promote urine flow.

4. What is the downside of using diuretics in acute renal failure?

Excessive diuresis may lead to volume depletion and renal hypoperfusion, adding insult to injury.

5. Why are high doses of loop diuretics needed in the setting of acute renal failure?

The formula espoused in Samuel Shem's novel *House of God:*

Age + blood urea nitrogen [BUN] = Lasix dose

is roughly correct! Furosemide and other loop diuretics act on the luminal side of tubular cells in the ascending limb of the loop of Henle. They arrive there following active secretion into the tubular lumen by proximal tubular cells. In patients with tubular necrosis, the latter process is impaired so that large doses of continuous infusions often are needed to achieve a diuretic effect.

6. How does "renal-dose" dopamine improve urine output in acute renal failure?

The benefit of dopamine in preventing or treating acute tubular necrosis and other forms of acute renal failure has not been clearly demonstrated. Nonetheless, administration of renal-dose (1–3 µg/kg/min) dopamine is a widespread practice in the managment of oliguric patients.

Renal-dose dopamine is thought to increase urine output through direct tubular effects. It may also help to increase the tubular delivery of diuretics and block aldosterone's salt-retaining effect in the distal tubule. Theoretically, renal-dose dopamine increases renal blood flow through specific renal dopaminergic receptors. Finally, dopamine may increase urine output through increased cardiac output as a result of beta-adrenergic stimulation of the heart.

7. What are the risks of administering renal-dose dopamine?

Even low-dose dopamine can induce tachycardia, cardiac arrhythmia, or myocardial ischemia. Dopamine also blunts hypoxemic ventilatory drive and can decrease minute ventilation. Because of its alpha-adrenergic effect, ischemia of the digits can occur. Bowel ischemia, although uncommon, can result in translocation of bacteria or bacterial products across the intestine. This is a particularly important risk in the face of increased susceptibility to infection seen in patients with acute renal failure.

8. What are the goals of renal replacement therapy (dialysis or continuous hemofiltration) in acute renal failure?

When conservative therapy fails to maintain fluid and electrolyte balance within safe ranges, or when uremic symptoms (including pericarditis) develop, renal replacement therapy is initiated. The goal of renal replacement therapy is to normalize the fluid-volume status, correct electrolyte balance, and control uremia. This simple statement masks the complexity of the decision making involved in starting renal replacement therapy. The exact method chosen, whether to start dialysis early or late in the course of acute renal failure, and the intensity of the renal replacement therapy are areas of controversy.

9. What are the advantages and disadvantages of intermittent versus continuous renal replacement therapies?

	Advantages	*Disadvantages*
Intermittent hemodialysis	Efficient and rapid removal of volume and small molecules Cost effective Readily available	Central venous access required Anticoagulation may be required May not be tolerated by hemodynamically unstable patients
Continuous hemofiltration	Excellent control of volume enabling liberal use of hyperalimentation, blood products, etc. Good removal of larger molecules Can be used in relatively hypotensive patients	Central venous access required Anticoagulation may be required Labor intensive and expensive
Peritoneal dialysis	No need for anticoagulation Cost-effective	Slow removal of uremic toxins Risk of peritonitis May be tolerated poorly in patients with splanchnic hypoperfusion

10. What about nutritional support for patients with acute renal failure?

Acute renal failure results in insulin resistance, changes in nitrogen balance due to increased protein turnover, exhaustion of antioxidant defenses, and hormonal alterations. Current recommendations for enteral or parenteral nutrition during acute renal failure are to give ~ 35 kcal/kg body weight/day, ~ 1.2 gm protein/kg body weight/day, and a ratio between glucose and lipid in the nonprotein part of energy of ~ 70/30. There is no proven difference between essential amino acid–enriched and routine formulas for hyperalimentation.

11. Does appropriate nutritional support result in improved morbidity and mortality?

Because of the severity of illness, complexity of care, and high incidence of comorbid conditions, the efficacy of nutritional therapy has *not* been demonstrated in patients with acute renal failure. Administration of large volumes of enteral nutrition to patients with renal failure can result in volume overload, more rapid increases in BUN, and alterations in critical plasma electrolyte levels. Careful attention must be given to controlling these factors when nutritional support is prescribed.

BIBLIOGRAPHY

1. Brady HR, Singer GG: Acute renal failure. Lancet 346:1533–1540, 1995.
2. Chertow GM, Sayegh MH, Allgren RL, Lazarus JM: Is the administration of dopamine associated with adverse or favorable outcomes in acute renal failure? Am J Med 101:49–53, 1996.
3. Klahr S, Miller SB: Acute oliguria. N Engl J Med 338:671–675, 1998.
4. Proceedings of the First International Course on Critical Care Nephrology. Kidney Int 64(suppl):S1–S90, 1998.
5. Shem S: The House of God. New York, Bantam Doubleday, 1978.
6. Solomon R, Werner C, Mann D, et al: Effects of saline, mannitol and furosemide on acute decreases in renal function induced by radiocontrast agents. N Engl J Med 331:1416–1420, 1994.
7. Thadhani R, Pascual M, Bonventre JV: Acute renal failure. N Engl J Med 334:1448–1460, 1996.
8. Weisberg LS, Kurnik PB, Kurnik BRC: Risk of radiocontrast nephropathy in patients with and without diabetes mellitus. Kidney Int 45:259–265, 1994.

11. PRERENAL AZOTEMIA

Edmond Ricanati, M.D.

1. What is prerenal azotemia?

Prerenal azotemia is an elevation of serum creatinine concentration or blood urea nitrogen (BUN) resulting from a reduction in renal blood flow and glomerular filtration rate. Prerenal azotemia is a physiologic response to diminished renal perfusion. Renal tubular function is normal and appropriate. By definition, the azotemia is not a consequence of parenchymal renal disease. However, patients with parenchymal renal disease may develop prerenal azotemia superimposed on a fixed decrease in glomerular filtration rate.

2. What are the most common pathologic causes of prerenal azotemia?
- Hypovolemia
  Dehydration
  Hemorrhage
  Renal fluid losses (diuretics)
  Gastrointestinal losses (vomiting, diarrhea)
  "Third spacing"
- Low cardiac output (e.g., congestive heart failure)
- Conditions associated with systemic vasodilatation
  Sepsis
  Neurogenic shock

3. Which medications can cause prerenal azotemia? Explain the mechanism(s) responsible for their adverse effects.

1. **Nonsteroidal anti-inflammatory drugs that inhibit renal prostaglandin biosynthesis** can trigger prerenal azotemia, particularly in patients with volume depletion. They act by interfering with the renal afferent arteriolar adaptive response to hypovolemia, namely afferent arteriolar vasodilation mediated by increased synthesis of prostaglandins (PGE_2 and PGI_2) in volume-depleted states.

2. **Angiotensin-converting enzyme (ACE) inhibitors or angiotensin II receptor blockers.** Angiotensin II maintains glomerular filtration pressure in renal hypoperfusion by preferentially constricting the efferent arterioles. Angiotensin inhibitors blunt this response and can result in a dissociation of the autoregulation of renal blood flow and glomerular filtration rate, leading to a significant reduction in glomerular filtration rate. This is a problem particularly in patients with bilateral renal artery stenosis but sometimes can be seen in volume-depleted patients.

3. **Other antihypertensive drugs** can cause prerenal azotemia if blood pressure is lowered excessively.

4. **Cyclosporine** causes intrarenal vasoconstriction that may be related to release of endothelin, a potent vasoconstrictor peptide released from the endothelial cells in the walls of the arterioles.

5. **Amphotericin B** causes intrarenal vasoconstriction and can lead to renal ischemia and prerenal azotemia with increasing doses of the drug. Amphotericin B is also directly toxic to the proximal epithelial cells.

4. What are the renal hemodynamic changes in hypovolemic states that preserve glomerular perfusion and filtration rate? How are they altered in prerenal azotemia?

When effective volume is diminished, several compensatory mechanisms are invoked to preserve glomerular filtration:

• Diminished glomerular perfusion stimulates stretch receptors in the afferent arterioles resulting in vasodilatation through a local myogenic response.
• Increased production of vasodilator substances (vasodilator prostaglandins such as PGE_2 and PGI_2 and possibly nitric oxide) maximally dilate the afferent arterioles.
• Increased intrarenal production of angiotensin II from renin causes a preferential constriction of the efferent arterioles resulting in increased filtration pressure.

Preglomerular arteriolar dilatation and postglomerular arteriolar constriction preserve glomerular perfusion and, by increasing filtration pressure, maintain a normal glomerular filtration rate. In prerenal azotemia, renal perfusion is significantly compromised, and the above autoregulatory mechanisms fail to maintain adequate glomerular perfusion and filtration pressure, resulting in the retention of creatinine and urea.

5. What clinical and laboratory findings distinguish prerenal azotemia from acute tubular necrosis?

In acute tubular necrosis, there is significant renal parenchymal damage due to severe renal ischemia or the administration of a nephrotoxic agent. Renal perfusion and tubular function are disrupted. In prerenal azotemia, renal tubular function is preserved. The major laboratory findings that distinguish prerenal azotemia from acute tubular necrosis are:

1. **Urine sediment**, which is normal in prerenal azotemia, reveals epithelial cells, epithelial cell casts, and muddy brown granular casts when examined at the time of the acute injury.

2. **Fractional excretion of sodium** (FENa; the percentage of filtered sodium that is excreted in the urine). In prerenal azotemia, there is intense retention of sodium, and the FENa is less than 1%. It is above 2% in acute tubular necrosis, an indication that there is tubular injury. The FENa is the most reliable index for the diagnosis of acute tubular necrosis (see Chapter 9, Etiology, Pathophysiology, and Diagnosis of Acute Renal Failure, for calculation of the FENa).

3. **Urine osmolality**. In acute tubular necrosis, there is early loss of concentrating ability. The urine osmolality is usually below 350 mOsm/kg. In prerenal azotemia, urine osmolality is usually above 500 mOsm/kg and reflects normal tubular function.

4. **BUN to plasma creatinine ratio**. This is in the normal range in acute tubular necrosis (10–15 to 1). In prerenal azotemia, it is usually greater than 20 to 1 and reflects the increase in urea absorption that follows the enhanced proximal reabsorption of sodium and water. This parameter is less reliable than the FENa and urine osmolality determinations.

None of the above criteria is helpful when prerenal azotemia is superimposed on underlying chronic renal disease. In chronic renal disease, sodium conservation and urine concentration are impaired, and the urine sediment may be abnormal.

6. When is the diagnostic utility of FENa of limited value?

The FENa is of limited value when prerenal azotemia is associated with
• Chronic renal failure in which high fractional excretion of sodium is required to maintain sodium balance
• Use of diuretics, which results in excessive urinary sodium loss
• Acute volume expansion, which promotes increased sodium excretion

There are a number of cases of acute renal failure other than prerenal azotemia in which fractional excretion of sodium may be less than 1%:
• Acute glomerulonephritis or vasculitis. In these conditions, glomerular filtration rate is reduced, but tubular function is preserved.
• Some cases of acute interstitial nephritis
• Some cases of acute renal failure due to radiocontrast media or heme pigments
• When prerenal azotemia is changing to acute tubular necrosis. This usually occurs within the first 48 hours of the ischemic event. Under these conditions, glomerular filtration rate is reduced, but tubular function is largely preserved.

7. What are the guidelines for treatment of prerenal azotemia?

1. Restore the normal circulating blood volume. In the absence of congestive heart failure, administration of fluids (usually normal saline) at a rate of 75–100 ml/hr is adequate. Hypovolemia due to hemorrhage or the presence of severe anemia should be corrected with blood transfusions.

2. The types of fluid administered and the rate at which replacement fluids are given will depend on the serum electrolytes (especially serum sodium, potassium, and the acid-base status of the patient) and the clinical status of the patient.

3. Monitor the adequacy of fluid replacement by the clinical examination of the patient and by the serial determinations of serum creatine concentrations, which reflect renal function. Follow daily weights, fluid intake, and urine output, as well as urine sodium excretion and serial measurements of the serum creatinine, BUN, serum electrolytes, and acid-base parameters. Hemodynamic monitoring may be necessary if clinical assessment of cardiovascular function and fluid status is difficult. Response to proper fluid replacement in prerenal azotemia is rapid; renal function usually returns to the previous baseline within 3–4 days.

8. What is the hepatorenal syndrome?

The hepatorenal syndrome is defined as progressive azotemia in a patient with advanced liver disease. In many ways, patients with hepatorenal syndrome appear to have intense prerenal azotemia. However, they usually fail to respond to conventional measures outlined in question 7 and usually exhibit a rapid downhill course characterized by oliguria, azotemia, and a high rate of mortality. Liver transplantation is currently the most effective treatment.

BIBLIOGRAPHY

1. Hricik DE, Dunn MJ: Angiotensin-converting enzyme inhibitor–induced renal failure: Causes, consequences, and diagnostic uses. J Am Soc Nephrol 1:845–858, 1990.
2. Klahr S, Miller SB: Acute oliguria. N Engl J Med 338:671–675, 1998.
3. Levy M: Hepatorenal syndrome. Kidney Int 43:737–753, 1993.
4. Miller TR, Anderson RJ, Linas SL, et al: Urinary diagnostic indices in acute renal failure: A prospective study. Ann Intern Med 47:89–96, 1978.

12. OBSTRUCTIVE UROPATHY

Lavinia A. Negrea, M.D.

1. What is obstructive uropathy?

Obstructive uropathy refers to structural or functional interference with normal urine flow anywhere along the urinary tract from the renal tubule to the urethra. Depending on the underlying disease process, obstruction may involve one or both kidneys. Obstruction of both kidneys generally results in some degree of renal failure.

2. What are the most common causes of obstructive uropathy?

The causes of obstructive uropathy vary with age and gender. In children, congenital abnormalities such as ureteropelvic junction obstruction (both sexes) and posterior urethral valves (boys) are the most common causes. Nephrolithiasis is the most common cause of obstructive uropathy in young men. In young women, the most common cause of obstruction is pregnancy, although this form of obstructive uropathy is rarely clinically significant. In the elderly, benign and malignant tumors, especially benign hypertrophy and carcinoma of the prostate, emerge as important causes of obstructive uropathy.

3. How does pregnancy cause obstructive uropathy?

Ureteral dilatation may be seen as early as the first trimester and probably reflects the hormonal effect of progesterone on ureteral peristalsis. In late pregnancy, ureteral dilatation has been attributed to pressure by the gravid uterus on the pelvic brim. The right ureter is more often affected than the left.

4. What is functional obstructive uropathy?

This term generally refers to neurologic disorders that lead to "neurogenic" bladder dysfunction. Disorders associated with upper motor neuron injury (e.g., cerebrovascular accidents) result in involuntary bladder contraction (spastic bladder) that can lead to obstructive uropathy. After lower motor neuron injuries or in patients with peripheral neuropathies (e.g., diabetic neuropathy), the bladder becomes atonic. Medications such as levodopa or disopyramide also can decrease bladder contractility and tone.

5. What changes in renal blood flow occur during obstruction?

An increase in renal blood flow to more than 40% above normal occurs within a few minutes of ureteral occlusion and is due to a decrease in renal vascular resistance. This effect is mediated by the local production of prostacyclin and prostaglandin E_2. In later stages of obstruction, renal blood flow decreases sharply below normal. Angiotensin II and thromboxane mediate this vasoconstrictive phase.

6. Why does glomerular filtration rate decrease during obstruction?

Early in obstruction, intrarenal tubular pressure proximal to the obstruction increases. The net glomerular filtration pressure (which equals glomerular filtration pressure minus intratubular pressure) then decreases, and glomerular filtration rate subsequently decreases. In later stages of obstruction, the glomerular filtration rate decreases due to the decrease in renal blood flow.

7. Does the glomerular filtration rate improve after the relief of obstruction?

The degree of improvement in glomerular filtration rate is influenced by the duration of obstruction. Normal renal function can be restored if the obstruction is corrected within 1 week. Approximately 20% of the glomerular filtration rate can be recovered after 4 weeks. Little or no recovery is expected after 6–8 weeks of continuous and complete obstruction.

8. What happens to urine output in obstructive uropathy?

Urine output varies from anuria (in complete obstruction) to significant degrees of polyuria. Polyuria is sometimes observed in patients with partial or incomplete obstruction. It represents a form of nephrogenic diabetes insipidus resulting from a concentrating defect that may be mediated by the direct effects of increased tubular pressure on the function of distal renal tubular cells.

9. Is pain always present in obstructive uropathy?

Pain due to obstruction is caused by distention of the collecting system. Its intensity is a reflection of the rapidity rather than the degree of obstruction. Acute blockage of the ureter may be associated with excruciating pain, whereas slowly developing obstruction may be completely painless.

10. What electrolyte abnormalities are associated with obstructive uropathy?

Obstructive uropathy often is associated with hyperkalemia or metabolic acidosis. Defects in the excretion of potassium or hydrogen sometimes reflect a state of resistance to mineralocorticoids such as aldosterone.

11. What is the most common complication of obstructive uropathy?

Urinary tract infection is by far the most common complication and results, at least partly, from decreased bacterial washout in the face of reduced urine flow. Eradication of infection is difficult as long as obstruction persists. As a corollary, relief of obstruction is critical to management of the concomitant infection.

12. What mechanisms account for hypertension in obstructive uropathy?

In chronic bilateral ureteral obstruction, hypertension is generally secondary to renal failure and extracellular fluid volume expansion. In acute unilateral obstruction, increased renin secretion is usually responsible for the hypertension.

13. What is postobstructive diuresis?

Postobstructive diuresis may occur from 2–8 days following relief of obstruction. It usually occurs after one has relieved sudden, complete obstruction and is often brief in duration. The diuresis is related to an expanded extracellular fluid volume, an osmotic diuresis resulting from rapid elimination of retained solutes, and a transient concentrating defect resulting from the mechanical effects of high intratubular pressure. Iatrogenic contributions include excessive volume replacement, particularly with isotonic solutions containing glucose or saline.

14. What are the merits and the limitations of the renal ultrasound in diagnosing obstruction?

Ultrasound is a noninvasive diagnostic test used initially in suspected obstruction. The main findings vary depending on the site of obstruction but can include dilation of the ureters or renal collecting systems. False-negative tests can occur, rarely, as a consequence of dehydration, recent onset of obstruction (within the first 1–3 days, when the collecting system is relatively noncompliant), or encasement of the collecting system by retroperitoneal fibrosis (idiopathic, drug-related, postradiation).

15. What are the advantages and disadvantages of an intravenous pyelogram in diagnosing obstructive uropathy?

Intravenous pyelography can identify both the presence and the location of obstruction. It is considered the procedure of choice in acute obstruction due to kidney stones. In patients with multiple renal cysts, it is superior to ultrasound in distinguishing hydronephrosis from parapelvic renal cysts. With increasing degrees of azotemia, the ability of intravenous pyelography to delineate the collecting system diminishes, and the risk of acute renal failure from exposure to radiocontrast increases.

16. What is the role of computed tomography (CT) scans in diagnosing obstruction?

The CT scan is an accurate technique for detection of urinary tract dilatation and is particularly helpful in identifying lesions extrinsic to the collecting system. However, administration of intravenous contrast often is required. The value of noncontrast helical (spiral) CT in the evaluation of obstruction is currently being investigated.

17. When is retrograde pyelography indicated in the diagnosis of obstructive uropathy?

Retrograde pyelography is used to diagnose an obstruction when other imaging techniques are equivocal, in patients with poor renal function, and in those allergic to radiocontrast dye.

18. What is a "furosemide renogram"?

A furosemide renogram is a radionuclide study in which images of the kidney are obtained before and after administration of the diuretic. By exaggerating urine flow, the study may demonstrate obstructive uropathy when other studies are equivocal. Loop diuretics other than furosemide can probably be employed with comparable results.

19. What percentage of end-stage renal disease is due to obstructive nephropathy?

Obstructive nephropathy accounts for about 2% of all of the patients with end-stage renal disease.

BIBLIOGRAPHY

1. Klahr S: Obstructive nephropathy. Kidney Int 54:286–300, 1998.
2. Klahr S: Obstructive nephropathy. In Jacobson HR, Striker GE, Klahr S (eds): The Principles and Practice of Nephrology. St. Louis, Mosby, 1991, pp 432–457.
3. Korbet SM: Obstructive uropathy. In Greenberg A (ed): Primer on Kidney Diseases, 2nd ed. San Diego, Academic Press, 1998, pp 348–356.
4. Schlueter W, Battle DC. Chronic obstructive nephropathy Semin Nephrol 8:17–28, 1988.
5. Yarger WE, Harris RH: Urinary tract obstruction. In Seldin DW, Giebisch G (eds): The Kidney: Physiology and Pathophysiology. New York, Raven Press, 1985, pp 1963–1978.

13. ASYMPTOMATIC PROTEINURIA

Jeffrey R. Schelling, M.D.

1. What is the normal amount of urinary protein excretion?

Protein excretion usually ranges between 40 and 80 mg per day, but most laboratories define 150 mg per day as the upper limit of normal.

2. How is asymptomatic proteinuria defined?

Asymptomatic proteinuria is urinary protein excretion greater than 150 mg, but less than 3.5 gm per day, not associated with symptoms or signs of the nephrotic syndrome (edema, hypoalbuminemia, hyperlipidemia, thrombotic complications). Despite the broad range of urinary protein excretion included in this definition, patients with asymptomatic proteinuria characteristically excrete less than 1 gm of protein per day. In general, the clinical conditions associated with asymptomatic proteinuria are of less serious consequence than those associated with the nephrotic syndrome.

3. Is the dipstick examination of urine a reliable measurement of protein excretion?

Under most circumstances, it is. However, there are certain exceptions that should be considered. First, urine dipsticks most reliably measure albumin, but even albumin is not consistently detectable until the concentration exceeds 20–30 mg/dl. Second, the dipstick exam is not useful for the detection of globulins, mucoproteins, and Bence Jones proteins. Finally, dipstick detection of protein provides only a semiquantitative assessment of proteinuria. A given protein concentration in a dilute urine reflects much greater protein excretion than does the same protein concentration in a concentrated urine. Therefore, the dipstick protein concentration should be assessed in the context of the urine specific gravity, which can be measured simultaneously during a routine urinalysis. Even normal amounts of urinary protein can register as 1+ on a dipstick if the urine is highly concentrated (specific gravity > 1.025).

4. What are the most reliable methods for quantitative measurement of urinary protein excretion?

The best method is a 24-hour urine collection for measurement of total protein. This assay should always be accompanied by measurement of the urine creatinine concentration to assess the adequacy of the urine collection. Women with normal muscle mass excrete approximately 15–20 mg creatinine/kg body weight/day, while men with normal muscle mass excrete about 20–25 mg creatinine/kg body weight/day. Values significantly less than these, regardless of the urine volume, indicate an inadequate urine collection, which will result in spuriously depressed estimates of urine protein excretion. Urine protein excretion can also be estimated from a spot urine sample by determining the ratio of urine protein (mg/dl) to urine creatinine (mg/dl) (see Chapter 4, Measurement of Urinary Protein).

5. What is glomerular permselectivity?

Glomerular permselectivity refers to a property of the glomerular capillary membrane whereby solutes, including proteins, are restricted from passage across the capillary wall into the urinary space. Exclusion of a protein from Bowman's space is based to some extent on its molecular size and conformation, but mostly results from its net negative charge. Negatively charged proteins are excluded from the glomerular ultrafiltrate due to their inability to pass through the negatively charged glomerular capillary basement and its surrounding endothelial and epithelial structures.

6. What are the common causes of asymptomatic proteinuria?

In contrast to nephrotic-range proteinuria, which is almost invariably due to glomerular disease, asymptomatic proteinuria may result from glomerular or tubular disorders. Glomerular proteinuria tends to be associated with excretion of high–molecular weight proteins, such as albumin and globulins, whereas tubular proteinuria characteristically involves excretion of smaller proteins as well. Some of the most common causes of each type of asymptomatic proteinuria are listed below:

Glomerular	Tubular
Functional proteinuria	Hereditary (Fanconi syndrome, Wilson's disease)
Orthostatic proteinuria	Chronic K^+ depletion
Early glomerular disease	Acute tubular necrosis
	Analgesic nephropathy
	Heavy metal toxicity (e.g., cadmium)
	Pyelonephritis
	Overflow proteinuria

7. What is functional proteinuria?

Functional proteinuria is transient protein excretion that is associated with a number of clinical conditions including fever, strenuous exercise, emotional stress, and congestive heart failure. The mechanism of increased protein excretion in these conditions is related, in part, to decreased renal plasma flow, which has been shown to facilitate albumin excretion. In conditions associated with high circulating levels of angiotensin II (e.g., heart failure, renovascular hypertension), proteinuria may be mediated by direct effects of angiotensin II on glomerular permselectivity.

8. What is orthostatic proteinuria?

Orthostatic or postural proteinuria is a condition in which patients excrete excess urine protein only when in the upright position. Orthostatic proteinuria occurs almost exclusively in young men and usually does not exceed 1 gm per 24 hours. To make a diagnosis, patients should be instructed to collect urine beginning in the morning and ending at bedtime (~ 16-hour collection). A second collection is then started at night and continued until the following morning (~ 8-hour collection). Both samples are then assayed for total protein, and values are extrapolated to 24 hours. A diagnosis of orthostatic proteinuria is made if the daytime (upright) protein excretion is elevated and the nighttime (recumbent) protein excretion is normal. If the protein content in both collections is increased, the patient has "persistent" proteinuria, which usually indicates the presence of structural glomerular or tubular renal disease. Long-term follow-up studies have revealed that the majority of patients with orthostatic proteinuria do not have associated glomerular pathology and exhibit spontaneous resolution of proteinuria over 5–10 years.

9. How does tubular disease lead to abnormal proteinuria?

Despite glomerular permselectivity, small amounts of protein normally are filtered at the glomerulus. However, most of the filtered protein is subsequently reabsorbed and catabolized by proximal tubular epithelial cells. In the presence of injured or diseased tubules, the capacity for protein reabsorption may be compromised, and much of the filtered protein load is excreted, rather than reabsorbed. Furthermore, some proteins, such as Tamm-Horsfall proteins, are actually produced by tubular epithelial cells.

10. What is overflow proteinuria?

Overflow or overproduction proteinuria is a clinical condition in which the plasma concentration of filtered protein exceeds tubular reabsorptive capacity. Overflow proteinuria is most commonly associated with paraproteinemias, such as multiple myeloma, monoclonal gammopathy, or light chain disease. Although the mechanism of proteinuria is primarily increased filtration rather than a specific glomerular defect, paraproteinemias can be associated with glomerular diseases such as light chain nephropathy or amyloidosis, which can then lead to subsequent glomerular proteinuria.

11. What is urinary protein selectivity?

Urinary protein selectivity refers to the ratio of urine immunoglobulin G (IgG) to albumin excretion. If the ratio is low, for example, less than 0.1, the proteinuria is considered to be selective. A ratio greater than 0.5 is considered nonselective. The only potential significance to establishing protein selectivity is to predict pathologic diagnoses. In particular, minimal change disease, which has a relatively benign clinical course, is associated with selective proteinuria, whereas more problematic glomerular diseases tend to exhibit nonselective proteinuria. Because minimal change disease occurs predominantly in children, urinary protein selectivity is measured more often by pediatric nephrologists than by adult nephrologists.

12. Should a patient with asymptomatic proteinuria undergo a diagnostic renal biopsy?

Under most circumstances, a renal biopsy is not necessary. However, if the proteinuria is persistent, a biopsy may be warranted, particularly (1) if the glomerular filtration rate is decreased, (2) if there is some clinical suspicion that the patient may have an undiagnosed systemic disease that may be causing the proteinuria (e.g., multiple myeloma, systemic lupus erythematosus), (3) if there is reasonable evidence that the biopsy will yield a diagnosis for which there is definitive treatment, or (4) to reassure the patient that the anticipated clinical course is benign.

BIBLIOGRAPHY

1. Ahmed Z, Lee J: Asymptomatic urinary abnormalities: Hematuria and proteinuria. Med Clin North Am 81:641–652, 1997.
2. Anderson S, Kennefick TM, Brenner BM: Renal and systemic manifestations of glomerular disease. In Brenner BM (ed): The Kidney, 5th ed. Philadelphia, W.B. Saunders, 1996, pp 1981–2010.
3. Ginsberg JM, Chang BS, Matarese RA, Garella S: Use of single voided urine samples to estimate quantitative proteinuria. N Engl J Med 309:1543–1546, 1983.
4. Hricik DE, Smith MC: Proteinuria and the Nephrotic Syndrome. Chicago, Year Book, 1986.
5. Kasiske BL, Keane WF: Laboratory assessment of renal disease: Clearance, urinalysis, and renal biopsy. In Brenner BM (ed): The Kidney, 5th ed. Philadelphia, W.B. Saunders, 1996, pp 1137–1174.
6. Kaysen GA: Proteinuria and the nephrotic syndrome. In Schrier RW (ed): Renal and Electrolyte Disorders, 4th ed. Boston, Little, Brown, 1992, pp 681–726.
7. Lafayette RA, Perrone RD, Levey AS: Laboratory evaluations of renal function. In Schrier RW, Gottschalk CW (eds): Renal and Electrolyte Disorders, 6th ed. Boston, Little, Brown, 1997, pp 330–354.
8. Oberhauer R, Haas M, Mayer G: Proteinuria as a consequence of altered glomerular permselectivity—clinical implications. Clin Nephrol 46:357–361, 1996.
9. Schelling JR, Sedor JR: Approach to the patient with proteinuria and nephrotic syndrome. In Kelley WN (ed): Textbook of Internal Medicine, 3rd ed. Philadelphia, Lippincott-Raven, 1997, pp 909–914.

14. ASYMPTOMATIC HEMATURIA

Jeffrey R. Schelling, M.D.

1. What is asymptomatic hematuria?

Hematuria can be either gross (obvious by visual inspection) or microscopic (detectable only by dipstick or microscopic examination) and may be associated with pain (e.g., in patients with infections, stones, or neoplasms). The term *asymptomatic hematuria* generally refers to painless hematuria that is usually, but not always, microscopic. In large cross-sectional studies, the prevalence of asymptomatic hematuria ranges from 2.5% to 13%.

2. How is a urinalysis performed to optimize detection of hematuria?

First, the voided specimen should be analyzed relatively soon after collection. A dipstick examination is conducted prior to centrifugation of the sample. The threshold for detection of red blood cells by dipstick is 3–5 cells per high-power (40×) field. At least 10 ml is mildly centrifuged (1000–2000 rpm, 2–5 min) to avoid destruction of casts. The supernatant is then poured off, and the pellet is resuspended in the remaining ~ 0.5 ml of urine. A drop of this suspension is then placed on a glass microscope slide and covered with a glass coverslip. A thorough search for red blood cells is then made using the 40× objective lens. Under normal circumstances, there should be less than 3–5 red blood cells per field. Discovery of more than 3–5 cells per field on at least two separate examinations warrants further investigation.

3. What are some causes of a false-positive dipstick reading for blood in the urine?

One should be suspicious of a false-positive dipstick for hematuria whenever the dipstick is positive and red blood cells are not visualized on microscopic examination. Conditions that lead to a false-positive dipstick for blood include exposure to certain:
- Foods: beets, food dyes, high concentrations of vitamin C
- Drugs: ibuprofen, sulfamethoxasole, nitrofurantoin, rifampin, phenytoin, L-dopa, quinine, Pyridium
- Red blood cell components: bile pigments, myoglobin, hemoglobin, porphyrins

While not technically a false-positive result, a urinalysis performed on a specimen obtained during menstruation may lead to the false conclusion that hematuria is present. Therefore, vigilance is required in the interpretation of urinalyses in women of childbearing age.

4. Can urinalysis determine the source of red blood cells in the urinary tract?

Hematuria can result from lesion(s) anywhere within the urinary tract, from the vascular supply of the kidney to the urethra. The presence of red blood cell casts is virtually pathognomonic for glomerular disease. Well-trained microscopists often can make a distinction between glomerular and collecting system pathologies on the basis of urine red blood cell morphology using phase contrast microscopy. In the case of glomerular disease, the red cells appear dysmorphic (i.e., crenated, wrinkled, or shrunken, with cytoplasm characterized by increased granularity and blebbing), due to filtration through the glomerulus or exposure to the hypertonic environment of nephrons that penetrate the medulla. Red blood cells that arise from lower tract disease appear relatively normal by microscopic examination. Because the predictive value is low, urine red blood cell morphology does not have broad clinical application. In addition, lower tract diseases (especially kidney stones and infections) are more likely to be accompanied by pain and macroscopic hematuria.

5. What are the common causes of asymptomatic hematuria?

Differential Diagnosis of Asymptomatic Hematuria

SYSTEMIC CAUSES	UPPER TRACT (KIDNEY) DISORDERS	LOWER TRACT DISORDERS
Fever	Vascular: infarction, embolism,	Stones
Strenuous exercise	venous thrombosis, arteriovenous	Tumors
Coagulopathies	malformation, vasculitis	Infections
Hemolytic disorders	Glomerular: IgA (immunoglobulin A)	Trauma
Factitious (e.g., men-	nephropathy, postinfectious glomerulo-	Vascular malformations
strual blood)	nephritis, proliferative glomerulonephritis,	Endometriosis
	thin basement membrane disease, lupus	
	nephritis, Henoch-Schönlein purpura,	
	Goodpasture's syndrome, Alport	
	syndrome, Fabry's disease	
	Tubulointerstitial: acute interstitial neph-	
	ritis, pyelonephritis, cystic diseases,	
	sickle cell nephropathy	

6. What diagnostic clues help to differentiate upper and lower tract disease?

Upper tract disease is usually asymptomatic, but associated respiratory, gastrointestinal, or skin infections may suggest IgA nephropathy or postinfectious or proliferative glomerulonephritis. Infectious or toxic exposures have been associated with glomerular and interstitial inflammation. A family history of hematuria is suggestive for Alport syndrome (particularly if accompanied by neurosensory deafness and ocular defects) or polycystic kidney disease. In patients who have asymptomatic *gross* hematuria, the portion of the urinary stream in which hematuria is observed may provide a clue to the site of lower tract disease. Blood in the initial stream is characteristic of urethral or male genital lesions. Blood at the end of the stream is most commonly observed with bladder pathology.

7. What is the significance of blood clots within the urinary tract?

A blood clot within the urinary tract is merely a sign of large amounts of bleeding. In general, urinary blood clots are observed with lower tract disease and are exceedingly rare with glomerular diseases. The presence of blood clots is not dangerous unless they obstruct urinary outflow.

8. What is the appropriate work-up for a patient with asymptomatic hematuria?

As previously mentioned, hematuria should be confirmed by at least two separate urinalyses. Although infectious causes generally present as symptomatic hematuria, a urine culture should be performed routinely to rule out an infectious etiology. If the urine culture is negative and the presence of red blood cell casts, proteinuria, or dysmorphic red cells is noted, a diagnosis of glomerular disease is suggested, and a renal biopsy should be considered. In the absence of such findings, a reasonable approach would include renal ultrasound to evaluate for tumors and cysts and urologic consultation for cystoscopy. Positive findings from these examinations would dictate further work-up, which might include additional radiologic imaging. In the setting of negative renal ultrasound and cystoscopic examinations, an argument could be made to proceed with a renal biopsy.

9. Should patients with idiopathic hematuria, with no evidence of urologic disease, undergo a renal biopsy?

Similar to arguments proposed for idiopathic proteinuria (see Chapter 13, Asymptomatic Proteinuria), it is not absolutely necessary, particularly because risk/benefit and cost-effectiveness studies have not been conducted. However, most nephrologists would probably recommend a renal biopsy in patients with persistent hematuria, particularly in the setting of declining glomerular filtration rate or concomitant proteinuria.

10. Should patients be routinely screened for hematuria?

Several large cross-sectional studies demonstrate a finite yield of urinary tract diseases from urine dipstick screening for hematuria. In particular, cases of urinary tract malignancies have been detected by such screening. For this reason, some studies recommend dipstick screening for patients older than 60 years of age. However, the cost-effectiveness of this screening strategy has not been determined. There are no data regarding the value of screening for hematuria to detect occult renal disease.

BIBLIOGRAPHY

1. Britton JP, Dowell AC, Whelan P, Harris CM: A community study of bladder cancer screening by the detection of occult urinary bleeding. J Urol 148:788–790, 1992.
2. Corwin HL: Urinalysis. In Schrier RW, Gottschalk CW (eds): Diseases of the Kidney, 6th ed. Boston, Little, Brown, 1997, pp 298–299.
3. Galla JH: Approach to the patient with hematuria. In Kelley WN (ed): Textbook of Internal Medicine, 3rd ed. Philadelphia, Lippincott-Raven, 1997, pp 906–909.
4. Glassock RJ, Cohen AH, Adler SG: Primary glomerular diseases. In Brenner BM (ed): The Kidney, 5th ed. Philadelphia, W.B. Saunders, 1996, pp 1412–1414.
5. Kasiske BL, Keane WF: Laboratory assessment of renal disease: Clearance, urinalysis, and renal biopsy. In Brenner BM (ed): The Kidney, 5th ed. Philadelphia, W.B. Saunders, 1996, pp 1137–1174.
6. Ritchie CD, Bevan EA, Collier SJ: Importance of occult hematuria found at screening. Br Med J 292:681–683, 1986.
7. Tisher CC, Croker P: Indications for and interpretation of the renal biopsy: Evaluations by light, electron, and immunofluorescence microscopy. In Schrier RW, Gottschalk CW (eds): Diseases of the Kidney, 6th ed. Boston, Little, Brown, 1997, pp 438–439.
8. Topham PS, Harper SJ, Furness PN, et al: Glomerular disease as a cause of isolated microscopic haematuria. Q J Med 87:329–335, 1994.

15. ACUTE GLOMERULONEPHRITIS

Diane M. Cibrik, M.D.

1. What are the clinical characteristics of acute glomerulonephritis?

Classically, the clinical syndrome of acute glomerulonephritis is characterized by the presence of hematuria, hypertension, edema, azotemia, and non–nephrotic-range proteinuria (< 3.0 gm of proteinuria per day). In severe cases, patients present with acute renal failure manifested by oliguria or severe renal insufficiency. Patients with acute glomerulonephritis are usually asymptomatic at presentation. However, those with severe cases may present with edema, signs or symptoms of uremia, or malignant hypertension.

2. What is clinically significant hematuria?

On microscopic examination of a centrifuged urine specimen, the finding of more than three red blood cells per high power field is considered to be clinically significant (see Chapter 14, Asymptomatic Hematuria).

3. What criteria aid in differentiating glomerular hematuria from hematuria of non-glomerular origin?

- Red blood cell casts in the urine
- Dysmorphic red blood cells in the urine
- Proteinuria associated with red cells in the urine

4. Can the urinary sediment be helpful in diagnosing acute glomerulonephritis?

Yes. The urine sediment of patients with acute glomerulonephritis generally contains dysmorphic (crenated) red blood cells, red cell casts, or heme-pigmented casts. Urinary casts are detectable in 50–80% of cases. In contrast, the urine from patients with nephrotic syndrome rarely contains casts.

5. What are the histologic features of acute glomerulonephritis?

The hallmarks of acute glomerulonephritis are glomerular inflammation mediated by infiltrating inflammatory cells and proliferation of resident mesangial, epithelial, or endothelial cells. In severe cases, extensive inflammation and proliferation can cause rupture of the glomerulus into Bowman's space resulting in crescent formation. Renal prognosis is poor when more than 50% of glomeruli are affected by crescent formation (see Chapter 16, Rapidly Progressive Glomerulonephritis).

Most renal pathology associated with acute glomerulonephritis is proliferative in character. In contrast, nonproliferative renal lesions tend to present clinically as nephrotic syndrome. Cellular proliferation within the kidney can be classified as either **focal** (involving a small percentage of glomeruli) or **diffuse** (involving the majority of glomeruli). As might be suspected, diffuse proliferative glomerulonephritis is associated with a poor renal prognosis when compared to focal glomerulonephritis.

6. What causes inflammation within the glomerulus?

Both humoral and cell-mediated immunity play a role in the pathogenesis of glomerular inflammation. In humoral immunity, antibodies can bind to glomerular antigens within the glomerular basement membrane (as in Goodpasture's syndrome) or to circulating antigens that become trapped within the glomerulus. In addition, circulating antigen-antibody complexes can become deposited within the glomerulus. T lymphocytes have been identified in the renal parenchyma of patients with glomerulonephritis and support a role for cell-mediated immunity.

48

Inflammatory mediators from infiltrating inflammatory cells or from resident glomerular cells also play a role in the pathogenesis of acute glomerulonephritis.

7. **What are the primary causes of acute proliferative glomerulonephritis?**
   - Mesangioproliferative glomerulonephritis
     IgA (immunoglobulin A) nephropathy
     IgM nephropathy
     Idiopathic
   - Membranoproliferative glomerulonephritis

8. **List the secondary causes of proliferative glomerulonephritis.**
   - Postinfectious glomerulonephritis
   - Lupus nephritis
   - Glomerulonephritis secondary to hepatitis B or C
   - Vasculitis (Wegener's granulomatosis, polyarteritis nodosa, Henoch-Schönlein purpura)

9. **What is the most common cause of glomerulonephritis worldwide?**
   IgA nephropathy.

10. **What is the role of complement in the pathogenesis and diagnosis of glomerulonephritis?**
   Many of the glomerulonephritides are associated with complement activation and hypocomplementemia. Activation of the alternative complement pathway results in low levels of circulating C3 and normal levels of C4. Activation of the classic pathway yields low levels of both C3 and C4. Activation of either pathway may lead to recruitment of inflammatory cells or to direct tissue injury.

11. **Which of the glomerulonephritides are associated with hypocomplementemia?**
   Acute postinfectious glomerulonephritis
   Membranoproliferative glomerulonephritis
   Lupus nephritis
   Subacute bacterial endocarditis
   Shunt nephritis
   Cryoglobulinemia

12. **What is the treatment for acute glomerulonephritis?**
   The treatment for acute glomerulonephritis depends on the underlying etiology of the renal disease. In some cases (e.g., poststreptococcal glomerulonephritis), therapy is supportive and focuses on management of the accompanying edema and hypertension. In contrast, patients with diffuse proliferative glomerulonephritis secondary to lupus may require aggressive treatment with steroids and cytotoxic drugs to prolong renal survival. For most of the mesangioproliferative glomerulonephritides, curative therapies are lacking.

BIBLIOGRAPHY

1. Cibrik DM, Sedor JR: Immunopathogenesis of renal disease. In Greenberg A (ed): Primer on Kidney Diseases, 2nd ed. San Diego, Academic Press, 1998, pp 141–149.
2. Glassock RJ, Cohen AH: The primary glomerulonephropathies. Dis Mon 42:329–383, 1996.
3. Hricik DE, Chung-Park M, Sedor JR: Glomerulonephritis. N Engl J Med 339:888–899, 1998.
4. Jennette JC, Falk RJ: Glomerular clinicopathologic syndromes. In Greenberg A (ed): Primer on Kidney Diseases, 2nd ed. San Diego, Academic Press, 1998, pp 127–141.
5. Madaio MP, Harrington JT: The diagnosis of acute glomerulonephritis. N Engl J Med 309:1299–1302, 1983.
6. Whitley K, Keane WF, Vernier RL: Acute glomerulonephritis. Med Clin North Am 68:259–279, 1984.

16. RAPIDLY PROGRESSIVE GLOMERULONEPHRITIS

Linda Zarif, M.D., and John R. Sedor, M.D.

1. Define rapidly progressive glomerulonephritis (RPGN).

Patients with RPGN have evidence of glomerular disease (proteinuria, hematuria, and red cell casts) accompanied by rapid loss of renal function over days to weeks. If untreated, RPGN often results in renal failure. The pathologic hallmark of RPGN is the presence of crescents on kidney biopsy.

2. What are crescents?

Crescent formation is a nonspecific response to severe injury of the glomerular capillary wall. As a result, fibrin leaks into Bowman's space, causing parietal epithelial cells to proliferate and mononuclear phagocytes to migrate into the glomerular tuft from the circulation (see Figure). Large crescents can compress glomerular capillaries and impair filtration. Although crescent formation can resolve, other chemotactic signals recruit fibroblasts, which ultimately may cause both the crescents and entire glomeruli to scar. Extensive scarring results in end-stage renal disease.

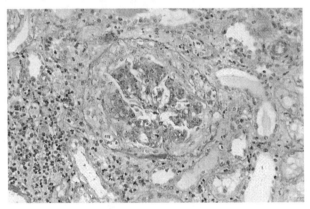

Micrograph from a patient with rapidly progressive glomerulonephritis showing a large crescent with a compressed glomerular capillary tuft. (From Hricik DE, Chung-Park M, Sedor JR: Glomerulonephritis. N Engl J Med 339:888–899, 1998, with permission.)

3. Do crescentic nephritis and RPGN describe the same disease process?

Although the terms *crescentic nephritis* and *RPGN* are used interchangeably, these diagnoses are not synonymous. RPGN describes a *clinical* syndrome of rapid loss of renal function in patients with evidence of glomerulonephritis. In contrast, crescentic nephritis is a *histopathologic* description of kidney biopsy specimens that demonstrate the presence of crescents in more than 50% of glomeruli. Biopsies of patients with RPGN very commonly reveal crescentic nephritis. However, RPGN can occur in the absence of crescentic nephritis, and extensive glomerular crescent formation rarely is identified in kidney biopsy specimens from patients without the clinical syndrome of RPGN.

4. How is primary RPGN classified?

RPGN can occur as a primary disorder in the absence of other glomerular or systemic diseases and is classified pathologically using immunofluorescence microscopy to describe the presence or absence of immune deposits and their character. Linear deposition of immunoglobulin along the glomerular basement membrane (GBM) is detected in approximately 20% of patients with primary RPGN without pulmonary hemorrhage. Granular immune complex deposition is detected in an additional 30% of patients with RPGN. In the remaining patients, no immune deposits ("pauci-immune") are detectable in glomeruli.

5. What diseases are associated with RPGN?

RPGN can complicate the clinical course of some primary glomerular diseases such as IgA nephropathy, membranous nephropathy, membranoproliferative glomerulonephritis, and hereditary nephritis (Alport syndrome). In addition, RPGN is associated with infectious and multisystem diseases including systemic lupus erythematosus, cryoglobulinemia, and system vasculitides. The Table below provides an overview of the classification of RPGN but is not intended to be exhaustive.

Classification of RPGN

Primary
Anti-GBM antibody disease (Goodpasture's disease)
Granular glomerular immune complex association
Pauci-immune glomerulonephritis
Superimposed on a primary glomerular disease

Secondary
Postinfectious
   Poststreptococcal glomerulonephritis
   Visceral abscess
Vasculitic
   Small vessel
      Microscopic polyangiitis
      Wegener's granulomatosis
      Churg-Strauss syndrome
      Systemic lupus erythematosus
      Henoch-Schönlein purpura
      Cryoglobulinemia
   Medium vessel
      Polyarteritis nodosa
   Goodpasture's syndrome
   Carcinoma
   Medication-associated
      Allopurinol
      Penicillamine

6. Describe the clinical manifestations of RPGN.

Unless complicated by systemic disease, RPGN is characterized by an insidious onset of generalized fatigue and malaise. Hematuria with dysmorphic red blood cells and red cell casts is usually detected on urinalysis. Moderate proteinuria, usually in the non-nephrotic range, is typical. Nephrotic-range proteinuria occurs in less than 30% of patients. Mild to severe azotemia is universally present.

7. Aside from urinalysis, which other laboratory tests are useful in defining the etiology of RPGN?

Certain serologic studies may be useful in narrowing the differential diagnosis. Complement levels (C3, C4) are usually normal in patients with either primary RPGN or RPGN associated with systemic disease, although patients with underlying systemic lupus erythematosus usually have depressed circulating C3 and C4 levels. In almost all patients, an antinuclear antibody level is a useful screen for lupus or other connective tissue diseases. Identification of circulating anti-GBM antibodies and antineutrophil cytoplasmic antibody (ANCA) can be useful in establishing a diagnosis in patients who present with RPGN. ANCA-positive patients frequently have a primary small-vessel vasculitis, although disease may be kidney-limited. The patient's clinical presentation also determines the predictive value of ANCA testing. For example, the predictive value of a positive ANCA test is considerably less significant in a patient who presents with hematuria, proteinuria, and a normal creatinine than in a patient with similar urinalysis findings in the presence of azotemia (see Chapter 35, Renal Vasculitis).

8. What are anti-GBM antibodies?

Anti-GBM antibodies are targeted toward the NC1 domain of the $\alpha 3$ chain of type IV collagen, which is a component of the GBM. Anti-GBM antibodies are found in approximately 90–95% of patients with Goodpasture's disease. On kidney biopsy, they form linear deposits of immunoglobulin along basement membranes detected by immunofluorescence (see figure in question 2).

9. Are Goodpasture's syndrome and anti-GBM glomerulonephritis (Goodpasture's disease) the same?

No. While both disease entities result from circulating anti-GBM antibodies, **Goodpasture's syndrome** describes a systemic disease with a clinical constellation of pulmonary hemorrhage, circulating anti-GBM antibodies, and glomerulonephritis. Anti-GBM glomerulonephritis, or **Goodpasture's disease**, is kidney-limited and describes a proliferative glomerulonephritis, which results from deposition of anti-GBM antibodies. Anti-GBM antibodies are the same in patients with Goodpasture's syndrome and Goodpasture's disease. Because alveolar basement membrane contains the epitope of type IV collagen that is recognized by anti-GBM antibodies, the variable presence of pulmonary disease seems to reflect whether alveolar basement membrane is accessible to the circulating anti-GBM antibodies. Alveolar injury from infections, smoking, toxins, or other underlying lung disease may predispose the lungs to deposition of anti-GBM antibodies.

10. What is the prognosis of RPGN?

Prognosis and response to treatment in patients with anti-GBM antibody or Goodpasture's disease have not been studied in large trials. Data from a number of trials with similar, but not identical, treatment strategies suggest that patient survivals are high (70–90%). However, only 40% of patients remain off dialysis at 1 year. Renal survival is particularly poor in patients with anti-GBM antibody disease who present with advanced renal insufficiency (creatinine > 6 mg/dl). Aggressive therapy with immunosuppressive drugs and plasma exchange may not be appropriate in this subgroup of anti-GBM antibody patients.

Although data on patients with kidney-limited, ANCA-positive RPGN are limited, treatment responses have been reported recently in several cohorts of patients with ANCA-associated necrotizing glomerulonephritis and either Wegener's granulomatosis or microscopic polyangiitis. Many patients (approximately 75%) achieve remission after induction therapy, but only 40–50% remain in long-term remission after 4–10 years. Entry serum creatinine is a strong predictor of renal survival in ANCA-positive patients. In contrast to patients with anti-GBM glomerulonephritis, patients with ANCA-associated glomerulonephritis can respond to therapy even if they have already required initiation of dialysis.

11. What are the treatment options for patients with RPGN?

RPGN needs to be treated aggressively and early in its course to reduce the likelihood of end-stage renal failure. Glucocorticoids and cyclophosphamide are the mainstays of treatment. The benefit of these agents is particularly great in patients with ANCA-associated vasculitis.

12. Is there any role for plasma exchange in the therapy for RPGN?

Plasma exchange is thought to remove circulating pathogenic autoantibodies from the circulation and is commonly used in the treatment of anti-GBM antibody disease. More recently, use of plasma exchange has been included in the therapy of patients with ANCA-associated glomerulonephritis who have presented with renal failure and require dialysis. Trials evaluating efficacy of plasma exchange for all causes of RPGN have been small. However, in view of the high risk of renal failure in patients with RPGN, plasma exchange may be an appropriate therapeutic modality for subsets of these patients.

BIBLIOGRAPHY

1. Bolton WK: Rapidly progressive glomerulonephritis. Semin Nephrol 16:517–526, 1996.
2. Cibrik DM, Sedor JR: Immunopathogenesis of renal disease. In Greenberg A (ed): Primer on Kidney Diseases, 2nd ed. San Diego, Academic Press, 1998, pp 141–149.
3. Falk RJ, Jennette JC: Anti-neutrophil cytoplasmic autoantibodies with specificity for myeloperoxidase in patients with systemic vasculitis and idiopathic necrotizing and crescentic glomerulonephritis. N Engl J Med 318:1651–1657, 1988.
4. Heilman RL, Offord KP, Holley KE, Velosa JA: Analysis of risk factors for patient and renal survival in crescentic glomerulonephritis. Am J Kidney Dis 9:98–107, 1987.
5. Hricik DE, Chung-Park M, Sedor JR: Glomerulonephritis. N Engl J Med 339:888–899, 1998.
6. Kalluri R, Sun MJ, Hudson BG, Neilson EG: The Goodpasture autoantigen: Structural delineation of two immunologically privileged epitopes of alpha3(IV) chain of type IV collagen. J Biol Chem 271:9062–9068, 1996.
7. Kerr PG, Lan HY, Atkins RC: Rapidly progressive glomerulonephritis. In Schrier RW, Gottschalk CW (eds): Diseases of the Kidney, 6th ed. Vol. 2. Boston, Little, Brown, 1997, pp 1619–1644.
8. Lal DPSS, O'Donoghue DJ, Haeney M: Effect of diagnostic delay on disease severity and outcome in glomerulonephritis caused by anti-neutrophil cytoplasmic antibodies. J Clin Pathol 49:942–944, 1996.
9. Mokrzycki MH, Kaplan AA: Therapeutic plasma exchange: Complications and management. Am J Kidney Dis 23:817–827, 1994.

17. NEPHROTIC SYNDROME

Diane M. Cibrik, M.D.

1. What is nephrotic syndrome?

The nephrotic syndrome is characterized by heavy proteinuria (> 3.5 gm per day) and varying degrees of hypoalbuminemia, edema, hyperlipidemia, and lipiduria. Proteinuria develops because the charge or size selectivity of the glomerular capillary wall becomes altered by an underlying glomerular disease (see Chapter 4, Measurement of Urinary Protein). In some cases, humoral and cellular immune responses are involved in altering glomerular permselectivity; in others, degenerative and sclerosing processes are responsible for the proteinuria.

2. What is the clinical presentation of patients with nephrotic syndrome?

Some patients are asymptomatic and are diagnosed only when proteinuria is discovered on routine urinalysis. The most common presenting symptom is edema, which can be severe (anasarca). In nephrotic patients, edema tends to be most noticeable in bodily areas where intravascular hydrostatic pressure is highest (e.g., ankles and feet) and where tissue hydrostatic pressure is lowest (e.g., genital tissues and periorbital area). Rarely, patients first present with thromboembolic events such as a pulmonary embolus or renal vein thrombosis. The presence of hypertension, azotemia, and hematuria at the time of presentation is variable and depends greatly on the underlying glomerular histology.

3. How does excessive proteinuria cause other features of the nephrotic syndrome?

Hypoalbuminemia: Urine protein losses together with tubular absorption and catabolism of filtered plasma proteins combine to overwhelm the synthetic capacity of the liver.

Edema: In the "underfill" theory, hypoalbuminemia leads to a reduction in intracapillary oncotic pressure resulting in net movement of fluid into the interstitial space. The subsequent decrease in plasma volume activates the release of renin and aldosterone leading to renal sodium retention that worsens the edema. Recent observations cast doubt on the validity of the underfill hypothesis. In most patients with nephrotic syndrome, plasma volume is normal or elevated. Moreover, renin and aldosterone levels are not uniformly increased. Results of some studies suggest that a defect in renal sodium excretion (overfill theory) is the primary cause of edema in nephrotic syndrome while the reduction in intravascular oncotic pressure promotes edema secondarily.

Hyperlipidemia: In response to a decrease in intravascular oncotic pressure, the liver nonspecifically increases its synthesis of a number of proteins including lipoproteins.

Lipiduria: Like other proteins, lipoproteins are filtered on the basis of defects in size or charge selectivity of the glomerular capillary membrane.

Thromboembolism: The nephrotic syndrome often is associated with a hypercoagulable state that has been attributed to a number of factors including platelet hyperaggregability, increased hepatic synthesis of procoagulant proteins, and urinary losses of anticoagulant factors such as protein S, protein C, and antithrombin III.

4. What is an oval fat body?

Oval fat bodies are sometimes seen on microscopic examination of urine from nephrotic patients. They are thought to be sloughed renal tubular cells that are filled with refractile fat droplets that have been reabsorbed from the glomerular filtrate.

5. What are the causes of nephrotic syndrome?

The glomerular diseases associated with nephrotic syndrome are generally categorized as either **primary** (idiopathic) or **secondary** to some systemic condition or disease. In children, minimal change disease (see Chapter 21, Minimal Change Disease) accounts for more than 80% of cases of nephrotic syndrome. In adults, the most common causes of idiopathic nephrotic syndrome are shown below:

Idiopathic Nephrotic Syndrome in Adults

COMMON CAUSES	SOMETIMES ASSOCIATED WITH NEPHROTIC SYNDROME
Membranous nephropathy	IgA (immunoglobulin A) nephropathy
Focal segmental glomerulosclerosis	Mesangioproliferative glomerulonephritis
Membranoproliferative glomerulonephritis	Fibrillary and immunotactoid glomerulonephritis
Minimal change disease	Crescentric glomerulonephritis

The frequency of the entities listed above is dependent on age and race. In adults over the age of 50 years, membranous nephropathy is the most common cause of idiopathic nephrotic syndrome. African Americans with nephrotic syndrome are more likely to have focal segmental glomerulosclerosis.

6. What are the most common causes of secondary nephrotic syndrome?
- Diabetic nephropathy
- Systemic lupus erythematosus
- Amyloidosis
- Human immunodeficiency virus (HIV) infection
- Malignancy (especially lymphoproliferative disorders and cancers of the breast, lung, stomach, and colon)
- Drugs (gold, penicillamine, nonsteroidal anti-inflammatory drugs)

At least 50% of patients with nephrotic syndrome have an identifiable secondary cause. Overall, diabetic nephropathy is the most common cause of nephrotic syndrome.

7. Is renal biopsy necessary in the management of patients with nephrotic syndrome?
In children, renal biopsy is not performed routinely because minimal change disease is the likely diagnosis. Instead, children more often are treated empirically with corticosteroids. Biopsy is reserved for those who do not respond to steroids or who present with atypical clinical features (see Chapter 21, Minimal Change Disease).

In adults, clinical findings alone are frequently inadequate to diagnose the cause of nephrotic syndrome. Although the indications for renal biopsy in nephrotic patients have been the subject of some debate, most nephrologists recommend biopsy for patients with idiopathic nephrotic syndrome. Biopsy usually is not performed when the underlying cause is clinically obvious (e.g., diabetes mellitus, systemic amyloidosis).

8. How is the nephrotic syndrome treated?
1. Treatment of the underlying disease (or the secondary cause)
2. Treatment of complications (e.g., edema, hyperlipidemia)
3. Nonspecific treatment of proteinuria

9. What are the treatment options for reducing proteinuria in nephrotic patients?
Persistence of heavy proteinuria is a predictor of progression to renal failure; conversely, reduction of urinary protein excretion may improve long-term prognosis. Antiproteinuric measures include:
1. Treatment with angiotension-converting enzyme (ACE) inhibitors or angiotensin II receptor antagonists
2. Cautious treatment with nonsteroidal anti-inflammatory drugs
3. Dietary protein restriction

The benefit of a low-protein diet is paradoxical. Some patients with nephrotic proteinuria may become frankly catabolic when dietary protein is restricted so this treatment modality also should be employed with caution.

10. How are thromboembolic complications treated in patients with nephrotic syndrome?
Anticoagulation (usually a short course of heparin followed by treatment with Coumadin) is recommended for patients with documented thromboembolic events and should be continued for as long as the patient has heavy proteinuria. The benefit of prophylactic anticoagulant or anti-platelet therapy remains controversial.

11. What diuretics should be used to treat edema in patients with nephrotic syndrome?
Nephrotic patients sometimes exhibit resistance to commonly available diuretics and frequently require treatment with high doses of loop diuretics (e.g., furosemide, torsemide, bumetanide). Resistance to loop diuretics can be explained by their binding to albumin and other proteins. These drugs enter the lumen of the nephron through active secretion by proximal tubular cells. When heavy proteinuria exists, the secreted drug is bound to protein in the tubular lumen, limiting its availability to bind with receptors in more distant portions of the nephron. Such resistance can be overcome by increasing the dose of the drug. Combinations of loop diuretics and thiazide-like diuretics are often needed to achieve adequate diuresis.

Excessive diuresis may precipitate volume depletion and acute renal failure—a phenomenon most commonly observed in patients with minimal change disease. Combined infusions of albumin and loop diuretics may be required to achieve diuresis in patients with severe hypoalbuminemia.

BIBLIOGRAPHY

1. Brater DC: Diuretic therapy. N Engl J Med 339:387–395, 1998.
2. Cibrik DM, Sedor JR: Immunopathogenesis of renal disease. In Greenberg A (ed): Primer on Kidney Diseases, 2nd ed. San Diego, Academic Press, 1998, pp 141–149.
3. Cotran RS, Kumar V, Robbins SL: Pathologic Basis of Disease, 5th ed. Philadelphia, W.B. Saunders, 1994.
4. Glassock RJ, Cohen AH: The primary glomerulopathies. Dis Mon 42:329–383, 1996.
5. Hricik DE, Smith MC: Proteinuria and the Nephrotic Syndrome. Chicago, Year Book, 1986.
6. Larson T: Evaluation of proteinuria. Mayo Clin Proc 69:1154–1158, 1994.
7. Orth SR, Ritz E: The nephrotic syndrome. N Engl J Med 338:1202–1211, 1998.
8. Palmer BF, Alpern RJ: Pathogenesis of edema formation in the nephrotic syndrome. Kidney Int 51(suppl 59):S21–S27, 1997.
9. Schelling JR, Sedor JR: Approach to the patient with proteinuria and nephrotic syndrome. In Kelley WN (ed): Textbook of Internal Medicine, 3rd ed. Philadelphia, Lippincott-Raven, 1997, pp 909–914.
10. Vander A: Renal Physiology, 5th ed. New York, McGraw-Hill, 1995.

18. NEPHROLITHIASIS

Miriam F. Weiss, M.D.

1. How common is nephrolithiasis?

Kidney stones are one of the most common medical problems. Renal colic is a frequent cause of hospitalization. In Western countries, 4–10 men and 1–5 women per 1,000 people per year will have a symptomatic episode relating to passing a stone. In men, the lifetime prevalence of nephrolithiasis is 10%. The chance of a second stone occurring within 5 years of the first one is 50%.

2. What is the chemical composition of kidney stones?

X-ray crystallography and infrared spectrometry can be used to determine the precise composition of a renal stone or fragment. Calcium is the primary ion in 70–80% of renal stones, either as calcium oxalate (~ 60%), calcium phosphate (~ 10%), or a mixture of calcium oxalate and calcium phosphate (~ 10%). Infection or struvite stones are also known as triple phosphate stones. These stones occur in about 10% of cases and contain calcium, magnesium, ammonium, and phosphate. Infection stones often grow to a large size and assume a "staghorn" or antler-like configuration as they fill the renal pelvis. They seldom pass spontaneously. Uric acid is the main constituent of about 10% of stones. Cystine and other substances make up less than 1% of stones.

3. How do stones form?

Urine is a complex mixture of many salts in solution. When urine is supersaturated with dissolved ions that can crystallize, nucleation occurs. Often nucleation and growth of the stone take place on the surface of another crystal, such as uric acid. The nuclei can aggregate into clumps that may adhere to the surface of the urothelium, particularly if there is inflammation or scarring in the urinary collecting system. Reducing the concentration of salts in the urine is the basis of many current medical treatments for nephrolithiasis.

In the majority of the population, stones do not form because of the presence of urinary inhibitor substances, a diverse group of molecules that prevent nucleation even in supersaturated urine. A partial list of these substances includes Tamm-Horsfall protein, uropontin, nephrocalcin, prothrombin F1 peptide, uronic acid-rich proteins, glycosaminoglycans, and citrate. Eventually, medical therapy for nephrolithiasis may focus on enhancing or replacing the function of these molecules.

4. Name the disease processes that can result in calcium stone formation.

Disease	Mechanism
Primary hyperparathyroidism	$\uparrow$ parathyroid hormone (PTH) causes hypercalciuria by $\uparrow$ bone resorption and stimulating $\uparrow$ renal synthesis of 1,25 dihydroxyvitamin D_3 [1,25 $(OH)_2D_3$], which results in $\uparrow$ gut absorption of calcium
Renal tubular acidosis	Acidemia causes release of bone buffers (calcium) and is associated with decreased urinary excretion of citrate Renal tubular acidosis associated with phosphate wasting can result in hypophosphatemia, which is a major stimulus to the $\uparrow$ synthesis of 1,25 $(OH)_2D_3$
Granulomatous disease (e.g., sarcoidosis, tuberculosis)	$\uparrow$ extrarenal synthesis of 1,25 $(OH)_2D_3$, which results in $\uparrow$ gut absorption of calcium
Milk-alkali syndrome	$\uparrow$ oral intake of calcium-containing antacids

Table continued on next page

Disease	*Mechanism*
Primary/enteric hyperoxaluria secondary to chronic bowel disease	Primary disease or ↑ gut oxalate absorption due to ↑ intestinal permeability to oxalate induced by steatorrhea or bile acids
Gout with hyperuricemia	Uric acid crystals precipitate in an acid urine; calcium oxalate crystals nucleate and aggregate on the surface of the uric acid crystals

5. **What are the pathophysiologic mechanisms underlying "idiopathic" hypercalciuria?**
   • Increased intestinal absorption of calcium. The etiology of increased intestinal absorption of calcium may be genetic. Several families with this disorder have been identified. Transient increases in serum calcium after a meal tend to suppress PTH levels in these patients.
   • Increased renal excretion of calcium (renal leak). The renal defect results in a decrease in serum calcium. Eventually secondary hyperparathyroidism develops, which stimulates the renal synthesis of $1,25 (OH)_2D_3$ and causes increased intestinal calcium absorption.

6. **Which type of stone is radiolucent?**
   Uric acid stones (see Figure). Uric acid stones will not be visible on a plain film of the abdomen.

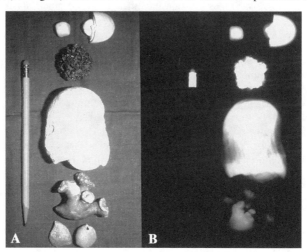

A, Recovered renal stones (from top to bottom): cystine, calcium oxalate, struvite, calcium phosphate, uric acid. Note the "staghorn" appearance of the calcium phosphate stone. Pencil provides size comparison. *B*, X-ray of *A*. All of the stones except the uric acid stone are radiopaque. The wood and graphite of the pencil, like the uric acid stones, are radiolucent. Note the lamellations present in the struvite stone.

7. **Do all patients with renal colic require urologic intervention?**
   Stones smaller than 5 mm in diameter may pass with hydration and medical management of pain. Up to 30% of stones require cystoscopy, extracorporeal shock wave lithotripsy, or surgery.

8. **List the key aspects of the medical management of acute renal colic.**
   • Most patients require narcotic analgesia. Passing a kidney stone hurts!
   • Use appropriate radiologic procedures to rule out ureteral obstruction. Prolonged obstruction can lead to kidney damage and may require urologic intervention.
   • Treat concurrent urinary infection.
   • Save the stone or its fragments for subsequent stone composition or analysis (strain all urine during an episode of renal colic).

9. What is the role for medical intervention in nephrolithiasis?

In patients with recurrent nephrolithiasis and all children who have passed a kidney stone, medical management is recommended. The goal of medical therapy is to prevent the formation of new stones and to reduce the rate of growth of existing stones. Medications, such as thiazide diuretics, allopurinol, and antibiotics, and dietary supplements, such as potassium citrate, all have efficacy. Recently, the costs of medical work-up and treatment (testing, follow-up, and medications) have been shown to be less than the cost of hospitalization and procedures associated with managing stones once they have formed.

10. What is the single most important therapeutic intervention in *any* patient with a history of nephrolithiasis?

Increase the urine output to greater than 2 L/day by increasing the oral intake of water (reduce urinary supersaturation).

11. What is medullary sponge kidney?

Medullary sponge kidney is a disorder in which the collecting ducts of the kidney are patulous and dilated. As a result, urine flow is slowed as it moves from the tubule into the renal pelvis. The disorder is usually asymptomatic. However, crystals forming in a supersaturated urine are more likely to adhere to the urothelium in the presence of low urinary flow, leading to increased nucleation, aggregation, and stone formation.

12. True or false: One way to reduce stone formation is to decrease the dietary intake of calcium?

False. Unless the patient has marked or excessive calcium intake (milk-alkali syndrome), absorption of calcium reflects underlying pathophysiology more than intake. It is more important to reduce the dietary intake of oxalate. Calcium in the diet may actually help to bind oxalate in the intestine and reduce its absorption.

13. What is the treatment for cystinuria and cystine stone formation?

Alkalize the urine to increase cystine solubility. Chelating agents, d-penicillamine, and alpha-mercaptopropionyl glycine (Thiola) reduce cystine excretion but have some toxic side effects.

14. Describe the outpatient work-up of a patient with nephrolithiasis.

Review the history and physical exam. If the patient was hospitalized during an episode of renal colic, review diagnostic x-rays. For example, the chest x-ray may demonstrate granulomatous disease. The following studies will confirm the results of stone analysis and lead to appropriate therapy of the underlying cause of nephrolithiasis.

Test	Result	Response
Urinalysis	Specific gravity > 1.020	Urine is too concentrated; encourage ↑ oral intake of fluids
	Urine pH > 6.0 with ↓ serum HCO_3	Suggests renal tubular acidosis (RTA)
	Pyuria	Send for urine culture and treat with appropriate antibiotic.
	Cystine crystals	Send urine for quantitative urine cystine.
Serum calcium	> 10.5 mg/dl	Consider primary hyperparathyroidism; send for PTH.
	< 10.5 mg/dl	Normal
Serum phosphate	< 2.8 mg/dl	If patient is calcium stone former, add KPO_4, 250 mg q.i.d., to thiazide regimen.

Table continued on next page

Test	Result	Response
Serum uric acid	> 8.0 mg/dl	If hyperuricosuria or uric acid stones also present, decrease dietary intake of purines and consider Rx with allopurinol.
Serum HCO_3	< 22 mEq/L	Consider RTA or incomplete distal RTA. Document with acid loading test. Treat with potassium citrate (1 mEq/kg/day).
24-hour urine	Volume < 1500 ml/24 hours	Increase oral fluid intake.
Creatinine	> 1.0–1.5 gm/24 hours	Adequate 24-hour urine collection.
	< 1.0 gm/24 hours	Collection may be inaccurate, affecting other values.
Urinary calcium	> 300 mg/24 hours (males); > 250 mg/24 hours (females); or > 4 mg/kg/24 hours	If stone analysis is consistent, begin hydrochlorothiazide, 25–50 mg q.d., and potassium citrate (20–40 mEq/day).
	> 150 mg/24 hours	If calcium stones are present, benefit from thiazide and potassium citrate is still seen.
Urinary uric acid	> 700 mg/day	Urinary alkalinization (potassium citrate, 50 mEq/day); allopurinol, 300 mg/day
	< 700 mg/day	If uric acid stones are present, begin treatment as above.
Urinary phosphate	Calculate tubular reabsorption of phosphate: $$TRP = \frac{U/P\ phosphate}{U/P\ creatinine} - 1.0$$	
	< 0.8	Renal wasting of phosphate may be secondary to renal tubular defect or hyperparathyroidism.
Urinary citrate	Normal range: 140–940 mg/24 hours	Low urinary citrate suggests RTA.
Urinary oxalate	> 25–50 mg/24 hours	Reduce dietary oxalate intake.
	> 50 mg/24 hours	Suggests hyperoxaluria secondary to gastrointestinal disease. Correct underlying cause and/or add cholestyramine to bind bile acids (8–10 gm/day PO).
	> 150 mg/24 hours	Primary hyperoxaluria. Treat with pyridoxine (150–400 mg/24 hours).

15. What is the relationship between bacteria and the formation of struvite stones?

Infection stones are formed largely through the action of bacterial urease. This urea-splitting enzyme is most commonly produced by gram-negative organisms such as *Proteus, Pseudomonas*, and *Klebsiella* and by gram-positive organisms such as *Streptococcus faecalis*. Bacterial urease generates increased amounts of ammonium with consequent urinary alkalinization. The characteristic lamellated structure of the struvite stone represents layers of bacterial products and mineral. The stone acts as a foreign body, difficult to penetrate with antibiotics. If possible, complete removal of the stone and appropriate antibiotic therapy are the most definitive therapy.

16. What are nanobacteria?

Recently, nanobacteria, as small as the largest viruses, have been found to live in urine. Antigens from these bacteria have also been found in a variety of human kidney stones. By precipitating calcium and other minerals around themselves, they may be the source of nucleation in urine.

BIBLIOGRAPHY

1. Coe FL, Parks JH: New insights into the pathophysiology and treatment of nephrolithiasis. J Bone Min Res 12:522–533, 1997.
2. Kajander EO, Ciftcioglu N: Nanobacteria: An alternative mechanism for pathogenic intra- and extracellular calcification and stone formation. Proc Natl Acad Sci U S A 95:8274–8279, 1998.
3. Kupin WL: A practical approach to nephrolithiasis. Hosp Pract 30:57–60, 63–64, 1995.
4. Pak CYC: Southwestern Internal Medicine Conference: Medical management of nephrolithiasis—A new, simplified approach for general practice. Am J Med Sci 313:215–219, 1997.
5. Parks JH, Coe FL: The financial effects of kidney stone prevention. Kidney Int 50:1706–1712, 1996.
6. Wasserstein AG: Nephrolithiasis: Acute management and prevention. Dis Mon 44:196–213, 1998.

19. URINARY TRACT INFECTION

Carolyn P. Cacho, M.D.

1. What are urinary tract infections and how are they classified?

The term *urinary tract infection* (UTI) refers to an infection occurring anywhere along the urinary tract from the perinephric fascia to the urethral meatus. UTIs have been classified based on the etiologic agent (e.g., bacterial, fungal, or mycobacterial), on the location in the genitourinary tract, and by complexity. In categorizing UTIs by location, a distinction generally is made between lower tract disease (e.g., cystitis, urethritis, prostatitis, and epididymitis) and upper tract disease (e.g., acute or chronic pyelonephritis). **Uncomplicated UTI** is an infection that occurs in a nonpregnant adult woman without structural or nephrologic dysfunction. This is the most common type of urinary tract infection and is usually responsive to appropriate antibiotic therapy. **Complicated UTI** includes infections at sites other than the bladder and those that occur in children, men, or pregnant women. They are more difficult to treat and may be associated with structural abnormalities of the urinary tract or with renal dysfunction.

2. What is the pathogenesis of UTI?

A urinary tract infection develops when the balance between the virulence and number of the infecting bacteria on the one hand and host defense mechanisms on the other is disrupted. The urinary tract can become infected by two major routes. Most infections occur by the **ascending route**. Bacteria, which have colonized the anus, distal urethra, or vagina, can enter and invade the proximal urethra and bladder. The mere presence of bacteria is not sufficient to cause infection, however. Invasion also depends on the virulence of the organism. Infection of the renal parenchyma generally occurs when bacteria in the bladder multiply and ascend up the ureters to the renal pelvis and kidney parenchyma. Vesicoureteral reflux or obstruction anywhere in the urinary tract enhances this process. A much less common route of infection of the urinary tract is the **hematogenous route**. For example, the kidneys can become infected in the presence of *Staphylococcus aureus* bacteremia or *Candida* fungemia.

3. Who gets UTIs?

UTIs are common and account for more than 7 million outpatient visits per year. In the neonatal period, UTIs are more common in boys than in girls. In childhood and throughout adulthood, females are at higher risk than males. Indeed, reports indicate that 20–50% of women will have at least one UTI in their lifetime. UTI continues to be a problem in the later stages of life for both men and women. The incidence of complicated UTI increases with advanced age because of the prevalence of urinary tract abnormalities such as prostatic disease, neurogenic disease, and a higher likelihood of urethral catheterization. Additionally, in postmenopausal women, lower levels of circulating estrogen may lead to decreased colonization of the vagina by lactobacilli, which lower vaginal pH and decrease adherence of pathogenic organisms to the uroepithelium. Age, however, is not the only risk factor predisposing to infection of the urinary tract. Recent sexual intercourse, use of a diaphragm with spermicide, pregnancy, and diabetes mellitus are all associated with increased incidence of UTI.

4. Which organisms most commonly cause UTI?

Seventy percent to 95% of UTIs are caused by *Escherichia coli*. Five percent to 20% of cases are caused by *Staphylococcus saprophyticus*. In patients with complicated UTI or who have risk factors such as hospitalization or diabetes mellitus, other fecal flora such as *Proteus mirabilis*, *Klebsiella* species, or *Enterococcus* may be the etiologic agents.

5. Can UTIs be prevented?

Yes. Prophylaxis of UTI should be considered in a number of clinical scenarios. In the woman with uncomplicated, recurrent UTIs, nonpharmacologic measures such as voiding immediately after intercourse, increasing fluid intake, and avoiding the use of a diaphragm with spermicide for contraception are often recommended but have not been confirmed in prospective studies to significantly decrease the risk of infection. On the other hand, consumption of cranberry juice has been shown to decrease bacteriuria and pyuria, likely by inhibiting the adherence of prefimbriated *E. coli* to uroepithelial cell surfaces by tannin compounds (proanthocyanidins) present in cranberries and blueberries.

A number of prophylaxis protocols using low doses of antibiotics are effective in the treatment of recurrent uncomplicated UTIs. These protocols use one of three strategies: continuous antibiotic prophylaxis, postcoital prophylaxis, or patient-administered self-treatment. In addition to antibiotic prophylaxis, institution of estrogen replacement therapy in postmenopausal women may favorably alter the vaginal flora and reduce the incidence of UTIs. Because pregnant women with bacteriuria have a twofold increase in the risk of premature delivery compared to those without bacteriuria, prevention of UTI is important in improving peripartum outcomes. Indications for prophylaxis in pregnant women include treatment of all women with a prepartum history of recurrent UTI, a single UTI early in pregnancy, and asymptomatic bacteriuria in early pregnancy. Both continuous and postcoital regimens have been shown to be effective (see question 13).

6. What are the signs and symptoms of UTI?

Symptoms include frequency, urgency, dysuria, hematuria, suprapubic tenderness, and flank pain. These classic signs and symptoms may be absent in elderly patients who sometimes present with gastrointestinal complaints (e.g., nausea and vomiting) or even with mental status changes.

7. How is UTI diagnosed?

In the patient with acute dysuria, cystitis must be distinguished from urethritis and vaginitis. A patient with frequency, dysuria, pyuria, and hematuria is likely to have a UTI, but the definite diagnosis depends on the demonstrated presence of white cells and bacteria in the urine. A urine dipstick test can rapidly demonstrate the presence of inflammation by the detection of leukocyte esterase. The leukocyte esterase test is generally positive when more than 10–20 leukocytes per milliliter are detected; however, this test does not specifically indicate bacterial infection. The presence of nitrites is highly specific for bacteria but is relatively insensitive, leading to many false negatives. In addition, the nitrite test is not positive in the presence of bacteria that do not produce nitrate reductase (e.g., *Staphylococcus, Enterococcus,* and *Pseudomonas* species). Gram stain of uncentrifuged urine is a useful diagnostic tool with a sensitivity and specificity that approach 90%. The presence of bacteria on Gram stain of uncentrifuged urine corresponds to a urine culture colony count of 10^5 organisms. The gold standard for establishing the diagnosis of a UTI is a urine culture detecting greater than 10^5 organisms per milliliter of urine. More recent data have shown that colony counts as low as 10^2 colony-forming units per milliliter in a female with acute symptoms is sufficient to establish this diagnosis. Similarly, in symptomatic men, the presence of 10^3 or greater colony-forming units per milliliter is sufficient to establish the diagnosis of a UTI.

8. How is an uncomplicated UTI treated?

While nonspecific therapies such as hydration, urine acidification, cranberry juice, and urinary tract analgesics play a limited role in the treatment of UTIs, the mainstay of treatment is antimicrobial therapy. Acute uncomplicated cystitis, such as commonly occurs in young women of childbearing age, has traditionally been treated with trimethoprim-sulfamethoxazole or amoxicillin for 7 days. Shorter 3-day and single-dose regimens have been developed in an effort to reduce cost, increase compliance, reduce the emergence of resistant organisms, and decrease the risk of adverse drug effects. The relative efficacy of single-dose therapy in comparison to 3-day therapy varies but appears to be related to the half-life of the antimicrobial agent. For example, a single dose of trimethoprim-sulfamethoxazole maintains adequate urine concentrations for approximately 48 hours when compared to 24 hours for the quinolones and 18 hours for the beta-lactams. The current recommendation is for a 3-day course of therapy with trimethoprim-sul-famethoxazole or a quinolone. Beta-lactam regimens are less desirable because of the high rate of resistance to these drugs.

9. What is the approach to treatment of UTI in the pregnant patient?
When UTI occurs in pregnancy, the chosen antimicrobial agent and duration of therapy should be effective in eradicating the infecting organism but also must be safe for the fetus. Trimethoprim-sulfamethoxazole should be avoided, especially in the third trimester, because of the potential for hyperbilirubinemia in the neonate. Quinolones have been studied inadequately and should probably also be avoided. The safest agents are the beta-lactams. However, as noted above, these agents have a short half-life, which makes short-course regimens less effective. Thus, most authorities currently recommend a 7-day course of amoxicillin, ampicillin, or a first-generation cephalosporin for treatment of cystitis in a pregnant woman.

10. How should adult males with UTI be treated?
Cystitis should always be considered a complicated UTI when it occurs in an adult male. Studies have shown that both single-dose and 3-day courses of therapy are unsuccessful in men and that cure rates are much higher when the antimicrobial (i.e., trimethoprim-sulfamethoxazole or a quinolone) is used for 7 or more days.

11. What is the approach to the geriatric patient with a positive urine culture?
Elderly patients frequently have asymptomatic bacteriuria. While initial studies shown a link between bacteriuria and mortality in this population, more recent studies have shown that the increase in mortality is related more to other comorbid factors than to bacteriuria per se. Accordingly, most experts currently recommend no treatment for elderly or institutionalized persons with asymptomatic bacteriuria. In the geriatric patient who is symptomatic with significant levels of bacteriuria, a 7-day course of therapy with trimethoprim-sulfamethoxazole, a quinolone, or a beta-lactam is suggested. Because renal function declines with age, the creatinine clearance should be estimated in order to adjust the dosage of these medications to the patient's level of renal function.

12. What is the approach to the patient with an upper tract UTI?
Like other forms of complicated UTI, treating acute pyelonephritis with a short course of therapy is inappropriate. Traditionally, these infections were treated for 4–6 weeks. However, recent studies show good recovery within 2 weeks of therapy. When the infection is mild and patients show no signs of dehydration or renal failure, admission to the hospital may not be required. A 14-day course of oral therapy with trimethoprim-sulfamethoxazole, a quinolone, or ampicillin-clavulanate is appropriate depending on culture results. Many patients with acute pyelonephritis, however, experience significant nausea, vomiting, or dehydration and may even exhibit overt signs of sepsis. In these cases, admission to hospital and initiation of therapy with intravenous antibiotics such as trimethoprim-sulfamethoxazole, a quinolone, or ampicillin plus an aminoglycoside is appropriate. A clinical response to therapy should be apparent in 24–48 hours. Once the patient is afebrile, the patient may be changed to oral therapy based on the results of urine culture. The 14-day course may be completed at home either with oral therapy or with intravenous antibiotics administered by a home care service.

13. What is the strategy for managing recurring UTIs?
Treatment of recurrent UTI poses a challenge. First, repeated urine cultures should be obtained to determine whether the patient is having a relapse or reinfection. A **relapse** occurs when the infecting agent has not been eradicated. This condition will yield a positive culture at the end of therapy. When the culture obtained after treatment is negative and the patient has another

infection, this is considered a **reinfection**. Relapses and reinfections are treated differently. If the patient is having a relapse, the appropriate initial step would be to administer antibiotics for a longer duration. If this strategy is unsuccessful, the likelihood that structural problems are contributing to the pathogenesis of infection is increased, and further work-up should be initiated. In patients who have frequent reinfections, risk factors should be investigated. When the infections are related to sexual intercourse, postcoital voiding may be helpful. Additionally, women experiencing this problem who use diaphragms or spermicides may benefit from alternative methods of birth control. When these nonantibacterial measures fail, antibiotic prophylaxis should be considered. Trimethoprim-sulfamethoxazole may be taken as a single dose immediately before or after intercourse. Similarly, in women with frequent recurrences of UTI that are not related to sexual intercourse or birth control methods and in whom a work-up to rule out structural causes of the UTI has proven negative, self-initiated therapy is often successful. Both single-dose and short-course regimens as previously described for acute cystitis (see question 8) can be helpful in a compliant patient who is able to determine that she has a UTI. In those patients who cannot reliably self-diagnose UTI and who have recurrent infections, a continuous low dose of antibiotics for a 6-month period may prevent further recurrences.

14. How should fungal infections be treated?

Immunocompromised and catheterized patients are at increased risk for fungal infections of the urinary tract. These infections are often mild and asymptomatic; however, on occasion, they may be complicated by fungus balls in the bladder and renal parenchymal infection with dissemination. When a catheterized patient develops candiduria, removal of the catheter is sufficient to treat the condition if the patient is asymptomatic. When the catheter cannot be removed, or when the patient is symptomatic, amphotericin B bladder washes or fluconazole is appropriate. Patients with severe fungal urinary tract infection should be treated with intravenous amphotericin B.

BIBLIOGRAPHY

1. Barnett BJ, Stephens DS: Urinary tract infection: An overview. Am J Med Sci 314:245–249, 1997.
2. Hooton TM, Stamm WE: Diagnosis and treatment of uncomplicated urinary tract infection. Infect Dis Clin North Am 11:551–581, 1997.
3. Rushton HG: Urinary tract infections in children: Epidemiology, evaluation, and management. Pediatric Clin North Am 44:1133–1169, 1997.
4. Sobel JD: Pathogenesis of urinary tract infection. Role of host defenses. Infect Dis Clin North Am 11:531–549, 1997.
5. Stapleton A, Stamm WE: Prevention of urinary tract infection. Infect Dis Clin North Am 11:719–733, 1997.
6. Svanborg C, Godaly GD: Bacterial virulence in urinary tract infection. Infect Dis Clin North Am 11:513–529, 1997.
7. Warren JW: Catheter-associated urinary tract infections. Infect Dis Clin North Am 11:609–622, 1997.

20. DISORDERS OF TUBULAR FUNCTION

Michael B. Ganz, M.D.

1. What filtered substances are reabsorbed in the proximal tubule?

The proximal tubule is responsible for most of the reabsorption of filtered sodium, glucose, amino acids, phosphate, uric acid, and bicarbonate. Genetic defects leading to defective reabsorption of individual substances can lead to isolated glucosuria, aminoaciduria, etc. Global proximal reabsorptive dysfunction can lead to full-blown **Fanconi syndrome**, characterized by renal bicarbonate wasting, glucosuria, aminoaciduria, phosphaturia, and uricosuria.

2. Describe the pathophysiology of glucosuria.

The appearance of glucose in the urine results either from hyperglycemia leading to increased delivery of glucose to the kidney or from a defect in the proximal tubular absorption of glucose. Under normal circumstances, filtered glucose is completely reabsorbed until the plasma glucose concentration exceeds 250 mg/dl. By definition, primary renal glucosuria refers to the presence of glucose in the urine when plasma glucose concentrations are below this level. Abnormalities in tubular glucose absorption can result from genetic defects (autosomal recessive with variable penetrance) or from spontaneous mutations affecting glucose transporters. Isolated primary renal glucosuria is a benign condition that is not associated with renal or other organ dysfunction.

3. What is aminoaciduria?

Normally, virtually all amino acids filtered through the glomeruli are reabsorbed by proximal tubular epithelial cells. The term *aminoaciduria* refers to excretion of more than 5% of the filtered load of an amino acid. In general, aminoaciduria can result either from overproduction of of an amino acid leading to "overflow" through the nephron or, much more commonly, from specific transport defects leading to faulty reabsorption. Separate transport mechanisms exist for neutral, basic, and acidic amino acids such that these groups of amino acids can be affected selectively or more globally in patients with Fanconi syndrome.

4. What is Hartnup disease?

Hartnup disease is a rare familial disorder (1 per 26,000 live births) characterized by defective reabsorption of the neutral amino acids. Affected individuals have a red, scaly rash, intermittent dystonia, diarrhea, and cerebellar ataxia. The phenotype is clinically similar to pellagra, which results from dietary deficiency of the essential amino acid tryptophan.

5. What is cystinuria?

Cystinuria is an inherited autosomal recessive disorder (occurring in 1 in 7,000 live births) that leads to excessive excretion of cystine and the production of cystine stones. Cystine is insoluble in urine and renal stone formation generally becomes clinically evident by the second or third decade of life. Treatment includes hydration (to dilute the urine), alkalinization, and administration of D-penicillamine—a drug that increases the solubility of cystine by forming mixed disulfides with cysteine.

6. What is hypophosphatemic rickets?

Although bone disease can occur in patients with chronic hypophosphatemia of any cause, the term *hypophosphatemic rickets* usually refers to osteomalacia that occurs in patients with isolated primary renal phosphate wasting or Fanconi syndrome.

7. What is renal tubular acidosis?

Renal tubular acidosis (RTA) results from defects either in proximal renal tubular reabsorption of bicarbonate (type II RTA) or in distal tubular hydrogen ion secretion (type I RTA). Type IV RTA is a variant that is observed in patients with the syndrome of hyporeninemic hypoaldosteronism. Pathophysiology, diagnosis, and treatment of RTAs are discussed in Chapter 61, Metabolic Acidosis.

8. What is type III RTA?

There is no such thing. Somebody thought it would be fun to confuse students of renal physiology!

9. How does aldosterone deficiency affect distal tubular function?

Aldosterone normally stimulates Na^+-K^+ and Na^+-H^+ exchange in the distal tubule. Deficiency of this hormone (or resistance to its action) generally results in hyperkalemia and acidosis. Certain diuretics (spironolactone, amiloride, triamterene) block the effects of aldosterone and can result in similar electrolyte and acid-base abnormalities.

10. What is Bartter's syndrome?

Bartter's syndrome consists of otherwise unexplained metabolic alkalosis and hypokalemia, sometimes associated with hypomagnesemia. Plasma renin and aldosterone levels are typically elevated but, in contrast to other states of hyperaldosteronism, blood pressure tends to be normal. The basic tubular defect underlying this syndrome is impaired absorption of chloride in the thick ascending limb of the loop of Henle. Treatment consists of potassium supplementation, potassium-sparing diuretics, and nonsteroidal anti-inflammatory drugs (e.g, indomethacin), which, by inhibiting prostaglandin synthesis, indirectly inhibit renin and aldosterone release.

11. What is Gitelman's syndrome?

Gitelman's syndrome is a rare disorder also characterized by metabolic alkalosis and hypokalemia. In contrast to Bartter's syndrome, this disorder is always associated with hypomagnesemia and also with hypocalciuria. Recent data suggest that this syndrome results from a defect in the gene for the thiazide-sensitive sodium-chloride cotransporter in the distal tubule.

BIBLIOGRAPHY

1. Battle DC, Sehy JT, Roseman MK, et al: Clinical and pathophysiologic spectrum of acquired distal renal tubular acidosis. Kidney Int 20:389–396, 1981.
2. Fox M, Their SO, Rosenberg LE, et al: Evidence against a single renal transport defect in cystinuria. N Engl J Med 270:556–562, 1964.
3. Gitelman HJ: Hypokalemia, hypomagnesemia, and alkalosis: A rose is a rose—or is it? J Pediatr 120:79–80, 1992.
4. Morris RC, Ives H: Inherited disorders of the renal tubule. In Brenner BM (ed): The Kidney, 5th ed. Philadelphia, W.B. Saunders, 1996, pp 1764 1827.
5. Scriver CR: Hartnup disease: A genetic modification of intestinal and renal transport of certain neutral alpha-amino acids. N Engl J Med 273:530–537, 1965.

III. Primary Glomerular Disease

21. MINIMAL CHANGE DISEASE

Ira D. Davis, M.D.

1. What is the most common cause of nephrotic syndrome in children?
According to the International Study of Kidney Disease in Children (ISKDC), minimal change disease (MCNS) occurs in 77% of children with nephrotic syndrome.

2. At what age is MCNS most commonly seen?
The median age for the diagnosis of MCNS is 2.5 years. MCNS accounts for approximately 90% of nephrotic syndrome cases in children younger than 10 years and less than 50% of cases in older children.

3. Does MCNS occur more often in males?
Yes. In young children, the male to female ratio for MCNS is 3:2. In teenagers and adults, MCNS occurs equally among males and females.

4. What is the histologic appearance of the kidney in MCNS?
By definition, the glomeruli in MCNS are normal in appearance on light microscopy. Immunofluorescence microscopy usually demonstrates no immunoglobulin (Ig) or complement deposition in the glomerulus, although minimal amounts of deposited IgM, IgA, IgG, or C3 are sometimes detected. Ultrastructural analysis reveals nonspecific widening and effacement of the visceral epithelial cell foot processes with loss of slit processes (referred to as foot-process fusion). This finding is seen in a variety of glomerular diseases associated with nephrotic syndrome and is not specific for MCNS.

5. Which clinical features favor the diagnosis of MCNS in a child with nephrotic syndrome?
Age between 1 and 8 years
Normal blood pressure
Normal serum creatinine concentration
Absence of microscopic hematuria

6. What is the standard therapy for treatment of the initial episode of nephrotic syndrome when MCNS is suspected?
High-dose prednisone at a dose of 60 mg/m²/day (maximum 80 mg/day) in 2–3 divided doses initially for 4–6 weeks is the accepted standard therapy for this disease. The prednisone is then decreased to a single dose of 40 mg/m² on alternate days for 1 month before discontinuing the prednisone using a slow taper over a 1–2 month period. In addition, a low-sodium diet is recommended to control edema.

7. What are the indications for albumin infusions and diuretics in MCNS?
Albumin infusions and diuretic therapy are often used to achieve fluid removal in the presence of significant edema. Salt-poor albumin (25%) infusions are commonly used in the presence of severe edema of the extremities associated with difficulty in ambulation, significant scrotal or labial edema, ascites associated with peritonitis, or respiratory distress due to pleural effusions or

tense ascites. Salt-poor albumin also may be used for intravascular volume expansion if significant hypovolemia has resulted from a fall in oncotic pressure due to hypoalbuminemia. Diuretics often are used in the presence of pitting edema of the extremities or genital edema, particularly when the patient's body weight has increased by at least 5% above baseline. Sodium restriction remains an essential component in managing edema in MCNS, even if diuretic therapy or albumin infusions are necessary.

8. What are the potential complications of albumin infusions and diuretics?

Albumin infusions should not be used in the presence of hypertension because exacerbation of a preexisting state of hypovolemia could worsen the hypertension or result in pulmonary edema. Excessive diuretic therapy has the potential to cause or worsen intravascular volume contraction, which may exacerbate a tendency to develop thromboembolic complications or acute renal failure.

9. Are antibiotics necessary in the management of the child with MCNS?

Use of antibiotics in patients with MCNS is controversial. Patients with nephrotic syndrome are prone to infections from encapsulated organisms such as *Streptococcus pneumoniae, Escherichia coli*, and *Haemophilus influenza*, most likely as a consequence of urinary loss of opsonizing antibodies. As a result, many nephrologists advocate prophylactic use of penicillin or amoxicillin in children with nephrotic syndrome. Administration of pneumococcal vaccine is also reasonable; however, it should be given during periods of remission when the patient is not receiving steroid therapy, which may impair antibody response to the vaccine.

10. How long does it take for a child with MCNS to go into remission when treated with prednisone?

Among patients with MCNS who are steroid responsive, 75–80% go into remission within 2 weeks of therapy, while 94% achieve a remission by 4 weeks of therapy.

11. Does MCNS recur or relapse?

Approximately 60–75% of children with MCNS will have at least one relapse of their nephrotic syndrome. Furthermore, 50% of patients with MCNS will have a frequently relapsing course defined as at least two relapses in a 6-month period. Frequent relapses during the initial 6 months after diagnosis of MCNS appear to predict which patients will have a frequently relapsing course during subsequent years.

12. What is steroid-dependent MCNS?

MCNS patients are considered steroid dependent if they achieve complete remission of their nephrotic syndrome during steroid therapy and relapse either while on a steroid taper or within 4 weeks of terminating steroid therapy.

13. What therapeutic options are available for children with recurrent episodes of MCNS?

Repeat courses of prednisone, 60 mg/m^2/day (maximum 80 mg/day) in 2–3 divided doses until the patient is in remission for 3 days, is commonly used for the first through third relapses. Once a remission is achieved, prednisone is tapered to a single dose of 40 mg/m^2 on alternate days for 1 month followed by either a rapid (over 2 months) or a slow (over 6–12 months) taper. Steroid-dependent patients or those with a frequent relapsing course and signs of steroid toxicity (i.e., growth retardation, obesity, cataracts, hypertension, hyperglycemia) may benefit from treatment with alkylating agents such as cyclophosphamide or chlorambucil. Other potential therapies include administration of cyclosporine or levamisole.

14. What is steroid-resistant MCNS?

Patients who do not achieve a remission after 4 weeks of prednisone, 60 mg/m^2/day in divided doses, and 4 weeks of a once-daily dose of prednisone, 60 mg/m^2/day, are considered steroid resistant. For children younger than 6 years, approximately 50% with steroid-resistant nephrotic syndrome have MCNS on renal biopsy and will eventually become steroid responsive. Less than 5% of steroid-resistant patients older than 6 years of age have MCNS. Pathologic lesions such as mesangial proliferative glomerulonephritis, focal segmental glomerulosclerosis, and membranoproliferative glomerulonephritis are more common in these patients.

15. Is a renal biopsy ever necessary in patients with a presumed diagnosis of MCNS?
Patients with a steroid-resistant course require a renal biopsy. Although controversial, most pediatric nephrologists perform a renal biopsy prior to initiating treatment with other medications, such as alkylating agents or cyclosporine, in the presence of steroid toxicity or frequently relapsing nephrotic syndrome. Renal biopsy also should be considered in patients older than 10 years and in those with hypertension, renal insufficiency, or gross hematuria.

16. What is the long-term prognosis for children with MCNS?
Patients with steroid-responsive MCNS have excellent survival and normal renal function. The frequency of relapses diminishes with advancing age. Patients with steroid-resistant nephrotic syndrome secondary to MCNS have a poorer long-term prognosis. Even when the initial renal biopsy shows MCNS, these patients often have mesangial proliferative glomerulonephritis or focal segmental glomerulosclerosis on follow-up biopsies. The latter lesions are associated with a 30–50% chance of progressing to end-stage renal disease within 5 years.

BIBLIOGRAPHY

1. Berns JS, Gaudio KM, Durante D, et al: Steroid-responsive nephrotic syndrome of childhood: A long-term study of clinical course, histopathology, efficacy of cyclophosphamide therapy, and effects on growth. Am J Kidney Dis 9:108–114, 1987.
2. Clark G, Barratt TM: Minimal change nephrotic syndrome and focal segmental glomerulosclerosis. In Holliday MA, Barratt TM, Avner ED (eds): Pediatric Nephrology, 3rd ed. Baltimore, Williams & Wilkins, 1994, pp 767–787.
3. International Study of Kidney Disease in Children: Early identification of frequent relapsers among children with minimal change nephrotic syndrome. J Pediatr 101:514–518, 1982.
4. International Study of Kidney Disease in Children: The primary nephrotic syndrome in children. Identification of patients with minimal change nephrotic syndrome from initial response to prednisone. J Pediatr 98:561–564, 1981.
5. International Study of Kidney Disease in Children: Nephrotic syndrome in children: Prediction of histopathology from clinical and laboratory characteristics at time of diagnosis. Kidney Int 113:159–165, 1978.
6. Robson WLM, Leung AKC: Nephrotic syndrome in childhood. Adv Pediatr 40:287–323, 1993.
7. Trompeter RS, Lloyd B, Hicks J, et al: Long-term outcome for children with minimal-change nephrotic syndrome. Lancet 1:368–370, 1985.
8. Tune BM, Mendoza SA: Treatment of the idiopathic nephrotic syndrome: Regimens and outcomes in children and adults. J Am Soc Nephrol 8:824–832, 1997.

22. FOCAL SEGMENTAL GLOMERULOSCLEROSIS

Linda Zarif, M.D., and John R. Sedor, M.D.

1. What is focal segmental glomerulosclerosis (FSGS)?

FSGS is a glomerular disease defined by a characteristic histologic pattern that occurs either as a primary kidney disease (primary FSGS) or as a result of a systemic illness (secondary FSGS).

2. What is the characteristic pathology of FSGS?

Light microscopy demonstrates mesangial collapse in some glomeruli ("focal") and scarring in parts of glomerular capillary tufts ("segmental"). Immunofluorescence microscopy often shows immunoglobulin (usually IgM) and complement (usually C3) deposition in scarred areas of the glomerulus but rarely in normal segments. Foot-process effacement is typically found by electron microscopy in both scarred and unscarred regions of the glomerulus, at least in patients with heavy proteinuria.

3. Are there variants of FSGS histology? Do the histopathologic variants predict the clinical course of the disease?

There are two important pathologic variants of FSGS. First, the **glomerular tip lesion** is characterized by swelling, vacuolation, and proliferation of epithelial cells and by sclerosis in the glomerular segments closest to the proximal tubule. Patients with this histology tend to exhibit a more benign course and to be more responsive to steroid therapy compared to patients with classic FSGS. A second variant is characterized by **focal** or **global glomerular capillary collapse** and sclerosis with visceral epithelial cell swelling. This lesion is associated with a less favorable prognosis and is more common in African-American patients and in patients with human immunodeficiency virus (HIV) nephropathy (see Chapter 30, HIV-Associated Renal Disorders). Severe tubulointerstitial disease associated with any of these glomerular lesions correlates with poor long-term renal survival.

4. What is the common clinical presentation of patients with FSGS?

The most common clinical manifestation is proteinuria. Protein excretion usually is in the nephrotic range in patients with idiopathic FSGS. Patients with secondary FSGS may have urine protein excretion of less than 3 gm per day. Hematuria is common and is found in up to 75% of patients. At the time of presentation, hypertension is found in 30–50% of patients, and renal insufficiency often coincides. Hyperlipidemia also may occur in nephrotic patients.

5. Is there a racial predilection for the development of FSGS?

Yes. FSGS is the most common cause of idiopathic nephrotic syndrome among African Americans. However, patients with FSGS constitute an increasingly larger fraction of nephrotic individuals in the general population. A survey of renal biopsies from 1995 to 1997 in adult patients with idiopathic nephrotic syndrome showed that FSGS is the most common lesion, accounting for 35% of all patients and for 50% of cases in African-American patients.

6. What are the causes of FSGS?

FSGS may be idiopathic or secondary (see Table). By definition, the term "idiopathic FSGS" is only used if evidence is lacking for other causes of focal glomerulonephritis that could result in focal scarring after healing.

Classification of FSGS	Cause
Primary	Idiopathic FSGS
	Classic
	Glomerular tip variant
	Collapsing or "malignant" variant
	Superimposed on minimal change nephropathy
	Familial
Secondary	Sickle-cell disease
	Unilateral renal agenesis
	HIV infection
	Vesicoureteral reflux
	Diabetes mellitus (rare)
	Postinflammatory scarring
	Morbid obesity

7. Describe the clinical course of FSGS.

In patients with idiopathic FSGS, prognosis and clinical course are greatly influenced by the severity of proteinuria. Persistent non–nephrotic-range proteinuria is associated with good long-term renal survival. In contrast, declining glomerular filtration rates characterize patients with persistent nephrotic-range proteinuria. In this latter group of FSGS patients, the prevalence of end-stage renal disease 10 years after initial diagnosis is greater than 50%. Patients with HIV-induced FSGS or the collapsing variant may progress to end-stage renal disease in months to 2–3 years. The course of secondary forms of FSGS will vary according to the severity and activity of the underlying disease.

8. Does FSGS recur after kidney transplantation?

Yes. The reported recurrence rates among patients with idiopathic FSGS range between 20% and 40%. Secondary FSGS may not recur depending on underlying disease and its activity after transplantation. Patients with high-grade proteinuria and a rapid course to renal failure are at highest risk for recurrence. Interestingly, FSGS recurs less often in African-American patients, despite the higher prevalence of progressive FSGS in this population.

9. What are the general principles of management for patients with FSGS?

1. Blood pressure should be normalized, if possible, in all hypertensive patients with FSGS.
2. All patients with nephrotic-range proteinuria and FSGS should be treated with angiotensin-converting enzyme (ACE) inhibitors, unless otherwise contraindicated. Nephrotic-range proteinuria of any cause is an independent risk factor for progression of chronic renal failure, and ACE inhibitors are the most potent antiproteinuric agents available.
3. Hyperlipidemia should be controlled with appropriate hyperlipidemic medications.
4. Salt restriction and diuretics can be used to control edema in nephrotic FSGS patients.

10. Should FSGS patients be treated with corticosteroids or other immunosuppressive drugs?

The therapy of FSGS remains controversial, and data for evidence-based decisions are lacking. Most studies of therapy for FSGS patients have employed regimens used for treatment of minimal change nephropathy and have reported a poor response to therapy. However, more recent studies of the treatment of FSGS patients with more prolonged courses of immunosuppressive therapy now report response rates of up to 60% and improved long-term renal survival.

11. What factors influence the decision to treat a patient who has FSGS?

The potential efficacy and side effects of therapy must be considered for each patient. The amount of proteinuria, presence and degree of renal insufficiency, and the extent of scarring on biopsy are appropriate variables to evaluate before administering anti-inflammatory drugs.

Nonspecific therapy (see question 9) is probably an appropriate first approach to therapy in patients with mild proteinuria and normal renal function. In contrast, patients with persistent nephrotic proteinuria and renal insufficiency should be considered for more aggressive therapy with steroids or other immunosuppressants.

12. Outline specific treatment options for patients with idiopathic FSGS.

Prednisone, 1 mg/kg/day for at least 2–4 months, is the most common treatment regimen for patients with FSGS and is usually continued for 1–2 weeks after induction of remission and then tapered slowly. A prolonged prednisone therapy of 5–8 months has been advocated by some experts. Some patients who initially respond to prednisone therapy may exhibit frequent relapses or become steroid dependent. Cyclophosphamide or other cytotoxic drugs can be added to the therapeutic regimen and may induce complete or partial remission in up to 75% of these individuals. In recent studies, cyclosporine has been reported to induce remission in steroid-dependent and steroid-resistant FSGS patients. However, relapse is common when cyclosporine is discontinued. In addition, cyclosporine itself can be nephrotoxic and should be used judiciously.

13. What factors are associated with steroid resistance?

Significant tubulointerstitial disease on renal biopsy, an elevated creatinine, and massive proteinuria of more than 10 gm daily suggest that the clinical response to steroid therapy may be poor. Patients with these risk factors may be candidates for early withdrawal from treatment if the steroids are tolerated poorly or cause significant side effects.

BIBLIOGRAPHY

1. Appel GB: Focal segmental glomerulosclerosis. In Greenberg A (ed): Primer on Kidney Diseases, 2nd ed. San Diego, Academic Press, 1998, pp 160–164.
2. Glassock RJ, Cohen AH, Adler SG: Primary glomerular diseases. In Brenner BM (ed): The Kidney, 5th ed. Philadelphia, W.B. Saunders, 1996, pp 1446–1452.
3. Haas M, Meehan SM, Karrison TG, Spargo BH: Changing etiologies of unexplained adult nephrotic syndrome: A comparison of renal biopsy findings from 1976–1979 and 1995–1997. Am J Kidney Dis 30:621–631, 1997.
4. Korbet SM: Primary focal segmental glomerulosclerosis. J Am Soc Nephrol 79:1333–1342, 1998.
5. Lewis EJ: Recurrent focal sclerosis after renal transplantation. Kidney Int 22:315–323, 1982.
6. Ponticelli C, Rizzoni G, Edefonti A, et al: A randomized trial of cyclosporine in steroid-resistant idiopathic nephrotic syndrome. Kidney Int 43:1377–1384, 1993.
7. Rydel JJ, Korbet SM, Borok RZ, Schwartz MM: Focal segmental glomerular sclerosis in adults: Presentation, course, and response to treatment. Am J Kidney Dis 25:534–542, 1995.
8. Schwartz MM, Korbet SM, Rydell J, et al: Primary focal segmental glomerulosclerosis in adults: Prognostic value of histologic variants. Am J Kidney Dis 25:845–852, 1995.
9. Seney FD Jr, Burns DK, Silva FG: Acquired immunodeficiency syndrome and the kidney. Am J Kidney Dis 16:1–13, 1990.
10. Tune BM, Mendoza SA: Treatment of idiopathic nephrotic syndrome: Regimens and outcomes in children and adults. J Am Soc Nephrol 8:824–832, 1997.

23. MEMBRANOUS GLOMERULOPATHY

Eduardo Lacson, Jr., M.D.

1. What is membranous glomerulopathy?

Membranous glomerulopathy is a morphologic entity defined by biopsy. Pathologic examination reveals subepithelial immune complex deposition within the glomerular basement membrane (see Figure) without associated mesangial hypercellularity or matrix expansion.

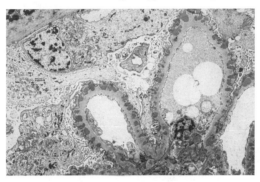

Electron micrograph from a patient with membranous glomerulopathy showing irregularly distributed electron-dense immune deposits in the subepithelial portion of the glomerular basement membrane.

2. What are some synonyms for membranous glomerulopathy?

Epimembranous, perimembranous, and *extramembranous glomerulonephritis* have been used interchangeably in the literature to refer to membranous glomerulopathy. Sometimes, it is called *membranous nephropathy* or *membranous glomerulonephritis.* The latter term is probably inappropriate because this entity is generally not associated with the cellular proliferation commonly associated with the term *nephritis.*

3. How common is membranous glomerulopathy?

Membranous glomerulopathy is one of the most common renal diseases associated with adult nephrotic syndrome. It accounts for 15–30% of all biopsies performed on adults with heavy proteinuria. Furthermore, in those older than 50 years of age, idiopathic membranous glomerulopathy encompasses 35–40% of cases. In contrast, it accounts for less than 5% of cases of nephrotic syndrome in children.

4. At what age does membranous glomerulopathy most commonly present?

The peak occurrence of membranous glomerulopathy is in the fifth decade. Most patients are diagnosed after the age of 30 years (80–95% of cases).

5. Is there any gender or racial predominance in membranous glomerulopathy?

Membranous glomerulopathy is more common in males with most series showing close to a 2:1 male to female ratio. No specific racial predominance has been identified.

6. What disease entities need to be excluded to make a diagnosis of primary idiopathic membranous glomerulopathy?

A secondary cause for membranous glomerulopathy can be found in 15–30% of adults and up to 80% of children (see Table). Of these, up to 75% of secondary cases are associated with systemic lupus erythematosus, hepatitis B, medications (e.g., gold, penicillamine), or malignancies.

Secondary Causes of Membranous Glomerulopathy

CAUSES	EXAMPLES	
Infections	Hepatitis B	Schistosomiasis
	Hepatitis C	Filariasis
	Malaria	Scabies
	Syphilis	Hydatid disease
	Leprosy	Castleman's disease
Autoimmune	Systemic lupus erythematosus	Hashimoto's thyroiditis
	Rheumatoid arthritis	Dermatitis herpetiformis
	Sjögren's syndrome	Myasthenia gravis
	Dermatomyositis	Guillain-Barré syndrome
	Sarcoidosis	Weber-Christian panniculitis
	Mixed connective tissue disease	Bullous pemphigoid/pemphigus
	Crohn's disease	Ankylosing spondylitis
	Anticardiolipin antibody syndrome	Graft vs. host disease
	Urticarial vasculitis	
Malignancies	Carcinoma (lung, colon, breast, stomach, esophagus, carotid body)	
	Melanoma	
	Leukemia/lymphoma (non-Hodgkin's type)	
Medications	Organic gold	Probenecid
	D-Penicillamine	Trimethadione
	Mercury-containing compounds	Nonsteroidal anti-inflammatory
	Captopril	drugs (ketoprofen, fenoprofen)
Genetic	Sickle cell disease	Sclerosing cholangitis
	Fanconi's syndrome	(?) Diabetes—increased incidence of membranous glomerulo-nephritis
Others	Kimura's disease	Systemic mastocytosis
	Gardner-Diamond syndrome	De novo in renal allografts
	Hydrocarbon exposure	

7. What is the most common clinical presentation of membranous glomerulopathy?

Membranous glomerulopathy presents with heavy proteinuria in more than 80% of patients, with a majority exhibiting the nephrotic syndrome (see Chapter 17, Nephrotic Syndrome). Some patients present with asymptomatic proteinuria, and even fewer will have accompanying microhematuria. The onset is insidious and is generally not associated with antecedent or concomitant infection.

8. Does membranous glomerulopathy present with renal failure?

Rarely. The patients will more often complain of edema and sometimes anasarca. Nonspecific symptoms such as nausea, anorexia, and malaise may be present. Hypertension and azotemia are usually absent on initial presentation but may develop in the course of membranous glomerulopathy.

9. How is the diagnosis of membranous glomerulopathy made?

Biopsy, as in most forms of primary glomerular disease, is necessary for definitive diagnosis. Although the clinical picture may suggest the possibility of membranous glomerulopathy, confirmation by biopsy is required. Again, one must carefully exclude secondary causes of membranous glomerulopathy by clinical evaluation for systemic disease.

10. Describe the biopsy findings in membranous glomerulopathy.

Examination	Findings
Light microscopy	Initially, the glomeruli and mesangial areas appear normal; later, capillary wall thickening appears as the disease progresses. Methenamine silver staining may reveal characteristic epithelial projections ("spikes") along the capillary walls, which represent new basement membrane material that surrounds the subepithelial deposits.
Immunofluorescence	Granular staining for IgG with some C3 (occasionally weak IgA and IgM)
Electron microscopy	May be classified under four stages (I–IV) with common features of variable subepithelial immune complex depositions and no obvious mesangial changes. The development, size, and frequency of the immune deposits determine the stage. Early and irregularly placed deposits are classified under stage I, while stage IV represents late, lightly staining, "burned out" deposits.

11. What causes primary membranous glomerulopathy?

The most commonly accepted mechanism in the pathogenesis of membranous glomerulopathy is in situ immune complex formation against antigens that have become implanted within the glomerular basement membrane. The antibody is thought to find its way to the subepithelial antigen, form immune complexes, and deposit there. Another theory proposes that preformed circulating immune complexes deposit in the subepithelial space. In some secondary forms of membranous glomerulopathy, the antigen has been discerned (e.g., hepatitis B surface and core antigens). A rat model known as Heymann's nephritis produces lesions similar to human membranous glomerulopathy. How immune complex deposition mediates proteinuria remains unclear. There appears to be a role for complement, especially the terminal complex C5b-C9, in lytic damage of glomerular epithelial cells.

12. What laboratory tests are useful in patients with membranous glomerulopathy?

Laboratory studies should include a chemistry profile to measure renal function and electrolyte status, a urinalysis to document proteinuria and hematuria, a 24-hour urine collection to quantitate the proteinuria and glomerular filtration rate, a serum albumin, and a lipid profile. Other ancillary tests may be used to rule out other etiologies as noted in question 6, depending on the clinical manifestations. Serum complement levels are usually normal.

13. How common is renal vein thrombosis in membranous glomerulopathy?

Although renal vein thrombosis has been described in cases of nephrotic syndrome, it appears to occur most frequently in idiopathic membranous glomerulopathy. The incidence, extent, and influence of renal vein thrombosis on the course of membranous glomerulopathy are not clear. Examination of a series of patients followed at the Mayo Clinic revealed that renal vein thrombosis occurred in half of 33 patients with membranous glomerulopathy. Apart from acute renal vein occlusion, this series did not reveal any influence of renal vein thrombosis on proteinuria and renal function over a period of 26–30 months during the study.

14. What is the incidence of end-stage renal disease in patients with membranous glomerulopathy?

The natural history of membranous glomerulopathy varies depending on several factors. The overall prognosis in children is excellent with less than 5% progressing to renal failure. Ten-year renal survival is over 80–90%. In adults, 20–40% undergo complete remission, and 20–35% undergo partial remission. Thus, depending on the series, 5-year renal survival is approximately 80–85%, 10-year renal survival is over 65–75%, and in one study, 15-year renal survival was 59%. Membranous glomerulopathy appears to have an indolent course among most patients.

However, 10–30% of patients do progress to end-stage renal disease over 10–20 years. Many patients succumb to one of the other diseases that accompany advanced age prior to reaching end-stage renal disease.

15. What factors indicate a poor prognosis in patients with membranous glomerulopathy?
The degree and duration of proteinuria appear to be the best indicators that have been validated in the literature so far. Patients with nephrotic-range proteinuria in excess of 8 gm/day for at least 6 months appear to have a 66% chance of developing renal insufficiency. Other indicators of poor prognosis include the presence of hypertension, older age, male sex, decreased renal function at presentation, and the presence of tubulointerstitial disease on biopsy.

16. What is the best therapy for primary membranous glomerulopathy?
This is the $64 million question. Most studies show an indolent course for membranous glomerulopathy indicating that the risks of therapy (e.g., side effects of steroids or alkylating agents) may outweigh the benefits. The use of steroids in multiple studies and meta-analyses appears to have lost favor in the primary management of adults with this disease. Some centers, however, continue to use alternate day prednisone therapy (60 mg/m² to a maximum of 80 mg) for children with variable success. Recently, for patients with poor prognostic signs or deteriorating renal function, some nephrologists have advocated the use of chlorambucil (0.15–0.2 mg/kg) alternating with steroid treatment (1 gm methylprednisolone for 3 days, then 0.5 mg/kg prednisone for 27 days) monthly for 6 months or cyclophosphamide (1–2 mg/kg/day) with or without steroids for 6–24 months. An Italian group reports a 92% 10-year renal survival with the chlorambucil and steroid regimen. These agents appear to have some benefits that have not yet been validated in large, multicenter, randomized, controlled trials.

17. Is there a role for cyclosporine in the treatment of membranous glomerulopathy?
Cyclosporine is increasingly being used in the treatment of membranous glomerulopathy with favorable short-term prognosis. However, long-term use and the associated increased risk for interstitial fibrosis, renal failure, and other side effects are a concern. This remains an alternative therapy for membranous glomerulopathy but will need further evaluation.

18. How about supportive care for membranous glomerulopathy patients?
Symptomatic therapy with diuretics and control of hypertension remains standard in the care of the patient with membranous glomerulopathy. Some have advocated low-protein diets, control of cholesterol intake, and use of lipid lowering agents. Angiotensin-converting enzyme (ACE) inhibitors have been used to decrease proteinuria. Some have tried nonsteroidal anti-inflammatory drugs (NSAIDs) as well. Prophylactic anticoagulation with warfarin, aspirin, or dipyridamole have been advocated, especially in patients with persistent nephrotic syndrome.

19. Does transplantation play a role in membranous glomerulopathy?
Yes, transplantation has an excellent prognosis for patients with membranous glomerulopathy who have reached end-stage renal disease. The risk for recurrence of membranous glomerulopathy is low, although it is slightly higher in patients whose original biopsy reveals crescent formation. Interestingly, de novo membranous glomerulopathy can occur in the allografts of patients whose primary disease was not membranous glomerulopathy, often presenting with otherwise unexplained nephrotic syndrome.

BIBLIOGRAPHY

 1. Adler SG, Nast CC: Membranous nephropathy. In Greenberg A (ed): Primer on Kidney Diseases, 2nd ed. San Diego, Academic Press, 1998, pp 164–169.
 2. Austin HA, Antonovych TT, Mackay K, et al: Membranous nephropathy. Ann Intern Med 116:672–681, 1992.
 3. Glassock RJ, Cohen AH, Adler SG: Membranous glomerulonephritis. In Brenner BM (ed): The Kidney, 5th ed. Philadelphia, W.B. Saunders, 1996, pp 1452–1458.

 4. Hogan SL, Muller KE, Jeanette JC, Falk RJ: A review of therapeutic studies of idiopathic membranous glomerulopathy. Am J Kidney Dis 25:862–875, 1995.
 5. Imperiale TF, Goldfarb S, Berns JS: Are cytotoxic agents beneficial in idiopathic membranous nephropathy? A meta-analysis of the controlled trials. J Am Soc Nephrol 5:1553–1558, 1995.
 6. Makker SP: Membranous glomerulopathy. In Holliday MA, Barratt TM, Avner ED (eds): Pediatric Nephrology, 3rd ed. Baltimore, Williams & Wilkins, 1994, pp 754–766.
 7. Pei Y, Cattran D, Greenwood C: Predicting chronic renal insufficiency in idiopathic membranous glomerulonephritis. Kidney Int 42:960–966, 1992.
 8. Ponticelli C, Zuchelli P, Passerini P, et al: A 10-year follow-up of a randomized study with methylprednisolone and chlorambucil in membranous nephropathy. Kidney Int 48:1600–1604, 1995.
 9. Reichert LJM, Koene RAP, Wetzels JFM: Prognostic factors in idiopathic membranous nephropathy. Am J Kidney Dis 31:1–11, 1998.
10. Sarasin FP, Schifferli JA: Prophylactic oral anticoagulation in nephrotic patients with idiopathic membranous nephropathy. Kidney Int 45:578–585, 1994.
11. Schieppati A, Mosconi L, Perna A, et al: Prognosis of untreated patients with idiopathic membranous nephropathy. N Engl J Med 329:85–89, 1993.
12. Wagoner RD, Stanson AW, Holley KE, Winter CS: Renal vein thrombosis in idiopathic membranous glomerulopathy and nephrotic syndrome: Incidence and significance. Kidney Int 23:368–374, 1983.
13. Wasserstein AG. Membranous glomerulonephritis. J Am Soc Nephrol 8:664–674, 1997.

24. IgA NEPHROPATHY

Donald E. Hricik, M.D.

1. What is IgA nephropathy?

IgA (immunoglobulin A) nephropathy is a common form of mesangioproliferative glomeru-lonephritis characterized pathologically by mesangial deposition of IgA (detected by immunofluorescence microscopy) and varying degrees of mesangial cell proliferation and expansion of mesangial matrix. Codeposits of IgG, IgM, or terminal components of the complement system are present in the majority of cases.

2. What is the cause of IgA nephropathy?

This disorder probably results from altered regulation of the production or structure of IgA. Circulating IgA immune complexes are detectable in many cases and roughly parallel the severity of the disease. Glomerular deposits in IgA nephropathy consist primarily of abnormally gly-cosylated polymeric forms of the isotype subclass IgA1. The underlying cause of the abnormalities are unknown. However, the common association of gross hematuria with infections of the respiratory or gastrointestinal tract suggests that abnormal production of IgA may be triggered by mucosal exposure to environmental antigens.

3. How common is IgA nephropathy?

The exact prevalence is difficult to determine because it is likely that the vast majority of cases are subclinical. Nevertheless, IgA nephropathy is now recognized as the most common form of glomerulonephritis worldwide. The prevalence varies considerably between and within countries, with high rates in the western Pacific rim and relatively low rates in the United States and northern Europe. The disorder occurs in all age groups with a peak incidence in the second and third decades. There is a male predominance of at least 2:1. IgA nephropathy is uncommon in African Americans.

4. What explains the geographic variation in the prevalence of IgA nephropathy?

Variations in the prevalence of the disease may reflect differences in genetic tendencies to develop the disorder. Because many patients with IgA nephropathy present with otherwise symptomless hematuria, it is also possible that geographic variations in prevalence rates reflect local health screening practices or locally accepted indications for renal biopsy.

5. How is IgA nephropathy related to Henoch-Schönlein purpura?

Henoch-Schönlein purpura is a systemic disease characterized by cutaneous purpura, arthritis, colitis, and glomerulonephritis. The glomerular findings in Henoch-Schönlein purpura are morphologically indistinguishable from those observed in primary IgA nephropathy so that these disorders often are considered to be related components of a pathophysiologic spectrum.

6. Are IgA levels elevated in patients with IgA nephropathy?

Plasma concentrations of IgA are elevated in up to 50% of cases. However, measurement of IgA levels is neither sensitive nor specific enough to be of use in the diagnosis of IgA nephropathy.

7. How do patients with IgA nephropathy present?

The most common clinical presentation (50–60% of cases) consists of episodic gross hematuria frequently associated with simultaneous respiratory or gastrointestinal infection. Persistent microscopic hematuria, typically discovered during screening examinations, occurs in 30% of cases. Finally, 10% of patients present either with acute glomerulonephritis or with nephrotic syndrome.

8. What treatments are available?

Curative therapy is lacking. However, a variety of therapies have been attempted in an effort to retard the progression of the disease. Angiotensin inhibitors are probably more effective than other antihypertensive agents in slowing the progression of IgA nephropathy. Steroids and cytotoxic drugs may have some benefit in reducing rates of urinary protein excretion, but it remains unclear whether these agents beneficially influence long-term renal function. Based on the premise that ω-3 fatty acids may limit the actions of cytokines and eicosanoids induced by glomerular depositions of IgA, fish oil has proved to be of benefit in some trials. Several other treatment regimens, including high-dose immunoglobulin therapy, phenytoin, antiplatelet agents, urokinase, dapsone, plasma exchange, and tonsillectomy, have been attempted without conclusive results.

9. What is the prognosis of patients with IgA nephropathy?

Although IgA nephropathy commonly presents with asymptomatic or "benign" hematuria, end-stage renal disease ultimately develops in 20–40% of patients 5–25 years after diagnosis. Risk factors for progression to end-stage renal disease include older age, male gender, hypertension, persistent heavy proteinuria, impaired renal function at the time of diagnosis, the absence of gross hematuria, the presence of glomerulosclerosis or interstitial fibrosis on renal biopsy, and presence of the DD genotype for the deletion polymorphism in the angiotensin-converting enzyme gene.

BIBLIOGRAPHY

1. Donadio JV, Bergstralh ES, Offord KP, et al: A controlled trial of fish oil in IgA nephropathy. N Engl J Med 331:1194–1199, 1994.
2. Emancipator SN: IgA nephropathy: Morphologic expression and pathogenesis. Am J Kidney Dis 23.451–462, 1994.
3. Galla JH: IgA nephropathy. Kidney Int 47:377–387, 1995.
4. Hricik DH, Chung-Park M, Sedor JR: Glomerulonephritis. N Engl J Med 339:888–899, 1998.
5. Ibels LS, Ayory AZ: IgA nephropathy: Analysis of the natural history, important factors in the progression of renal disease, and a review of the literature. Medicine 73:79–102, 1994.
6. Julian BA, Waldo FB, Fifai A, Mestecky J: IgA nephropathy, the most common glomerulonephritis worldwide. A neglected case in the United States? Am J Med 84:129–132, 1988.
7. Mestecky J, Tomana M, Crowley-Nowick PA, et al: Defective galactosylation and clearance of IgA1 molecules as a possible etiopathogenic factor in IgA nephropathy. Contrib Nephrol 104:172–182, 1993.
8. Rostoker G, Desvaux-Belghiti D, Pilatte Y, et al: High-dose immunoglobulin therapy for severe IgA nephropathy and Henoch-Schonlein purpura. Ann Intern Med 120:476–484, 1994.
9. Schena FP: A retrospective analysis of the natural history of primary IgA nephropathy worldwide. Am J Med 89:209–215, 1990.
10. Schena FP, Montenegro M, Scivittaro P: Meta-analysis of randomized controlled trials in patients with IgA nephropathy (Berger's disease). Nephrol Dial Transplant 5:47–52, 1990.

25. MEMBRANOPROLIFERATIVE GLOMERULONEPHRITIS

Eduardo Lacson, Jr., M.D., and Ira D. Davis, M.D.

1. What is membranoproliferative glomerulonephritis (MPGN)?

MPGN is a morphologic entity defined by mesangial proliferation and thickening of the glomerular capillary walls as seen on light microscopy. The capillary wall thickening is due to immune deposits and interposition of mesangial matrix that results in double contours ("tram tracks") of the glomerular basement membrane, best appreciated on silver-stained specimens. Both primary and secondary forms of MPGN occur.

2. What are some synonyms for MPGN?

Mesangiocapillary glomerulonephritis
Lobular glomerulonephritis
Hypocomplementemic persistent glomerulonephritis

3. Describe the three types of primary MPGN.

The three types are shown in the table below and differ with reference to pathology and prevalence. The pathologic differentiation is based definitively on electron microscopic findings.

Pathology of MPGN

TYPE	LIGHT MICROSCOPY	IMMUNO-FLUORESCENCE	ELECTRON MICROSCOPY
Type I (most common)	Focal mesangial deposits with a nodular quality and double contours best seen with the Jones methenamine silver stain	IgG and C3 predominate in a granular mesangial and subendothelial pattern	Mesangial proliferation with immune deposition; mesangial cell "interposition" noted between the GBM and endothelium; subendothelial electron-dense deposits surrounded by new basement membrane producing double contours
Type II or dense deposit disease (least common)	Less uniform hypercellularity with band-like thickening of the lamina densa containing intra-membranous PAS positive, silver positive deposits	C3 only in a linear or double-contoured distribution along the GBM with occasional nodular mesangial deposition	Highly electron-dense deposits replacing the lamina densa to create smooth and ribbon-like depositions; nodular mesangial deposits present
Type III (uncommon)	Combined double contour and "spikes" denoting presence of subendothelial and subepithelial deposits seen best with silver stain	Mostly C3 with variable IgG deposition in the subendothelial, subepithelial, and mesangial areas	Electron-dense deposits in mixed subendothelial and subepithelial lesions producing "tram tracks" on the inner aspect and "spikes" on the outer aspect

PAS = periodic acid–Schiff stain, GBM = glomerular basement membrane

4. What secondary causes of MPGN must be excluded in order to call it a primary glomerular disease?

Secondary Causes of MPGN

CAUSES	EXAMPLES	
Infections	Hepatitis B	Malaria
	Hepatitis C + cryoglobulinemia	Schistosomiasis
	Infective endocarditis	Epstein-Barr virus
	Visceral abscesses	Human immunodeficiency
	Infected ventriculoatrial shunts	virus (HIV)
	Angiofollicular lymph node	Mycoplasma
	syndrome (Castleman's disease)	
Autoimmune	Systemic lupus erythematosus	
	Rheumatoid arthritis	
	Sjögren's syndrome	
	Scleroderma	
	Sarcoidosis	
	Celiac disease	
Chronic liver disease	Cirrhosis of any etiology	
Thrombotic micro-	Hemolytic uremic syndrome–thrombotic thrombocytopenic purpura	
angiopathies	Antiphospholipid antibody syndrome	
	Sickle cell nephropathy	
	Chronic allograft failure	
	Radiation nephritis	
Malignancies	B-cell lymphomas	
	Chronic lymphocytic leukemia	
	Other carcinoma (rarely)	
Genetic disorders	Alpha$_1$-antitrypsin disease	
	Complement deficiency (C2 or C3) with or without partial lipodystrophy	
	Kartagener's syndrome	
	Renal artery dysplasia	
	Buckley's syndrome	
Dysproteinemias	Cryoglobulinemia	
	Light chain deposition disease	
	Waldenström's macroglobulinemia	

5. What causes primary MPGN?

The pathogenesis is largely speculative. However, intermittently low complement levels (70% of cases) and circulating immune complexes (found in 50%) do support the role of immune complex deposition in the etiology of MPGN type I. The pathophysiology of types II and III remains unknown.

6. What is the most common clinical presentation of MPGN?

Fifty percent of patients present with nephrotic syndrome, 30% present with asymptomatic proteinuria (with or without recurrent gross or microscopic hematuria), and 20% present with acute glomerulonephritis. Type I MPGN especially tends to present with nephrotic syndrome. Some patients report a respiratory illness preceding the overt signs and symptoms of renal disease.

7. What age groups are most commonly affected by MPGN?

MPGN occurs most commonly between the ages of 7 and 30 years. Seventy percent of cases present in the second decade.

8. Is there any gender or racial predominance in MPGN?

There is near equal incidence between males and females although, in some series, there is a slight female predominance in type I disease. Although it is seen in most races, MPGN appears to predominate among caucasians.

9. How is the diagnosis of MPGN made?

Biopsy, biopsy, biopsy! As stated in question 1, this is a morphologic diagnosis, and definitive diagnosis can only be made with renal tissue and confirmed by electron microscopy.

10. What laboratory tests are useful in patients suspected of having MPGN?

Helpful tests include a chemistry profile to assess renal function and electrolyte status, a urinalysis to document proteinuria and hematuria, a renal ultrasound to exclude obstruction, serum complements to support the diagnosis (usually a low C3), and a 24-hour urine specimen to quantitate proteinuria and glomerular filtration rate. Other ancillary tests to rule out secondary causes of MPGN will be needed depending on the clinical presentation.

11. Does complement pattern have a bearing in diagnosis?

Type I MPGN is most often associated with panhypocomplementemia including decreased levels of C3, C4, and C5. Patients with type II MPGN tend to have only low C3, suggesting activation of the alternative complement pathway. Type III has low C3 or C5 but usually normal C4. This is only a rough guide, and there is a moderate degree of overlap in the complement patterns associated with the three entities.

12. What is the C3 nephritic factor?

This term refers to an antibody that is responsible for binding C3 convertase. As a result, the C3 convertase becomes stable and resistant to degradation by C3b inactivator, thus increasing its half-life tenfold. Consequently, it acts on the C3b amplification loop, markedly lowering C3 levels. C3 nephritic factor is found mostly in type II MPGN (40–50%) but also is present in up to 20% of MPGN type I and some cases of MPGN type III.

13. What are poor prognostic signs for patients with MPGN?

Rapidly progressing renal failure, severe hypertension, and persistent nephrotic syndrome are poor prognostic signs. Renal biopsy findings of glomerular crescents and interstitial fibrosis are also associated with a poor prognosis leading to chronic renal failure.

14. What is the treatment for MPGN?

No consensus has been reached regarding the ideal treatment for MPGN. Most children are given a trial of prednisone at 2 mg/kg/day every other day based on the protocol first described at the University of Cincinnati. A randomized, controlled trial by the International Study of Kidney Disease in Children failed to show a significant beneficial effect of steroids and indicated a high incidence of steroid toxicity, including hypertension. Some studies have suggested benefit using antiplatelet agents such as aspirin and dipyridamole. A low-protein diet has been advocated by some authors. Control of blood pressure is advocated to help retard progression of renal disease. The empiric use of angiotensin-converting enzyme (ACE) inhibitors to decrease proteinuria is also practiced by many physicians.

15. What are renal survival rates in primary MPGN?

Although older studies reported a 50% 10-year survival, recent studies quote survival rates of 60–85% in 10 years. The Cincinnati group reports a 20-year renal survival rate of 59% on alternate-day steroid therapy.

16. Does transplantation play a role in MPGN patients who reach end-stage renal disease?

Yes, transplantation is an option for patients with this disease. However, recurrence rates in post-transplant patients with MPGN type I and type II are 30% and 80%, respectively.

Furthermore, the recurrent disease causes graft failure in 40% of type I and 10–20% of type II MPGN patients. Risk of recurrence in type III disease is not known.

17. Are there any new treatments on the horizon for MPGN?
Plasmapheresis, angiotensin II receptor antagonists, cyclosporine, and mycophenolate mofetil have been used for MPGN, but experience with these agents is largely anecdotal. Newer therapies will undoubtedly arise as we gain more understanding of the biomolecular basis and pathogenesis of this disease.

BIBLIOGRAPHY

1. Cameron JS, Turner JR, Heaton J, et al: Idiopathic mesangiocapillary glomerulonephritis. Am J Med 74:175–192, 1983.
2. Curtis JJ, Wyatt RI, Bhathena D, et al: Renal transplantation for patients with type I and type II membranoproliferative glomerulonephritis. Am J Med 66:216–225, 1979.
3. D'Agati V: Membranoproliferative glomerulonephritis. In Greenberg A (ed): Primer on Kidney Diseases, 2nd ed. San Diego, Academic Press, 1998, pp 153–160.
4. Donadio JV, Offord KP: Reassessment of treatment results in membranoproliferative glomerulonephritis, with emphasis on life-table analysis. Am J Kidney Dis 14:445–451, 1989.
5. Glassock RJ, Cohen AH, Adler SG: Mesangiocapillary glomerulonephritis. In Brenner BM (ed): The Kidney, 5th ed. Philadelphia, W.B. Saunders, 1996, pp 1458–1466.
6. Jackson EC, McAdams AJ, Strife CF, et al: Differences between membranoproliferative glomerulonephritis types I and III in clinical presentation, glomerular morphology, and complement perturbation. Am J Kidney Dis 9:115–120, 1987.
7. McEnery PT: Membranoproliferative glomerulonephritis: The Cincinnati experience—cumulative renal survival from 1957 to 1989. J Pediatr 116:S109–S114, 1990.
8. McEnery PT, Coutinho MJ: Membranoproliferative glomerulonephritis. In Holliday MA, Barratt TM, Avner ED (eds): Pediatric Nephrology, 3rd ed. Baltimore, Williams & Wilkins, 1994, pp 739–753.
9. McEnery PT, McAdams AJ, West CD: The effect of prednisone in a high-dose, alternate-day regimen on the natural history of idiopathic membranoproliferative glomerulonephritis. Medicine 64:401–424, 1986.
10. Nakamura T, Obata J, Onizuka M, et al: Candesartan prevents the progression of mesangioproliferative nephritis in rats. Kidney Int Suppl 63:S226–S228, 1997.
11. West CD: Idiopathic membranoproliferative glomerulonephritis in childhood. Pediatr Nephrol 6:96–103, 1992.

IV. Secondary Glomerular Disease

26. DIABETIC NEPHROPATHY

Jeffrey R. Schelling, M.D.

1. What renal pathologic lesions are characteristic in diabetic nephropathy?

Nodular glomerulosclerosis, which is characterized by the presence of eosinophilic Kimmelstiel-Wilson nodules at the glomerular periphery, is the most pathognomonic finding of diabetic nephropathy but is present in only about 10–20% of patients with diabetic renal disease. Other characteristic pathologic features of diabetic nephropathy include a thickened glomerular basement membrane, glomerular epithelial cell foot-process fusion, and glomerular enlargement due to extracellular mesangial matrix expansion. With advanced disease, tubular atrophy and interstitial fibrosis can be observed.

2. What are the risk factors for progression of diabetic nephropathy?

In general, only about one out of three type I or type II diabetics will proceed to develop significant diabetic nephropathy, but identification of susceptible patients has been problematic. Over the past decade, several longitudinal studies have suggested that microalbuminuria, defined as urine albumin excretion ranging between 30 and 300 mg/24 hours, predicts progression to overt proteinuria and then renal insufficiency. By definition, microalbuminuria is urine protein concentration below the detection limits of standard urine dipsticks. However, use of a more sensitive laboratory assay to detect microalbuminuria has become standard. In patients who do develop microalbuminuria, it is generally observed 5–10 years after the onset of diabetes, with nephrotic-range proteinuria occurring at 10–15 years and severe renal insufficiency with progression to end-stage renal disease occurring within 15–20 years. Once dipstick-positive proteinuria is detected, progression of renal disease is virtually certain, unless the patient dies from another cause first.

Multiple intervention trials also have demonstrated that blood pressure and glycemic control delay the progression of renal disease (see question 5), indicating that hypertension and hyperglycemia, in the context of diabetes, may also pose risks for progressive diabetic nephropathy. There is fairly tight concordance of retinopathy and neuropathy with nephropathy in patients with type I diabetes. Discordance in expression of these manifestations of diabetic end-organ damage is more common in type II diabetics. Finally, there is increased concordance for diabetic nephropathy within families and in certain racial groups (African Americans, Native Americans), suggesting a genetic component to diabetic renal disease. The specific genes that regulate the expression of diabetic nephropathy have yet to be discovered, however.

3. Is renal biopsy necessary in the diagnosis of patients with suspected diabetic nephropathy?

Although the histologic features of diabetic nephropathy are well described, the diagnosis is usually made using clinical criteria, and patients require biopsy only if the clinical presentation is unusual. A biopsy diagnosis is commonly warranted if the duration of diabetes is less than 10 years, in the absence of accompanying retinopathy or neuropathy, or for clinical suspicion of an alternative diagnosis. An estimated 25% of patients with type II diabetic nephropathy may also have another concomitant renal lesion. Other renal pathology is much rarer in patients with type I diabetic nephropathy.

4. What are the typical urinalysis findings in patients with diabetic nephropathy?

The hallmark of the urinalysis in diabetic nephropathy is proteinuria. The predominant protein in the urine is albumin. A minority of patients with diabetic nephropathy will demonstrate microscopic hematuria. The presence of cellular casts should prompt careful consideration of other diagnoses, but cellular casts have been described in patients with diabetic renal disease.

5. What treatments should be considered to slow the progression of diabetes mellitus nephropathy?

1. **Blood pressure control**. Blood pressure control is one of the mainstays in the treatment of diabetic nephropathy. In particular, antihypertensive treatment with angiotensin-converting enzyme (ACE) inhibitors may be preferential to other antihypertensive regimens, at least in patients with type I diabetes mellitus. Lowering blood pressure with an ACE inhibitor–containing regimen has been associated with enhanced slowing of diabetic nephropathy progression when compared to equivalent blood pressure control with regimens that do not contain an ACE inhibitor. The mechanism by which ACE inhibitors achieve this "renoprotective" effect is debated. ACE inhibitors reduce both systemic and intraglomerular pressures. An alternative or additional renoprotective mechanism of ACE inhibition may be through inhibition of glomerular sclerosis and interstitial fibrosis, because in vitro studies have shown that angiotensin II promotes extracellular matrix deposition and fibrosis. Most studies that have demonstrated benefit from ACE inhibitor therapy in diabetic nephropathy have enrolled patients with mild to moderate renal disease (e.g., serum creatinine < 2.0 mg/dl). It remains to be determined if conclusions from these studies can be extrapolated to patients with more advanced renal disease.

Even in patients who do not tolerate ACE therapy, blood pressure control is critical. Large, prospective, randomized trials are currently ongoing to determine the optimum target blood pressure. Lowering blood pressure, to below the standard target of less than 140/90 mmHg for the general population, may provide more benefits in diabetics with evidence of renal disease.

2. **Glycemic control**. It has always been sensible to attempt tight blood glucose control in diabetics, but only recently have well-designed studies definitively demonstrated that this approach results in slowing of diabetic renal disease progression. In the Diabetes Control and Complications trial, tight glycemic control, which was achieved with multiple daily insulin injections, was associated with a 40–50% decrease in the incidence of proteinuria.

3. **Dietary protein restriction**. Use of dietary protein restrictions as a therapeutic maneuver was initially identified using animal models of diabetic renal disease. The purported mechanism of action was reduction in glomerular capillary pressures. Initial human studies confirmed these results, although these data have been difficult to corroborate. In the Modification of Diet in Renal Disease study, which was designed to answer this question, there was no clear benefit to patients with established renal disease after 3 years of dietary protein restriction. However, type I diabetics were excluded from this study, and the type II diabetic cohort comprised only 3% of the study population.

6. Should ACE inhibitor therapy be instituted in normotensive patients with diabetic nephropathy?

Because ACE inhibitors are believed to slow the progression of diabetic nephropathy, in part, by nonhemodynamic mechanisms, a number of large clinical trials have been conducted to address the efficacy of ACE inhibitor therapy on renal disease progression in normotensive diabetics. In general, all of the major studies have demonstrated that ACE inhibitors reduce proteinuria. Not all studies evaluated the effect of ACE inhibitors on glomerular filtration rate, but in those that did, there was a consistent benefit of ACE inhibitor therapy. Therefore, it seems reasonable to recommend ACE inhibitor therapy to normotensives with diabetic nephropathy. In general, the ACE inhibitor regimens were well tolerated. However, because diabetics are at risk for hyporeninemic hypoaldosteronism and atherosclerotic renal artery stenosis, periodically monitoring serum electrolytes and creatinine after instituting the ACE inhibitor regimen is probably wise.

7. Should calcium channel blockers be recommended for the treatment of hypertension in diabetic nephropathy?

Fairly good evidence exists to support the use of the nondihydropyridine classes of calcium channel blockers (verapamil and diltiazem family) for the treatment of hypertension in diabetic nephropathy. In animal models of diabetic renal disease, as well as human studies, benefit has been shown both with respect to preservation of glomerular filtration rate and diminution of proteinuria. The data are much less compelling with dihydropyridine calcium channel blocker, particularly the older generation short-acting agents (e.g., nifedipine). Most studies have shown no effect on, or even increases in, proteinuria with these agents. Ongoing studies designed to determine the effects of second-generation dihydropyridine calcium channel blockers in diabetic nephropathy should soon be completed. Finally, some evidence suggests an additive benefit of antihypertensive regimens with combined ACE inhibitor and nondihydropyridine calcium channel blockers in diabetic nephropathy.

8. How does the development of diabetic nephropathy alter the management of blood glucose?

Because the kidney both metabolizes and excretes glucose, the half-life of endogenously and exogenously administered insulin is prolonged in the setting of decreased glomerular filtration rate. Therefore, to avoid hypoglycemia, the dose of oral hypoglycemic agents or insulin often needs to be decreased in patients with diabetic nephropathy.

9. What are the renal replacement therapy options in patients with end-stage renal disease from diabetic nephropathy?

Diabetic nephropathy is now the most common cause of end-stage renal disease, accounting for one in three patients entering renal replacement therapy programs. Similar to other causes of chronic renal disease, the optimum treatment is kidney transplantation. The 10-year survival rate in some series is as high as 40%, which is superior to mortality figures for diabetics on dialysis (see question 10). The data should be viewed with some caution, though, because there is a selection bias toward transplantation of diabetics with fewer comorbid medical problems. As with other types of glomerular disease, diabetic nephropathy may recur in the transplant allograft. A combined kidney and pancreas transplantation may be the most preferable treatment for diabetic nephropathy, although this is an option at only a few medical centers. Because of the relatively small supply of donor organs and the high incidence of comorbid conditions in diabetics, which may preclude a transplant, the majority of patients with diabetic end-stage renal disease are treated with either hemodialysis or peritoneal dialysis (see Figure). Outcome studies comparing hemodialysis versus peritoneal dialysis have yielded mixed results. Therefore, either modality is generally considered acceptable. The rates of peritoneal dialysis catheter infection and malfunction are higher in diabetics versus nondiabetics. Finally, mortality with all forms of renal replacement therapy is higher in diabetics compared to nondiabetics.

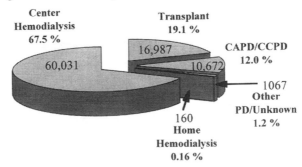

Distribution of patients with end-stage renal disease caused by diabetes mellitus to various renal replacement modalities. (From Friedlander MA, Hricik DE: Optimizing end-stage renal disease therapy for the patient with diabetes mellitus. Sem Nephrol 17:331–345, 1997, with permission.)

10. What is the mean life expectancy of diabetics on dialysis, and what are the major causes of death?

The life expectancy of diabetics with end-stage renal disease depends on age and comorbid conditions. In general, however, the mean life expectancy on hemodialysis is approximately 2–3 years. The leading cause of death is cardiovascular disease, which reflects the increased incidence of both macrovascular and microvascular disease in the setting of diabetes. Infection or sepsis is the second most common cause of death. Mortality is similar in diabetics on peritoneal dialysis, although cardiovascular disease and infection are roughly equal as the most common cause of death.

BIBLIOGRAPHY

1. Bloembergen WE, Port FP, Mauger EA, Wolfe RA: A comparison of mortality between patients treated with hemodialysis and peritoneal dialysis. J Am Soc Nephrol 6:177–183, 1995.
2. Diabetes Control and Complications Trial Research Group: The effect of intensive treatment of diabetes on the development and progression of long-term complications in insulin-dependent diabetes mellitus. N Engl J Med 329:977–986, 1993.
3. EUCLID Study Group: Randomized placebo-controlled trial of lisinopril in normotensive patients with insulin-dependent diabetes and normoalbuminuria or microalbuminuria. Lancet 349:1787–1792, 1997.
4. Fenton SSA, Schaubel DE, Desmeules M, et al: Hemodialysis versus peritoneal dialysis: A comparison of adjusted mortality rates. Am J Kidney Dis 30:334–344, 1997.
5. Friedlander MA, Hricik DE: Optimizing end-stage renal disease therapy for the patient with diabetes mellitus. Sem Nephrol 17:331–345, 1997.
6. Klahr S, Levey AS, Beck GJ, et al: The effects of dietary protein restriction and blood-pressure control on the progression of chronic renal disease. Modification of Diet in Renal Disease Study Group. N Engl J Med 330:877–884, 1994.
7. Kloke HJ, Branten AJ, Huysmans FT, Wetzels JF: Antihypertensive treatment of patients with proteinuric renal diseases: Risks or benefits of calcium channel blockers? Kidney Int 53:1559–1573, 1998.
8. Lewis EJ, Hunsicker LG, Bain RP, Rohde RD: The effect of angiotensin-converting enzyme inhibition on diabetic nephropathy. N Engl J Med 329:1456–1462, 1993.
9. Maki DD, Ma JZ, Louis TA, Kasiske BL: Long-term effects of antihypertensive agents on proteinuria and renal function. Arch Intern Med 155:1073–1080, 1995.
10. Mogensen CE, Christensen CK: Predicting diabetic nephropathy in insulin-dependent patients. N Engl J Med 311:89–93, 1984.
11. Ravid M, Brosh D, Levi Z, et al: Use of enalapril to attenuate decline in renal function in normotensive, normoalbuminuric patients with type 2 diabetes mellitus. A randomized, controlled trial. Ann Intern Med 128:982–988, 1998.
12. Reichard P, Nilsson B-Y, Rosenqvist U: The effect of long-term intensified insulin treatment on the development of microvascular complications of diabetes mellitus. N Engl J Med 329:204–309, 1993.
13. Zatz R, Dunn BR, Meyer TW, et al: Prevention of diabetic glomerulopathy by pharmacologic amelioration of glomerular capillary hypertension. J Clin Invest 77:1925–1930, 1986.

27. LUPUS NEPHRITIS

Marcia R. *Silver,* M.D.

1. What proportion of patients with systemic lupus erythematosus (SLE) develop lupus nephritis?

The kidney is the most common site of major organ system involvement in SLE. About 40% of patients with SLE develop lupus nephritis. Nearly 100% of those with major organ system involvement, such as lupus cerebritis, pneumonitis, or vasculitis, will have lupus renal disease as well.

2. How are the lesions of lupus nephritis classified?

Based on pathologic findings, the World Health Organization (WHO) developed the following classification:

World Health Organization Classification of Lupus Nephritis Lesions

CLASS	DESCRIPTION
I	Normal glomeruli
II	Pure mesangial alterations (mesangial widening with or without hypercellularity)
III	Focal segmental glomerulonephritis (associated with mild or moderate mesangial alterations)
IV	Diffuse glomerulonephritis (severe mesangial, endocapillary, or mesangiocapillary proliferation and/or extensive subendothelial deposits with mesangial deposits present invariably and subepithelial deposits present often)
V	Diffuse membranous glomerulonephritis (but if associated with proliferative lesions, go to class IV)
VI	Advanced sclerosing glomerulonephritis

3. Do nonglomerular renal diseases occur in patients with SLE?

The possibility that a patient with SLE may develop renal disease that is not included in the WHO classification of lupus nephritis must always be considered. The frequent use of nonsteroidal anti-inflammatory drugs for management of arthritis may result in renal impairment. Pure interstitial nephritis may occur. A renal thrombotic microangiopathy has been described in the presence of antiphospholipid antibodies and in the absence of other findings of renal vasculitis or antibody-mediated glomerulonephritis.

4. What are the usual presenting signs and symptoms of lupus nephritis?

Many patients are asymptomatic. Early detection (highly desirable!) may be accomplished through regular monitoring of the urinalysis in patients with SLE, looking for hematuria, casts, or proteinuria. Hypertension also may be a clue to the presence of renal disease. Edema may occur in patients with nephrotic-range proteinuria. Uremic signs and symptoms are very late findings—the renal disease is rarely reversible at this stage.

5. What is the prognosis of patients with lupus nephritis?

Overall survival for patients with SLE is about 70% at 10 years. Infection and renal failure are the most common causes of death. Outcomes are worse in blacks, Hispanics, Asians, poor people, and patients with evidence of disease affecting major organs such as the brain, kidneys, lungs, or heart.

Outcomes for patients with lupus nephritis appear to have improved substantially over the past 4 decades. In the 1950s and 1960s, the 5-year survival rate for all patients with lupus was about 45%, and the rate for patients with class IV lupus nephritis was about 20%. Since the early 1990s, 5-year survival for all patients with lupus nephritis has increased to approximately 80%. Some of these dramatic improvements, based on historical controls, may be the result of more aggressive and judicious use of immunosuppressive agents to treat lupus, but they also may be due to increased sensitivity and availability of serologic tests for the disease leading to earlier diagnosis and diagnosis of patients with milder disease. Also, patients who develop end-stage renal disease (ESRD) can now be managed successfully with dialysis and transplantation. Of great interest is the repeated observation that extrarenal manifestations of lupus tend to become quiescent when lupus patients develop ESRD. This improvement is usually sustained in patients who receive a kidney transplant. It is possible that the immunosuppressive effects of ESRD have a salutary impact on those extrarenal manifestations and that, after transplantation, the immunosuppressive agents required to prevent rejection of the transplanted organ may act similarly.

6. How is the diagnosis of lupus nephritis made? When should a renal biopsy be performed?
   The presence of an abnormal urinalysis, hypertension, elevated serum creatinine concentration, edema, or other elements of the nephrotic syndrome (see Chapter 17, Nephrotic Syndrome) should trigger a thorough evaluation for the presence of lupus nephritis or other forms of kidney disease. The indications for renal biopsy in patients with SLE are controversial. Some experts think that patients with an established diagnosis of SLE who develop typical findings consistent with lupus nephritis can be treated empirically, avoiding the risks and expense of renal biopsy. Renal biopsy would still be indicated for those who fail to respond to initial treatment or for those with an atypical clinical presentation. Others opine that every patient suspected of having lupus nephritis requires a biopsy to determine the nature of the renal pathology. The benefits of this approach include (1) assuring that one is not dealing with allergic interstitial nephritis or pure antiphospholipid syndrome, disorders that are associated with different diagnostic and management implications; (2) promptly determining the pathologic classification of the lupus nephritis, so that the best therapy can be selected and instituted early in the course of the disease (see question 7); and (3) allowing assessment of the degree of chronicity (scarring and other irreversible changes) on the biopsy, findings that may serve to temper the aggressive use of immunosuppressive agents. Also, up to 40% of patients with lupus nephritis may show changes in renal pathology on repeat biopsy, especially in the setting of changing clinical findings (e.g., new red cell casts, new hypertension, or new nephrotic syndrome).

7. Does the classification scheme help the nephrologist make management decisions?
   Yes. Patients with class II (pure mesangial) and class V (pure membranous) lesions appear to have a better prognosis than those with proliferative lesions (classes III and IV). Treatment with potentially toxic immunosuppressive regimens is usually reserved for patients with more aggressive lesions.

8. How should lupus nephritis be managed?
   Vigorous management of hypertension delays the progression of all forms of renal disease. The goal should be a blood pressure of 120/80 or less in most patients. Measures to decrease proteinuria (such as use of angiotensin-converting enzyme [ACE] inhibitors) probably are also beneficial in delaying the progression of any renal disease, including all forms of lupus nephritis. Although clinical data are somewhat limited, many nephrologists also believe that vigorous management of persistent hyperlipidemia may have a beneficial effect on renal and cardiovascular outcomes.
   The data supporting the widely accepted notion that steroids are of significant benefit in lupus would not likely meet today's standards for evidence-based medicine. Nevertheless, the limited randomized trials of management of lupus nephritis include only a few hundred patients worldwide and generally compare some form of aggressive management with steroids with "steroid-sparing" alternative immunosuppressive agents such as cyclophosphamide or azathioprine. Evidence from a number of such trials suggests that the prognosis of patients with proliferative lupus nephritis (class III or IV) is substantially improved by treatment with cyclophosphamide

and reduced doses of prednisone as compared with prednisone alone. Pulse intravenous cyclophosphamide is about as effective as daily oral cyclophosphamide but has become popular because of reduced gonadal and bladder toxicities. The data on azathioprine are mixed, with some evidence suggesting that it may be as effective as cyclophosphamide, perhaps with less long-term toxicity. In particular, it seems not to interfere with fertility or pregnancy, often an important issue for the many young women suffering with this disease. Mycophenolate mofetil is a newer agent that may be of benefit in patients who are unresponsive to cyclophosphamide, although human data thus far have been limited to case reports. Pulse methylprednisolone may be less toxic and equally efficacious compared to prolonged therapy with high doses of oral steroids in managing acute exacerbations of lupus renal disease. A randomized, controlled trial of plasmapheresis in severe lupus nephritis showed no benefit.

BIBLIOGRAPHY

1. Austin HA III, Klippel JH, Balow JE, et al: Therapy of lupus nephritis: Controlled trial of prednisone and cytotoxic drugs. N Engl J Med 314;614–619, 1986.
2. Balow JE, Boumpas DT, Fessler BJ, Austin HA III: Management of lupus nephritis. Kidney Int 49:S88–S92, 1996.
3. Berden JHM: Lupus nephritis. Kidney Int 52:538–558, 1997.
4. Cameron JS: The long-term outcome of glomerular diseases. In Schrier RW, Gottschalk CW (eds): Diseases of the Kidney, 6th ed. Boston, Little, Brown, 1997, pp 1919–1982.
5. Donadio JV Jr, Glassock RJ: Immunosuppressive drug therapy in lupus nephritis. Am J Kidney Dis 21:239–250, 1993.
6. Glicklich D, Acharya A: Mycophenolate mofetil therapy for lupus nephritis refractory to intravenous cyclophosphamide. Am J Kidney Dis 32:318–322, 1998.
7. Hricik DE, Chung-Park M, Sedor JR: Glomerulonephritis. N Engl J Med 339:888–899, 1998.
8. Levey AS, Lan SMPII, Corwin III, et al: Progression and remission of renal disease in the lupus nephritis collaborative study. Results of treatment with prednisone and short-term oral cyclophosphamide. Ann Intern Med 116:114–123, 1992.
9. Lewis EJ, Hunsicker LG, Lan SP, et al: A controlled trial of plasmapheresis therapy in severe lupus nephritis. N Engl J Med 326:1373–1379, 1992.
10. Sloan RP, Schwartz MM, Korbet SM, et al: Long-term outcome in systemic lupus erythematosus membranous glomerulonephritis. Lupus Nephritis Collaborative Study Group. J Am Soc Nephrol 7:299–305, 1996.

28. POSTINFECTIOUS GLOMERULONEPHRITIS

Ira D. Davis, M.D.

1. What common infections are associated with postinfectious glomerulonephritis?

Acute pharyngitis, upper respiratory infections, and skin infections are the most frequent infections associated with postinfectious glomerulonephritis. This entity also may be seen following infection of ventriculoatrial or ventriculoperitoneal shunts or in association with acute and subacute bacterial endocarditis.

2. What is the most common cause of acute postinfectious glomerulonephritis?

Specific nephritogenic strains of group A beta-hemolytic streptococci are the most common organisms associated with acute glomerulonephritis. These strains differ from the strains associated with rheumatic fever.

3. What other infectious agents are associated with acute postinfectious glomerulonephritis?

Other infectious organisms that cause acute postinfectious glomerulonephritis include a variety of bacteria and viruses. *Staphylococcus aureus* is often seen in cases of shunt infections, while *Staphylococcus epidermis* and various streptococcal species are frequently seen in glomerulonephritis associated with subacute bacterial endocarditis. Viruses associated with acute postinfectious glomerulonephritis include enteric cytopathic human orphan (ECHO) viruses, human immunodeficiency virus (HIV), adenovirus, and influenza A. Acute glomerulonephritis also has been reported following Rocky Mountain spotted fever, cat-scratch fever, trichinosis, and toxoplasmosis.

4. What is the pathogenesis of acute poststreptococcal glomerulonephritis?

Acute poststreptococcal glomerulonephritis is an immune-complex–mediated glomerular disease, although the precise nature of the antigen-antibody complex remains undefined. Unique streptococcal antigens associated with nephritogenic strains of streptococci have been found in immune complexes in the glomerulus. Glomerular immune deposits result from deposition of circulating immune complexes or binding of immunoglobulin to streptococcal antigens "planted" in glomerular structures, leading to in situ development of immune complexes.

5. What are the typical pathologic changes of the glomerulus in acute postinfectious glomerulonephritis?

The glomeruli are often enlarged, swollen, and bloodless with an intense diffuse cellular infiltrate of polymorphonuclear leukocytes, eosinophils, and monocytes. Capillary lumina are occluded by proliferating mesangial and endothelial cells and infiltrating leukocytes, resulting in a diffuse proliferative glomerulonephritis on light microscopy. The typical immunofluorescence finding is fine granular deposition of IgG and C3 in capillary walls, sometimes referred to as a "starry sky" pattern. Predominant immunoglobulin or C3 deposition in the axial or stalk region of the glomerulus is another immunofluorescent pattern. Characteristic findings on electron microscopy include "hump" electron-dense deposits on the epithelial side of the basement membrane (see Figure, top of next page) and less discrete deposits in the mesangium and endothelial side of the basement membrane.

6. When do symptoms of renal disease occur in relation to the timing of the infection in acute postinfectious glomerulonephritis?

A latency period of a few days to 3 weeks is typically seen in cases of acute glomerulonephritis following a streptococcal infection. The latency periods following pharyngitis and impetigo infections are typically 10 and 21 days, respectively.

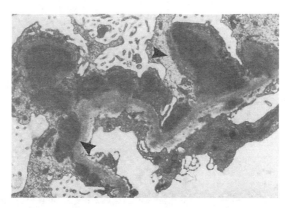

Large, nodular, subepithelial immune deposits (*arrows*), referred to as "humps," in an electron micrograph taken from a patient with poststreptococcal glomerulonephritis. (From Hricik DE, Chung-Park M, Sedor JR: Glomerulonephritis. N Engl J Med 339:888–899, 1998, with permission.)

7. What are the most common presenting complaints of patients with acute postinfectious glomerulonephritis?

These patients commonly present with the abrupt onset of edema and cola-colored (or tea-colored) urine. Other symptoms may include malaise, lethargy, anorexia, fever, abdominal pain, weakness, and headache.

8. How common is hypertension in acute postinfectious glomerulonephritis?

Hypertension occurs in over 75% of children requiring hospitalization for acute glomerulonephritis. Approximately 5% of hospitalized patients develop severe hypertension that may be associated with encephalopathy (see Chapter 59, Hypertensive Emergencies). Hypertension usually resolves within 3–4 weeks of disease onset.

9. What is the etiology of hypertension in acute postinfectious glomerulonephritis?

The primary cause is expansion of the extracellular fluid compartment due to an increased avidity of the kidney for sodium and water. Interestingly, the renin-angiotensin-aldosterone axis appears to be suppressed. Because some patients are resistant to diuretics, other unknown factors also contribute to the development of hypertension in this disorder.

10. How often is the complement component C3 depressed in patients with acute postinfectious glomerulonephritis?

C3 levels and total hemolytic complement activity (CH_{50}) are depressed in 90% of patients and usually return to normal within 8 weeks. By contrast, patients with membranoproliferative glomerulonephritis or lupus nephritis exhibit depressed levels of C3 (often associated with a low C4) that persist for more than 8 weeks following the initial presentation with acute glomerulonephritis.

11. How often are the streptozyme test and antistreptolysin O (ASO) titers elevated in patients with acute poststreptococcal glomerulonephritis?

Streptozyme test positivity and elevated ASO titers occur in 90% and 70% of patients, respectively. However, early treatment of the infection may limit the ability of the patient to mount a serologic response to the streptococcal infection.

12. Does treatment of the infection clear the glomerulonephritis?

No. Once the immunologic response to the offending organism occurs, treatment with antibiotics does not limit pathologic injury to the kidney.

13. Does acute postinfectious glomerulonephritis recur?

Long-term studies suggest that recurrent active disease, manifested primarily by gross hematuria, occurs in approximately 10% of patients. This usually occurs within 1 year of the initial episode of acute glomerulonephritis.

14. What other renal diseases must be considered in the differential diagnosis of acute postinfectious glomerulonephritis?

Acute exacerbation of a chronic glomerulonephritis
Henoch-Schönlein purpura
IgA nephropathy
Thin basement membrane disease
Hereditary nephritis (Alport's syndrome)

15. What is the long-term prognosis of patients with acute postinfectious glomerulonephritis?

The long-term prognosis in children is very good, with complete recovery in most cases. However, chronic renal disease may occur in as many as 1–2% of patients. This favorable prognosis contrasts with reports of postinfectious glomerulonephritis in the adult population in which over 50% of patients may have evidence of persisting renal disease.

BIBLIOGRAPHY

1. Baldwin DS, Melvin C, Gluck MC, et al: The long-term course of poststreptococcal glomerulonephritis. Ann Intern Med 80:342–358, 1974.
2. Brouhard BH, Travis LB: Acute postinfectious glomerulonephritis. In Edelmann CM, Bernstein J, Meadow SR, et al (eds): Pediatric Kidney Disease. Boston, Little, Brown, 1992, pp 1199–1221.
3. Cole BR, Salinas-Madrigal L: Acute proliferative glomerulonephritis and crescentic glomerulonephritis. In Holliday MA, Barratt TM, Avner ED (eds): Pediatric Nephrology, 3rd ed. Baltimore, Williams & Wilkins, 1994, pp 697–718.
4. Dodge WF, Spargo BH, Travis LB, et al: Poststreptococcal glomerulonephritis. A prospective study in children. N Engl J Med 286:273–278, 1972.
5. Hricik DE, Chung-Park M, Sedor JR: Glomerulonephritis. N Engl J Med 339:888–899, 1998.
6. Perlman LV, Herdman RC, Kleinman H, et al: Poststreptococcal glomerulonephritis. A ten-year follow-up of an epidemic. JAMA 194:175–182, 1965.
7. Potter EV, Lipschultz SA, Abidh S, et al: Twelve to seventeen-year follow-up of patients with poststreptococcal acute glomerulonephritis in Trinidad. N Engl J Med 307:725–729, 1982.
8. Rodriguez-Iturbe B, Garcia R: Acute glomerulonephritis. In Holliday MA, Barrett TM, Vernier RL (eds): Pediatric Nephrology, 2nd ed. Baltimore, Williams & Wilkins, 1987, pp 407–419.

29. HEPATITIS-ASSOCIATED GLOMERULONEPHRITIS

Ashwini R. Sehgal, M.D.

1. What types of hepatitis are associated with glomerulonephritis?
Chronic infection with hepatitis B or C is associated with glomerulonephritis. Hepatitis A does not result in chronic infection and is not associated with glomerulonephritis.

2. How does hepatitis viral infection cause glomerulonephritis?
Immune complexes containing hepatitis B or C antigens, either deposited from the circulation or formed in situ, are frequently found in affected glomeruli. These may elicit an inflammatory response involving complement activation and infiltration by monocytes and neutrophils. These leukocytes can release oxidants and proteases that damage both endogenous glomerular cells and the glomerular basement membrane resulting in altered permeability.

3. Name the types of glomerular disease associated with hepatitis B and C.

	TYPE OF GLOMERULAR DISEASE	
	MOST COMMON	LESS COMMON
Hepatitis B	Membranous nephropathy	Polyarteritis nodosa Membranoproliferative glomerulonephritis
Hepatitis C	Essential mixed cryoglobulinemia	Membranoproliferative glomerulonephritis Membranous nephropathy

4. How common is hepatitis-associated glomerulonephritis?
In the United States, the prevalence of renal disease associated with hepatitis B is relatively low. By contrast, hepatitis C infection is found in 80–90% of patients with essential mixed cryoglobulinemia, in 10–20% of patients with membranoproliferative glomerulonephritis, and in less than 10% of patients with membranous nephropathy.

5. How are hepatitis B and C acquired?
In developed countries, hepatitis B is acquired from sexual activity, intravenous drug use, or occupational exposure (e.g., needle sticks). Hepatitis C is usually acquired from intravenous drug use or blood transfusions. In about 25% of cases, the mode of transmission of hepatitis B or C is unclear.

6. What is the natural history of hepatitis B and C infection?
While acute hepatitis B infection tends to be symptomatic, less than 5% of patients go on to develop chronic hepatitis. By contrast, acute hepatitis C infection is generally mild and asymptomatic. However, persistent viremia is typical, and chronic hepatitis C infection eventually develops in two thirds of patients.

7. How long does it take for hepatitis-associated glomerulonephritis to develop?
Hepatitis B–associated glomerulonephritis develops several months to several years after acute hepatitis B infection. Hepatitis C–associated glomerulonephritis generally develops more than 10 years after acute hepatitis C infection.

8. What is the liver function of patients with hepatitis-associated glomerulonephritis?
Most patients with hepatitis B–associated glomerulonephritis have elevated transaminase levels. However, transaminase levels may also be normal, and a history of acute hepatitis may be absent in these patients.

9. How is hepatitis-associated glomerulonephritis diagnosed?
• Serologic evidence of hepatitis antigens or antibodies
• Kidney biopsy findings of an immune complex glomerulonephritis with glomerular deposits containing hepatitis antigens

10. Describe the pathologic findings in hepatitis-associated glomerulonephritis.
The glomerular lesions in hepatitis C–associated cryoglobulinemia are diverse, but membranoproliferative glomerulonephritis accounts for 80% of cases. Hepatitis-associated membranoproliferative glomerulonephritis, with or without cryoglobulinemia, is histologically similar to idiopathic type I membranoproliferative glomerulonephritis (see Chapter 25, Membranoproliferative Glomerulonephritis). Light microscopy shows increased mesangial matrix and cellularity and basement membrane thickening; immunofluorescence shows immunoglobulin M (IgM), IgG, and C3 deposits in the mesangium and in capillary walls. Electron microscopy shows mesangial and subendothelial immune deposits. Hepatitis C–associated membranoproliferative glomerulonephritis differs from idiopathic membranoproliferative glomerulonephritis in that additional deposits with ultrastructural features characteristic of cryoglobulins sometimes fill the capillary lumen.
Hepatitis-associated membranous nephropathy is histologically similar to idiopathic membranous nephropathy (see Chapter 23, Membranous Glomerulopathy). Light microscopy shows normal cellularity with basement membrane thickening, immunofluorescence shows IgG and C3 deposits in capillary walls, and electron microscopy shows subepithelial immune deposits and effacement of podocyte foot processes. Hepatitis B–associated membranous nephropathy differs from idiopathic membranous nephropathy in that additional subendothelial or mesangial deposits are frequently present as well. Hepatitis B–associated polyarteritis nodosa results in necrotizing inflammation of medium-sized arteries and is similar to polyarteritis nodosa not associated with hepatitis (see Chapter 35, Renal Vasculitis).

11. What is the prognosis of hepatitis-associated glomerulonephritis?
Hepatitis B–associated membranous nephropathy generally resolves spontaneously in children but tends to be progressive in adults. Hepatitis C–associated glomerulonephritis is generally slowly progressive.

12. How is hepatitis-associated glomerulonephritis treated?
Optimal therapy for these disorders has yet to be defined. Antiviral therapy with interferon may be helpful, although relapses often occur once treatment is stopped. The use of immunosuppressive treatment is risky because steroid and cyclophosphamide use may result in increased viral replication that can accelerate progression of liver disease.

13. Can patients with hepatitis B or C receive a renal transplant?
Renal transplantation may be performed in patients with asymptomatic hepatitis B or hepatitis C infection. However, the presence of hepatitis B infection may adversely affect allograft survival. Furthermore, there is a risk of accelerated liver disease when patients with hepatitis B are treated with immunosuppressive drugs. Most transplant centers are willing to offer a kidney transplant to patients who are hepatitis B surface antigen–positive, so long as they have normal liver function tests and no serologic evidence for active viral replication (i.e., a positive hepatitis E antigen or high DNA titers). Experience with renal transplantation in patients with hepatitis C is limited. Some studies suggest that the risk of chronic liver disease after a kidney transplant is comparable to the risk in patients who remain on dialysis.

BIBLIOGRAPHY

1. D'Amico G: Renal involvement in hepatitis C infection: Cryoglobulinemic glomerulonephritis. Kidney Int 54:650–671, 1998.
2. Fishman JA, Rubin RH, Koziel MJ, Periera BJ: Hepatitis C virus and organ transplantation. Transplantation 62:147–154, 1996.
3. Gumber SC, Chopra S: Hepatitis C: A multifaceted disease. Ann Intern Med 123:615–620, 1995.
4. Johnson RJ, Couser WG: Hepatitis B infection and renal disease: Clinical, immunopathogenetic, and therapeutic considerations. Kidney Int 37:663–676, 1990.
5. Johnson RJ, Willson R, Yamabe H, et al: Renal manifestations of hepatitis C virus infection. Kidney Int 46:1255–1263, 1994.
6. Praditpornsilpa K, Eiam-Ong S, Sitprija V: Hepatitis virus and kidney. Singapore Med J 37:639–644, 1996.
7. Stehman-Breen C, Johnson RJ: Hepatitis C virus–associated glomerulonephritis. Adv Intern Med 43:79–97, 1998.
8. Willson RA: Extrahepatic manifestations of chronic viral hepatitis. Am J Gastroenterol 92:4–17, 1997.

30. HIV-ASSOCIATED RENAL DISORDERS

Hany S. Y. Anton, M.D.

1. What parenchymal renal diseases have been associated with human immunodeficiency virus (HIV) infection?
- Focal glomerulosclerosis (most common)
- Immune-complex mediated glomerulonephritis (sometimes with glomerular immunoglobulin A [IgA] deposits)
- Membranoproliferative glomerulonephritis (often associated with hepatitis C)
- Membranous glomerulopathy
- Acute tubular necrosis (associated with sepsis)
- Interstitial nephritis (due to drug allergies or cytomegalovirus [CMV] infection)
- Thrombotic thrombocytopenic purpura

2. How does the pathology of HIV-associated focal glomerulosclerosis differ from other causes?
Focal segmental glomerulosclerosis associated with HIV infection is usually the collapsing variant characterized by retraction of glomerular capillary walls leading to occlusion of capillary lumina (see Chapter 22, Focal Segmental Glomerulosclerosis). Although mesangial expansion can be seen in less advanced cases, cellular proliferation typically is absent. Patchy foci of mononuclear interstitial infiltrates are common, and often interstitial fibrosis is out of proportion to the extent of glomerular involvement. As in other forms of focal sclerosis, immunofluorescence microscopy typically reveals IgM and C3 in sclerotic segments of glomeruli. Overall, the light and immunofluorescence microscopy findings are quite similar to those observed in "heroin nephropathy," a form of focal glomerulosclerosis that occurred in intravenous drug users long before the discovery of HIV. On electron microscopy, however, HIV-associated focal glomerulosclerosis often can be differentiated from heroin nephropathy, idiopathic focal segmental glomerulosclerosis, and other secondary forms of focal glomerulosclerosis based on the finding of typical tubuloreticular inclusion bodies within glomerular and peritubular capillary endothelial cells.

3. What is the clinical presentation of patients with HIV nephropathy?
HIV-associated renal disease was first described in patients with advanced acquired immunodeficiency syndrome (AIDS). It is now known, however, that nephropathy can develop at any stage of HIV infection. In fact, in some reports, the onset of nephropathy has been most common in otherwise asymptomatic patients. Heavy proteinuria is the clinical hallmark, at least in patients with focal glomerulosclerosis. In many, but not all, cases development of nephrotic-range proteinuria is accompanied by rapid deterioration of renal function within 3–6 months. Hypertension and edema are less common in patients with HIV nephropathy than in patients with other forms of focal glomerulosclerosis. More than 80% of patients are either normotensive or frankly hypotensive at the time of presentation.

4. What are the risk factors for nephropathy in patients with HIV infection?
The incidence of HIV-associated focal glomerulosclerosis is clearly affected by race with a 12 to 1 predominance in blacks when compared to nonblacks. Recent data suggest that there is no predilection for intravenous drug abusers or homosexual patients. The IgA variant of HIV-associated glomerular disease is more common in white patients than in blacks.

5. What is the incidence of HIV nephropathy?
Autopsy studies suggest an incidence ranging between 3% and 10% in patients infected with HIV. There is wide geographic variation in the reported incidence, probably reflecting differences in the racial makeup of HIV-infected populations.

6. What are the most common causes of acute renal failure in patients infected with HIV?

In one large series, acute tubular necrosis (usually occurring in the setting of sepsis) accounted for 75% of cases of acute renal failure in HIV patients; obstructive uropathy accounted for 17% of cases.

7. What is the treatment for HIV nephropathy?

Controlled trials are lacking. However, in uncontrolled trials, a number of treatment modalities have been associated with a reduction in urine protein excretion, an improvement in renal function, or a decrease in the rate of decline in renal function. These treatments include:

Antiviral agents (e.g., zidovudine [AZT])
Corticosteroids
Cyclosporine (rare reports)
Angiotensin-converting enzyme (ACE) inhibitors

8. What is the experience with renal replacement therapy in patients with HIV nephropathy who progress to end-stage renal disease?

Both hemodialysis and peritoneal dialysis have been used to treat HIV patients with end-stage renal disease. Not surprisingly, the average time between onset of end-stage renal disease and death is far shorter in the HIV population than in other dialysis patients. Most transplant centers currently do not offer renal transplantation to patients infected with HIV, irrespective of the underlying cause of renal failure. However, the risks, benefits, and cost-effectiveness of transplanting such patients has not been fully explored.

9. What electrolyte abnormalities occur in patients infected with HIV?

A number of acid-base and electrolyte abnormalities have been reported in this patient population. In many cases, the abnormalities can be attributed to comorbid conditions (e.g., specific infections) or drug therapy. These abnormalities include:

- Hyponatremia (including syndrome of inappropriate secretion of antidiuretic hormone [SIADH] associated with pulmonary or intracranial disease)
- Hypernatremia (e.g., from drug-induced diabetes insipidus [foscarnet, amphotericin])
- Hypokalemia (e.g., from chronic diarrheal disorders or infections)
- Hyperkalemia (including drug effects [trimethoprim-sulfa, pentamidine])
- Hypocalcemia (including drug effects [foscarnet, pentamidine])
- Hypercalcemia (e.g., related to granulomatous infections or lymphoma)
- Hyperphosphatemia (e.g., in renal failure or secondary to foscarnet)
- Hyperuricemia (including drug effects [pyrazinamide, rifampin, didanosine {DDI}])

BIBLIOGRAPHY

1. D'Agati V, Appel GB: Renal pathology in human immunodeficiency virus infection. Semin Nephrol 18:406–421, 1998.
2. Dave MB, Shabih K, Blum S: Maintenance hemodialysis in patients with HIV-associated nephropathy. Clin Nephrol 50:367–374, 1998.
3. Humphreys MC: Human immunodeficiency virus-associated glomerulosclerosis. Kidney Int 48:311–320, 1995.
4. Kimmel PL, Bosch JP, Vassolotti JA: Treatment of human immunodeficiency (HIV)–associated nephropathy. Semin Nephrol 18:446–458, 1998.
5. Klotman PE: Early treatment with ACE inhibition may benefit HIV-associated nephropathy patients. Am J Kidney Dis 4:719–720, 1998.
6. Smith MC, Austen JL, Carey JT, et al: Prednisone improves renal function and proteinuria in human immunodeficiency virus-associated nephropathy. Am J Med 101:41–48, 1996.
7. Spital A: Should all human immunodeficiency virus-infected patients with end-stage renal disease be excluded from transplantation? Transplantation 65:1187–1191, 1998.

V. Other Parenchymal Renal Diseases

31. RENAL DYSPLASIA

Beth A. Vogt, M.D.

1. What is renal dysplasia?

Renal dysplasia is a congenital renal anomaly in which one or both kidneys develop abnormally in utero. A dysplastic kidney is composed of primitive ducts surrounded by sheaths of fibromuscular and undifferentiated cells, often with islands of cartilage. Renal dysplasia includes a spectrum of defects having certain features in common. Most dysplastic kidneys are associated with collecting system abnormalities that can produce unilateral, bilateral, or segmental urinary obstruction. Renal cystic changes also may be present.

2. How common is renal dysplasia?

The exact incidence of renal dysplasia is unknown. However, renal dysplasia accounts for 15–20% of children with chronic renal insufficiency and end-stage renal disease.

3. What causes renal dysplasia?

The exact cause of renal dysplasia is unknown. Current theories include:
• Mutations in renal developmental genes
• Altered interaction of the ureteric bud with extracellular matrix
• Abnormalities of renal growth factors
• Antenatal urinary tract obstruction

4. What other types of urinary tract developmental anomalies are associated with renal dysplasia?

Posterior urethral valves, prune-belly (Eagle-Barrett) syndrome, ureteropelvic junction obstruction, and ureterovesicular junction obstruction are all associated with renal dysplasia. The timing and severity of the obstruction in utero are believed to correlate with the severity of renal dysplasia.

5. What other conditions are associated with renal dysplasia?

Although most cases of renal dysplasia are sporadic, a minority are associated with other anomalies or congenital syndromes. Some examples include VACTERL (*v*ertebral, *a*nal, *c*ardiac, *t*racheal, *e*sophageal, *r*enal, and *l*imb) syndrome; branchio-oto-renal syndrome; CHARGE (*c*oloboma of the eye, *h*eart anomaly, choanal *a*tresia, *r*etardation, and *g*enital and *e*ar anomalies) syndrome; trisomies 13, 18, and 21; and Jeune's syndrome.

6. What is the clinical course of patients with renal dysplasia?

Although the function of dysplastic kidneys is quite variable, children with bilateral involvement generally develop progressive renal insufficiency during early childhood. Nephrogenic diabetes insipidus, salt wasting, and distal renal tubular acidosis are commonly seen in children with renal dysplasia. Hematuria, heavy proteinuria, and hypertension can occur but are unusual clinical features.

7. What is the multicystic dysplastic kidney (MCDK)?

An MCDK is the most severe form of renal dysplasia. Just as in a dysplastic kidney, the normal renal parenchyma is replaced by cartilage and disorganized epithelial structures in the form of primitive ducts. In addition, the MCDK is characterized by the presence of multiple cysts of varying size and atresia of the renal pelvis and ureter.

8. Is an MCDK functional?
In general, MCDK has no appreciable function. In fact, on a radionuclide renal scan, no tracer appears in the area of an MCDK.

9. How common is MCDK?
The incidence of unilateral MCDK has been estimated to be 1 out of 4300 live births. MCDK is the most common cause of a unilateral abdominal mass in the neonatal period.

10. What causes MCDK?
MCDK is believed to result from an abnormal induction of the metanephric blastema by the ureteric bud. Although some families appear to have a genetic predisposition to MCDK and other urologic abnormalities, MCDK usually occurs as a sporadic event.

11. What other conditions are associated with MCDK?
VACTERL syndrome
Branchio-oto-renal syndrome
Williams syndrome
Beckwith-Wiedemann syndrome
Trisomy 18

12. What other urinary tract malformations are associated with MCDK?
Other urinary tract abnormalities are present in about 50% of patients with MCDK. Contralateral vesicoureteral reflux is present in 10–30% of individuals with MCDK. Other associated abnormalities include ureteropelvic junction obstruction, renal agenesis, renal hypoplasia, renal dysplasia, horseshoe kidney, ureterocele, bladder wall diverticulum, ectopic kidney, crossed fused renal ectopia, patent urachus, and posterior urethral valves.

13. How are MCDKs discovered?
Prior to the advent of fetal ultrasonography, the most common presentation of MCDK was discovery of an abdominal mass in a healthy newborn infant. Currently, most MCDKs are detected by antenatal ultrasonography and may be detected as early as the second trimester.

14. What other conditions mimic MCDK?
A severe ureteropelvic junction obstruction may be difficult to distinguish from MCDK.

15. What is the natural history of bilateral MCDK?
Bilateral MCDK usually results in stillbirth or death shortly after birth due to the consequences of pulmonary hypoplasia and renal failure.

16. What is the natural history of a unilateral MCDK?
The majority of unilateral MCDKs undergo spontaneous involution, a process that may begin even before birth. The contralateral kidney, if unaffected by other urologic malformations, grows larger than expected due to compensatory hypertrophy.

17. Are there any complications related to unilateral MCDK?
Hypertension has been reported in less than 2% of patients with MCDK and, in several cases, has been cured by surgical removal of the MCDK. In the past 20 years, there have been fewer than 10 reports of renal malignancy in patients with MCDK including Wilms' tumor, embryonal cell tumor, and renal cell carcinoma.

18. How should an MCDK be managed?

When an MCDK is suspected, radionuclide renal scan should be performed to confirm the diagnosis. Voiding cystourethrogram should also be performed to rule out contralateral vesicoureteral reflux or bladder abnormality. Thereafter, optimal management of MCDK is controversial. Some clinicians advocate conservative management with surveillance renal ultrasounds and ongoing monitoring of blood pressure. In view of the small but real risk of hypertension and malignancy, others advocate surgical removal in infancy.

BIBLIOGRAPHY

1. Atiyeh B, Husmann D, Baum M: Contralateral renal abnormalities in multicystic-dysplastic kidney disease. J Pediatr 121:65–67, 1992.
2. Becker N, Avner ED: Congenital nephropathies and uropathies. Pediatr Clin North Am 42:1319–1341, 1995.
3. Holliday MA, Barratt TM, Avner ED: Pediatric Nephrology, 3rd ed. Baltimore, Williams & Wilkins, 1994.
4. Lennert T, Tetzner M, Er M: Multicystic renal dysplasia: Nephrectomy versus conservative management. Contr Nephrol 67:183–187, 1988.
5. Orejas G, Malaga S, Santos F: Multicystic dysplastic kidney: Absence of complications in patients treated conservatively. Child Nephrol Urol 12:35–39, 1992.
6. Robson WLM, Leung AKC, Thomason MA: Multicystic dysplasia of the kidney. Clin Pediatr 34:32–40, 1995.
7. Susskind MR, Kim KS, King LR: Hypertension and multicystic kidney. Urology 34:362–366, 1989.
8. Woolf AS: Clinical impact and biological basis of renal malformations. Semin Nephrol 15:361–372, 1995.

32. CYSTIC DISEASES OF THE KIDNEYS

Linda Zarif, M.D., and John R. Sedor, M.D.

1. What are the major types of renal cystic diseases?

Renal cystic disease can result from congenital diseases (e.g., renal cystic dysplasia and medullary sponge kidney), hereditary diseases with onset during fetal life (e.g., autosomal recessive medullary multicystic kidney disease), or hereditary diseases with onset during late childhood or early adulthood (e.g., autosomal dominant polycystic renal disease). Renal cysts also can be acquired later in life. Renal cysts are common and often are discovered as an incidental finding on a radiologic exam obtained for another purpose. Sometimes, renal cysts cause significant disease (see Table).

Renal Cystic Disease

Congenital (results from abnormal development and not necessarily heritable)	Multiple anomaly syndromes (usually from toxic insult in vitro) Cystic renal dysplasia Multilocular cysts Pyelocalyceal cysts

Hereditary	Fetal, infantile, or juvenile onset diseases
	    Autosomal recessive polycystic kidney disease
	    Autosomal dominant polycystic kidney disease
	    Medullary sponge kidney
	    Autosomal recessive medullary cystic disease (juvenile
	        nephronophthisis)
	    Hereditary and familial dysplasia
	    Tuberous sclerosis
	Adult onset
	    Autosomal dominant medullary cystic disease (medullary
	        cystic disease complex)
	    von Hippel-Lindau disease

Acquired cystic disease	Simple cysts: single or multiple Acquired cystic disease in patients with end-stage renal disease Renal lymphangiomatosis Hilar and perinephric pseudocysts

Adapted from Welling LW, Grantham JJ: Cystic renal diseases. In Brenner BM (ed): The Kidney, 5th ed. Philadelphia, W.B. Saunders, 1996, pp 1828–1863.

2. Which renal cystic diseases are the most common?

Simple cysts are the most common renal cystic abnormality and can be single or multiple. Simple cysts are rare in children but increase in incidence with age and are found in approximately 20% of 40-year-old individuals. Autosomal dominant polycystic kidney disease (ADPKD) is the most common heritable cystic kidney disease, occurring in about 1 in 400 to 1 in 1000 individuals.

3. What is the genetic basis of ADPKD?

Two different genes for this disease have been identified. ADPKD1 is located on the short arm of chromosome 16 and is responsible for 85–90% of the disease in the white population. ADPKD2 is located on chromosome 4. A third gene, which has not been cloned, may also cause a small number of cases.

4. Does ADPKD have extrarenal manifestations?

Yes. ADPKD is a systemic disease that has multiple chemical manifestations, including renal cysts of varying sizes, hepatic cysts, pancreatic cysts, colonic diverticula, intracranial aneurysms and thoracic and abdominal aortic aneurysms. In addition, hypertension prior to the development of end-stage renal disease is common. Certain manifestations of ADPKD tend to cluster in families. For example, some families of ADPKD patients have a high incidence of intracranial aneurysms while other families do not. Most patients express manifestations of the disease after the age of 30, with highest incidence of onset occurring between ages 45 and 65.

5. What are the clinical features of autosomal recessive polycystic renal disease (ARPKD)?

ARPKD is a rare disease with incidence ranging from 1 in 6000 to 1 in 40,000. A gene for this disease is located on chromosome 6. The disorder is often diagnosed by ultrasonography in utero, when large echogenic kidneys and oligohydramnios are demonstrated. Renal cysts in ARPKD patients result from tubular ectasia of the collecting ducts. Liver abnormalities are universally identified in ARPKD patients. Severe liver fibrosis is the most common associated hepatic disease, but cholangitis and portal hypertension with variceal bleeding also can occur. In 75% of cases, ARPKD results in death in the perinatal period. The remainder of ARPKD patients present with milder disease later in infancy or childhood or even in early adulthood and may have a much better prognosis.

6. Which imaging studies are used to diagnose cystic diseases of kidneys?

Renal ultrasound is a commonly used, noninvasive screening tool. Computed tomography (CT) with contrast is another highly sensitive study that provides more accurate information about involvement of the pancreas, liver, and spleen. A CT scan can detect cysts as small as 1.5 cm.

7. What are the most reliable diagnostic criteria to differentiate ADPKD from ARPKD?

Differentiating ARPKD and ADPKD in children may be difficult. The best distinguishing criterion is a history of PKD in families with definitive inheritance patterns. Despite the identification of several ADPKD genes, genetic testing is not common in clinical practice as yet. Another reliable method to differentiate between these two inherited renal cystic diseases is to perform renal ultrasonography on parents. A negative renal ultrasound in both parents strongly supports a diagnosis of ARPKD in the proband but cannot rule out a de novo ADPKD mutation. Hepatic fibrosis with biliary dysgenesis occurs in virtually 100% of ARPKD patients but is rare in ADPKD patients. Hepatic biopsy may be necessary to differentiate ARPKD and ADPKD in children and young adults with PKD and no family history. The ultrasonographic appearance of the kidney in the index patient may also be a useful tool to distinguish ARPKD and ADPKD. Discrete fluid-filled cysts scattered in renal cortex and medulla favor a diagnosis of ADPKD (see Figure, top of next page). In contrast, the typical sonogram in the ARPKD patient shows enlarged kidneys with increased cortical and medullary echogenicity. Discrete cysts are generally identified only in ARPKD patients with late onset of disease.

8. Is it possible to have a normal renal ultrasound and still have ADPKD?

Yes. Up to 24% of adult ADPKD patients younger than 30 years and up to 40% of children younger than 5 years with ADPKD may have a normal renal ultrasound.

9. What are the most common clinical complications of ADPKD?

1. **Pain:** Abdominal or flank pain commonly occurs and usually results from rupture of cysts, hemorrhage into cysts, passage of kidney stones, or infection of cysts.

2. **End-stage renal disease (ESRD):** About 50% of patients have progressed to ESRD by the age of 60 years. Male gender, African ethnicity, the presence of hypertension, early age of onset, and recurrent infections are predictors of a poor prognosis.

3. **Hematuria:** Either microscopic or macroscopic hematuria results from bleeding into a cyst or passage of a kidney stone.

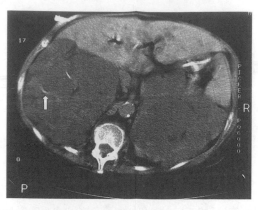

A CT scan of 70-year-old woman with ADPKD. The kidneys are massively enlarged and compress other intra-abdominal viscera. Cyst walls are indistinct because the cysts have accumulated fluid and increased in size; the arrow indicates a portion of a remaining cyst wall.

4. **Hypertension:** Elevated blood pressure occurs in 30% of children and in 60% of adults prior to development of ESRD. Over 80% of adult ADPKD patients with ESRD are hypertensive.

5. **Nephrolithiasis:** Kidney stones occur in up to 34% of ADPKD patients and most likely result from urinary stasis and decreased excretion of citrate, an inhibitor of stone formation. Stones in ADPKD patients are most commonly composed of uric acid or calcium oxalate. Renal parenchymal calcifications or nephrocalcinosis also may occur. Therapy for stones in these patients is similar to treatment of kidney stones in patients without PKD.

6. **Recurrent urinary tract infections:** Recurrent urinary tract infections are a major problem for ADPKD patients, especially women. Cysts can become infected, essentially resulting in abscesses that are difficult to treat because these cysts no longer freely communicate with tubular lumens. A prolonged course of parenteral antibiotics may be required to treat these infections (see question 11).

7. **Stroke:** Five percent to 10% of ADPKD patients have intracranial aneurysms, which tend to cluster in families. Rupture of aneurysms usually occurs after the age of 30 years and in aneurysms larger than 10 mm in diameter. Individuals from ADPKD families with a history of aneurysm rupture may be candidates for screening using cerebral magnetic resonance imaging (MRI) or magnetic resonance angiography (MRA).

10. What are the indications for nephrectomy in ADPKD?
Nephrectomy is performed as a last resort and may be indicated in ADPKD patients with the following complications: (1) severe recurrent urinary tract infections that have not been eradicated after an appropriate course of antibiotic therapy; (2) intractable pain; (3) renal neoplasm; (4) compression of inferior vena cava or other intra-abdominal organs; (5) persistent gross hematuria; and (6) nephrolithiasis that is not successfully treated by lithotripsy or percutaneous nephrostolithotomy.

11. Which antibiotics should be used for treatment of urinary tract infection in ADPKD patients?
Most cysts are no longer connected to the tubule from which they originated. In contrast to patients with simple renal parenchymal infection (pyelonephritis), ADPKD patients with cyst infections usually present as treatment failures after an appropriate course of antibiotic therapy. Antibiotics chosen to treat urinary tract infections in PKD patients should penetrate well into the cysts. Quinolones (e.g., ciprofloxacin and norfloxacin), trimethoprim, chloramphenicol, and clindamycin are lipid-soluble antibiotics with good penetration into cysts. Ampicillin and aminoglycosides penetrate less well but can be used if the bacterial susceptibilities necessitate use of these drugs.

12. Which ADPKD patients should be screened for intracranial aneurysms?

Most authorities agree that ADPKD patients who have a family history of aneurysmal bleeding or who present with appropriate symptoms (such as new headache, change in headache pattern, nerve paresis, paralysis, meningeal irritation, or strokes) should undergo evaluation for intracranial aneurysm. ADPKD patients engaging in activities such as contact sports, working as pilots, or undergoing major surgery, which could result in hemodynamic instability and severe hypertension, should also be considered for radiographic screening with MRI or MRA.

13. What are the clinical characteristics of tuberous sclerosis?

Tuberous sclerosis is a disease complex characterized by epilepsy, mental retardation, skin abnormalities including adenoma sebaceum and "ash leaf" spots, and hamartomas of multiple organs. Patients with tuberous sclerosis may or may not have renal cysts. Renal hamartomas (angiomyolipomas) can be identified in as many as 50% of patients and should be distinguished from renal cysts. Renal cysts and hamartomas commonly are found in the same patients. The presence of renal cysts in the absence of renal hamartomas is relatively uncommon, occurring in only 18% of patients. Two defective genes on chromosomes 9 and 16 have been identified. Tuberous sclerosis frequency is approximately 1 in 10,000.

14. What are the major characteristics of von Hippel-Lindau disease?

Up to 75% of patients have numerous, irregularly distributed renal cysts. Other clinical features of this disorder include retinal angiomas, cerebellar and spinal hemangioblastomas, pancreatic cysts, renal cell carcinomas, and pheochromocytomas. The disease is inherited by autosomal dominant transmission, and the defective gene responsible for von Hippel-Lindau disease is on the short arm of chromosome 3. Its onset usually is in the third or fourth decade.

15. What are distinguishing radiographic characteristics of simple cysts?

Most simple cysts are found on radiographic exams of the urinary tract and abdomen that are obtained for other indications. They appear on ultrasound as smooth-walled, fluid-filled structures without internal debris. Simple cysts are acquired and increase in incidence with age. Although usually single and unilateral, simple cysts can be multiple and bilateral. Suggested CT criteria to differentiate a simple cyst from a more serious lesion include a homogenous attenuation value near water density, lack of enhancement after injection with radiocontrast, no measurable wall thickness, and a smooth interface with normal kidney parenchyma. In the absence of fever, leukocytosis, hematuria, or pain, no further evaluation of simple cysts is indicated.

16. What is nephronophthisis-medullary cystic kidney disease complex?

This hereditary disease has several variants that invariably progress to ESRD. The most common variants are familial juvenile nephronophthisis, an autosomal recessive disease that causes ESRD in affected individuals by age 20 years, and medullary cystic kidney disease, an autosomal dominant disease that affects young adults between the ages of 20 and 50 years. Both variants are characterized by multiple renal cysts arising from distal and collecting tubules located primarily at the corticomedullary junction and in the medulla. The cysts are characteristically small (approximately 2 cm) and contain fluid. However, almost 25% of patients will have no grossly identifiable cysts due to the small size of these cysts. Renal biopsy demonstrates tubular atrophy, cysts lined by a single epithelial layer, and nonspecific glomerular hyalinosis. The clinical manifestations of the disease reflect dysfunction of affected nephron segments, predominantly reduced concentrating ability, polyuria, polydipsia, hypovolemia, and hyponatremia early in the course of the disease. Subsequently, glomerular filtration declines as the glomerular hyalinosis develops and progresses. The best imaging modality for diagnosis is thin-section CT scan of kidneys.

17. How does medullary sponge kidney differ from other cystic diseases?

Medullary sponge kidney is a benign disease that results from a congenital anomaly. It is characterized by small and large cysts, which are limited to medulla and do not involve the cortex. Many patients are asymptomatic, but some individuals present with kidney stones, recurrent urinary tract infections, and hematuria. The diagnosis can be made only by intravenous pyelography. It has an excellent prognosis in most patients.

18. What is acquired cystic kidney disease (ACKD)?
ACKD is an acquired disorder, characterized by the development of multiple renal cysts in patients with progressive, noncystic renal disease. A minimum of five cysts is required for diagnosis. CT scan is more sensitive than ultrasound in establishing this diagnosis. ACKD occurs in up to 40% of patients who have been on hemodialysis for 3 years and in 80–90% of patients on dialysis for 5–10 years. Patients with significant renal failure, who have not yet started on dialysis, may also have ACKD.

19. Are renal tumors more common in patients with ESRD than in patients with ACKD?
Yes. The development of renal cell neoplasms, ranging from adenomas to renal cell carcinomas, is the most serious complication of ACKD. Patients with ACKD have a fiftyfold increased risk of renal carcinoma compared to the general population. ACKD-associated renal cell carcinoma predominates in males, is frequently bilateral (9%) and multicentric (50%), and often occurs in ESRD patients at an age younger than that of patients with renal cell carcinoma but without renal failure.

20. How are tumors in ACKD patients managed?
Tumors larger than 3 cm are treated by nephrectomy. Management of tumors smaller than 3 cm in patients with back pain or hematuria is controversial, but many authorities recommend nephrectomy because these tumors often are renal cell carcinomas. Asymptomatic patients with tumors smaller than 3 cm can also be followed with serial CT examinations.

BIBLIOGRAPHY

1. Chapman AB, Rubinstein D, Hughes R, et al: Intracranial aneurysms in autosomal dominant polycystic kidney disease. N Engl J Med 327:916–920, 1992.
2. Elzouki AY, al-Suhaibani H, Mirza K, al-Sowailem AM: Thin-section computed tomography scans detect medullary cysts in patients believed to have juvenile nephronophthisis. Am J Kidney Dis 27:216–219, 1996.
3. Fick GM, Duley IT, Johnson AM, et al: The spectrum of autosomal dominant polycystic kidney disease in children. J Am Soc Nephrol 4:1654–1660, 1994.
4. Fick GM, Gabow PA: Hereditary and acquired cystic disease of the kidney. Kidney Int 46:951–964, 1994.
5. Gabow PA: Polycystic and acquired cystic disease. In Greenberg A (ed): Primer on Kidney Diseases, 2nd ed. San Diego, Academic Press, 1998, pp 313–318.
6. Griffin M, Torres VE, Kumar R: Cystic kidney diseases. Curr Opin Nephrol Hypertension 6:276–283, 1997.
7. Harris PC, Ward CJ, Peral B, Hughes J: Polycystic disease: Part 1: Identification and analysis of the primary defect. J Am Soc Nephrol 3:1871–1877, 1993.
8. Hildebrandt F, Jungers P, Grunfeld J-P: Medullary cystic and medullary sponge renal disorders. In Schrier RW, Gottschalk CW (eds): Diseases of the Kidney, 6th ed. Boston, Little, Brown, 1996, pp 499–520.
9. Truong LD, Krishnan B, Cao JT, et al: Renal neoplasm in acquired cystic kidney disease. Am J Kidney Dis 26:1–12, 1995.
10. Welling LW, Grantham JJ: Cystic renal diseases. In Brenner BM (ed): The Kidney, 5th ed. Philadelphia, W.B. Saunders, 1996, pp 1828–1863.
11. Wolf JS Jr: Evaluation and management of solid and cystic renal masses. J Urol 159:1120–1133, 1998.

33. OTHER HEREDITARY RENAL DISEASES

Beth A. Vogt, M.D.

1. What is Alport syndrome?

Alport syndrome is an inherited progressive nephropathy associated with persistent microscopic hematuria and sensorineural deafness. It is a generalized disorder of basement membranes resulting from mutations in basement membrane collagen.

2. How is Alport syndrome inherited?

Classic Alport syndrome (85% of cases) is inherited as an X-linked dominant trait. Other reported modes of inheritance include autosomal dominant (15% of cases) and autosomal recessive (very uncommon).

3. What is the genetic abnormality in Alport syndrome?

The classic or X-linked dominant form of Alport syndrome usually results from a point mutation in the collagen 4A5 gene on the X chromosome. The substitution of another amino acid for a glycine residue alters the structure of the collagen 4A5 chain, preventing normal incorporation of A3 and A4 chains into basement membranes. Mutations in the collagen 4A3 and A4 genes on chromosome 2 have been reported in autosomal recessive Alport syndrome.

4. How many children with asymptomatic microscopic hematuria will have Alport syndrome?

An estimated 10% of children with persistent microscopic hematuria evaluated by a nephrologist have Alport syndrome.

5. What are the clinical findings in males with Alport syndrome?

Microscopic hematuria is usually present by the age of 10 years in all affected males. Episodes of macroscopic hematuria may be seen in children with Alport syndrome but become less common after adolescence. Proteinuria and renal insufficiency can occur as early as the second decade of life but may not be present until well into adulthood. Bilateral, high-frequency, sensorineural hearing loss is seen in 80% of males with Alport syndrome and is usually detectable by audiologic screening by 6–7 years of age.

6. What are the clinical findings in females with Alport syndrome?

Females with Alport syndrome have a much milder course than males. Microscopic hematuria is present but may be intermittent in nature. Significant proteinuria and renal insufficiency are unusual and, if present, occur later in life. Approximately 20% of females with Alport syndrome have sensorineural hearing loss.

7. What other abnormalities may be associated with Alport syndrome?

Ocular abnormalities such as anterior lenticonus and perimacular flecks are identified in 15–40% of patients with Alport syndrome and are associated with early progression to end-stage renal disease. Esophageal leiomyomatosis and platelet abnormalities are occasionally seen.

8. What are the characteristic renal biopsy findings in Alport syndrome?

Light microscopy shows segmental or global glomerulosclerosis, interstitial fibrosis, and tubular atrophy. Immunofluorescence shows nonspecific deposition of immunoglobulin G (IgG), IgM, and C3. The pathognomonic renal biopsy finding in Alport syndrome, however, is diffuse thickening of the glomerular basement membrane with splitting of the lamina densa on electron microscopy. In young patients, both thickening and thinning of the glomerular basement membrane may be present, causing difficulty in distinguishing Alport syndrome from thin basement membrane nephropathy.

9. What treatment is available for Alport syndrome?

At present, there is no definitive therapy for Alport syndrome. Treatment remains supportive in nature and should focus on control of hypertension, management of the consequences of progressive renal insufficiency, and early identification of all affected family members. Renal transplantation is successful in most patients.

10. What is post-transplant antiglomerular basement membrane nephritis?

Post-transplant antiglomerular basement membrane nephritis is a condition that occurs in 5–7% of transplanted males with Alport syndrome. The cause of this condition is not well understood but may represent an immunologic response by the recipient to the presentation of a previously unrecognized glomerular basement membrane antigen in the donor kidney. The subset of patients at highest risk for this complication are males with significant deafness who develop end-stage renal disease before 30 years of age. Allograft failure occurs in more than 75% of patients with this phenomenon.

11. What is thin basement membrane nephropathy?

Thin basement membrane nephropathy, also known as benign familial hematuria or benign familial nephritis, is an inherited condition characterized by persistent microscopic hematuria with minimal or no proteinuria and normal renal function.

12. What is the inheritance pattern of thin basement membrane nephropathy?

Thin basement membrane nephropathy appears to follow an autosomal dominant pattern of inheritance. However, a 50% de novo mutation rate has been suggested. The genetic basis of thin basement membrane nephropathy is not clearly understood, although recent studies have identified a mutation in the collagen 4A4 gene. This finding suggests that thin basement membrane nephropathy and Alport syndrome may be related disorders.

13. What are renal biopsy findings in thin basement membrane nephropathy?

The pathognomonic renal biopsy finding in thin basement membrane nephropathy is irregular thinning of the glomerular basement membrane on electron microscopy, with attenuation of the lamina densa. Light and immunofluorescence microscopic analyses are usually normal.

14. How many children with asymptomatic microscopic hematuria have thin basement membrane nephropathy?

An estimated 30% of children with persistent asymptomatic microscopic hematuria have thin basement membrane nephropathy.

15. What is the natural history of thin basement membrane nephropathy?

In the majority of patients, thin basement membrane nephropathy is a benign condition in which progressive renal insufficiency does not occur. Rare patients, however, have been reported to develop significant proteinuria and chronic renal insufficiency.

16. What are juvenile nephronophthisis and medullary cystic disease?

Juvenile nephronophthisis and medullary cystic disease are distinct entities. Both disorders are characterized by inherited progressive tubulointerstitial nephropathy with eventual progression to end-stage kidney disease. In general, individuals with juvenile nephronophthisis present in childhood or adolescence while those with medullary cystic disease present in adulthood.

17. What is the genetic basis of juvenile nephronophthisis–medullary cystic disease (JN-MCD) complex?

Juvenile nephronophthisis is inherited in an autosomal recessive fashion. A gene for juvenile nephronophthisis (NPH-1) was recently mapped to the short arm of chromosome 2, but the function of this gene is unknown. Medullary cystic disease is inherited in an autosomal dominant fashion, but the genetic defect remains unknown.

18. What are the clinical findings in JN-MCD complex?

The symptoms of the JN-MCD complex include polyuria, polydipsia, weakness, pallor, short stature, failure to thrive, and insidious onset of chronic renal insufficiency. Hematuria, proteinuria, urinary tract infection, and hypertension are very uncommon.

19. What extrarenal findings have been associated with JN-MCD complex?

Twenty-five percent to 33% of patients with juvenile nephronophthisis have retinal degeneration, which is detectable by 10 years of age. This condition can be confirmed by electroretinogram and is associated with progressive loss of vision. In this subset of patients with juvenile nephronophthisis, other abnormalities including mental retardation, cerebellar ataxia, skeletal abnormalities, and congenital hepatic fibrosis may be seen. Extrarenal findings have not been reported in medullary cystic disease.

20. What are the ultrasound findings in JN-MCD complex?

The renal ultrasound of patients with JN-MCD complex shows small, hyperechoic kidneys with small medullary cysts, 1–2 mm in diameter, at the corticomedullary junction. These cysts correspond to the distal convoluted and medullary collecting tubules. Absence of medullary cysts does not rule out the diagnosis of JN-MCD complex.

21. What are the renal biopsy findings in JN-MCD complex?

Renal biopsy findings in advanced juvenile nephronophthisis or medullary cystic disease show tubulointerstitial atrophy, interstitial fibrosis, and thickening of the tubular basement membrane. Electron microscopy reveals thickening and loss of definition of the tubular basement membrane.

22. What is the treatment for JN-MCD complex?

There is currently no definitive treatment for juvenile nephronophthisis or medullary cystic disease. Treatment is focused on supportive therapy for progressive renal insufficiency, control of hypertension, and early identification of affected family members. Renal transplantation is successful, and recurrent disease in the renal allograft has not been reported.

BIBLIOGRAPHY

1. Antignac C, Arduy CH, Beckman JS, et al: A gene for familial juvenile nephronophthisis (recessive medullary cystic kidney disease) maps to chromosome 2p. Nature Genet 3:342–345, 1993.
2. Bodziak KA, Hammond WS, Molitoris BA: Inherited diseases of the glomerular basement membrane. Am J Kidney Dis 23:605–618, 1994.
3. Holliday MA, Barratt TM, Avner ED: Pediatric Nephrology, 3rd ed. Baltimore, Williams & Wilkins, 1994.
4. Kashtan CE, Michael AF: Alport syndrome. Kidney Int 50:1445–1463, 1996.
5. Lemmink HH, Nillesen WN, Mochizuki T, et al: Benign familial hematuria due to mutation of the type IV collagen a4 gene. J Clin Invest 98:114–118, 1996.
6. Nieuwhof CMG, De Heer F, De Leeuw P, et al: Thin GBM nephropathy, Premature glomerular obsolescence is associated with hypertension and late onset renal failure. Kidney Int 51:1596–1601, 1997.
7. Waldherr R, Lennert T, Weber H-P, et al: The nephronophthisis complex. Virchows Arch 394:235–254, 1982.

34. REFLUX NEPHROPATHY

Beth A. Vogt, M.D.

1. What is vesicoureteral reflux?

Vesicoureteral reflux is defined as retrograde propulsion of urine into the upper urinary tract during bladder contraction. Currently, vesicoureteral reflux is believed to result from ectopic insertion of the ureter into the bladder wall, which results in a shorter intravesicular ureter that acts as an incompetent valve during micturition.

2. How common is vesicoureteral reflux?

The exact incidence and prevalence of vesicoureteral reflux is not known. Population studies show a less than 2% incidence of reflux in healthy children without a history of urinary tract infection. However, at least one third of children evaluated for their first urinary tract infection have vesicoureteral reflux.

3. What is the difference between primary and secondary vesicoureteral reflux?

Primary vesicoureteral reflux refers to reflux that is not associated with other abnormalities of the urinary tract. Secondary vesicoureteral reflux refers to reflux associated with dysfunctional voiding syndromes (e.g., detrusor instability, detrusor-sphincter dyssynergia), obstructive uropathy (e.g., posterior urethral valves), or neurogenic bladder (e.g., myelodysplasia).

4. Is there a genetic basis for primary vesicoureteral reflux?

Although a gene for primary vesicoureteral reflux has not been described, a genetic predisposition clearly is present in some patients. For example, there is a 30% chance that a sibling of a child with vesicoureteral reflux will also have the disorder. Furthermore, 60–70% of offspring of individuals with a history of vesicoureteral reflux will also exhibit evidence of reflux.

5. How is vesicoureteral reflux discovered?

Vesicoureteral reflux is most commonly discovered by a cystogram performed as part of the evaluation of a patient with urinary tract infection. Screening identifies a smaller number of patients who have a family history of vesicoureteral reflux. Occasionally, reflux is discovered in patients evaluated by cystography for voiding dysfunction. Recently, an increasing number of cases have been discovered during evaluation of hydronephrosis detected in the antenatal period.

6. What tests can be performed to detect vesicoureteral reflux?

Both radiographic (using contrast dye and x-rays) and radionuclide (using a radioisotope and nuclear scanning) voiding cystourethrograms (VCUG) can detect the presence or absence of vesicoureteral reflux. Both tests involve catheterization of the bladder, a procedure that causes discomfort and anxiety, especially in children. To date, ultrasound-based tests to evaluate patients for vesicoureteral reflux have not been reliable.

7. What are the advantages and disadvantages of radiographic VCUG?

The radiographic VCUG offers the ability to accurately grade reflux (see question 10). In addition, the radiographic VCUG allows visualization of the urethra, an advantage particularly important for boys in whom the diagnosis of posterior urethral valves must be excluded. The primary disadvantage of this procedure is increased exposure to radiation as compared to the radionuclide VCUG.

8. What are the advantages and disadvantages of radionuclide VCUG?

The primary advantage to radionuclide VCUG is reduction in radiation exposure ($\frac{1}{100}$ of the radiation associated with the radiographic VCUG). In addition, radionuclide VCUG is more sensitive at detecting intermittent reflux. Disadvantages of this procedure include the inability to accurately grade reflux or to image the urethra.

9. Which VCUG should be used to evaluate vesicoureteral reflux?

In general, radiographic VCUG should be used for the first assessment of vesicoureteral reflux in an infant or child following urinary tract infection. This test allows careful grading of reflux and good visualization of the urethra in boys. The radionuclide VCUG is most useful as a follow-up study and as a screening test for siblings and children of patients with vesicoureteral reflux. Some clinicians advocate the use of the radionuclide VCUG for evaluation of first urinary tract infections in girls because visualization of the urethra is less important than in boys.

10. How is vesicoureteral reflux graded?

Vesicoureteral reflux is graded on a I–V scale (see Figure) according to the International Reflux Study Committee.

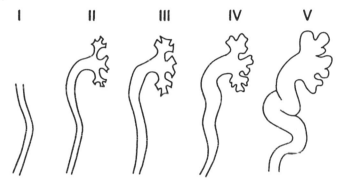

Classification of vesicoureteral reflux based on the degree of dilatation affecting the ureter and renal collecting system.

11. What is intrarenal reflux?

Intrarenal reflux refers to retrograde flow of urine from the renal pelvis into the papillary collecting ducts and renal tubules. Intrarenal reflux occurs primarily in specific renal papillae ("refluxing papillae") that are present in many, but not all, human kidneys and tend to be most common at the upper and lower poles. In patients with vesicoureteral reflux, cortical scarring tends to occur in association with areas of intrarenal reflux.

12. What are the complications of vesicoureteral reflux?

Vesicoureteral reflux can be associated with hypertension, renal scarring, and chronic renal failure. Hypertension is present in at least 10% of patients with reflux nephropathy and is most frequent in patients with bilateral, high-grade reflux and extensive renal scarring. At least 30% of patients have renal scarring at the time of diagnosis. The risk of progressive scarring is greatest in children younger than 5 years. Reflux nephropathy accounts for about 25% of cases of end-stage renal disease in children and for 5–15% of cases in adults.

13. What is the natural history of primary vesicoureteral reflux?

Primary vesicoureteral reflux tends to resolve over time as the intravesical segment of the ureter elongates with growth. The incidence of spontaneous resolution is greatest in patients with the lowest grades of reflux (80% of grade I; 60% of grade II, 50% of grade III). In contrast, rates of spontaneous resolution are quite low in patients with grade IV or grade V reflux. In general, 20% of patients with low-grade reflux will experience spontaneous resolution per year, although complete resolution may not occur until adolescence.

14. How should vesicoureteral reflux be managed?

In the past, surgical therapy was offered to most patients diagnosed with vesicoureteral reflux. With the recognition that spontaneous resolution commonly occurs, a more conservative approach is now recommended. All patients with reflux should be treated with daily prophylactic antibiotics to prevent urinary tract infection. Surveillance urine cultures should be obtained every 3–4 months to ensure sterility of the urine. VCUGs should be obtained every 12–18 months to assess for spontaneous resolution of reflux.

15. What is the current recommendation for antibiotic prophylaxis?

Most clinicians advocate the use of oral amoxicillin for infants younger than 2 months of age. For infants older than 2 months of age and children, low-dose trimethoprim-sulfamethoxazole, administered once daily, is recommended.

16. When should surgical ureteral reimplantation be considered?

Surgical ureteral reimplantation should be considered in children with high-grade (grade IV or V) reflux because of the lower probability of spontaneous resolution. Children with breakthrough urinary tract infections despite antibiotic prophylaxis may be considered for surgical treatment to reduce the risk of further renal scarring. Adolescents with unresolved reflux may also be considered for surgery because of the lower probability of spontaneous resolution.

17. Are there any new treatments for vesicoureteral reflux on the horizon?

Endoscopic injections of material (e.g., Teflon, collagen) into the ureterovesicular junction have been used to impede retrograde propulsion of urine. With further testing, such injections may emerge as a nonsurgical treatment for vesicoureteral reflux.

BIBLIOGRAPHY

1. Arant BS: Vesicoureteral reflux and renal injury. Am J Kidney Dis 5:491–511, 1991.
2. Becker GJ, Kincaid-Smith P: Reflux nephropathy: The glomerular lesion and progression of renal failure. Pediatr Nephrol 7:365–369, 1993.
3. Elder JS, Peters CA, Arant BS, et al: Pediatric Vesicoureteral Reflux Guidelines Panel summary report on the management of primary vesicoureteral reflux in children. J Urol 157:1846–1851, 1997.
4. Greenfield SP, Wan J: Vesicoureteral reflux: Practical aspects of evaluation and management. Pediatr Nephrol 10:789–794, 1996.
5. Homsy YL: Dysfunctional voiding syndromes and vesicoureteral reflux. Pediatr Nephrol 8:116–121, 1994.
6. Noe HN: The current status of screening for vesicoureteral reflux. Pediatr Nephrol 9:638–641, 1995.

35. RENAL VASCULITIS

Linda Zarif, M.D., Marcia R. Silver, M.D., and John R. Sedor, M.D.

1. List the major types of vasculitis.

The vasculitides are a group of diseases in which tissue ischemia and necrosis occur as a consequence of inflammation of blood vessels, either as a primary event or secondary to a systemic disease. Different vasculitides have a predilection for vessels of different sizes (see Table).

Vessel Size	Vasculitides
Large-vessel	Giant cell vasculitis: Granulomatous arteritis of aorta and major branches. Temporal artery involvement is common. Headache and polymyalgia rheumatica common in patients older than 50 years.
	Takayasu's arteritis: Involves aorta and major branches in patients younger than 50 years.
Medium-vessel	Polyarteritis nodosa: Necrotizing inflammation of medium-sized vessel. Affects renal arteries but not capillaries. No glomerulonephritis on biopsy. Often involves visceral vessels such as hepatic and mesenteric artery.
	Kawasaki syndrome: More common in young children. Associated with mucocutaneous lymph node syndrome.
Small-vessel	Pauci-immune vasculitis with antineutrophil cytoplasm antibody (ANCA)
	Wegener's granulomatosis: Necrotizing granulomatous inflammation of upper and lower respiratory tract. Sinusitis, nasal ulcers, and hemoptysis are common, often associated with glomerulonephritis.
	Churg-Strauss syndrome: Eosinophil-predominant inflammation of respiratory tract. Asthma and blood eosinophilia are common.
	Microscopic polyangiitis: Necrotizing glomerulonephritis, necrotizing arteritis of small- and medium-sized vessels are common.
	Immune complex vasculitis
	Henoch-Schönlein purpura: IgA deposits typically identified in small vessels of skin, gut, and glomeruli
	Essential cryoglobulinemic vasculitis: Cryoglobulin immune deposits of small vessels. Skin and glomeruli most commonly affected.
	Systemic lupus erythematosus
	Other vasculitides related to connective tissue disease

Adapted from Jennette JC, Falk RJ, Rassy K, et al: Nomenclature of systemic vasculitides: The proposal of an international consensus conference. Arthritis Rheum 37:187–192, 1994.

2. What are the distinctive features of the common vasculitides?

Clinical criteria based on the size of the vessel involved were defined at the Chapel Hill Consensus Conference on the Nomenclature of Systemic Vasculitis (see above table). Patients with large-vessel vasculitis usually present with signs and symptoms of tissue ischemia. In contrast, evidence for inflammation (purpura, hemoptysis, red cell casts, and hematuria) are more commonly identified in patients with small-vessel vasculitis.

3. How does primary vasculitis differ from secondary vasculitis?

Primary vasculitis comprises a distinct group of diseases in which the blood vessels are the primary site of injury. Vasculitis also may occur as a secondary response to infection or a multisystem autoimmune disease. Viral infections with hepatitis B and C (see Chapter 29, Hepatitis-Associated Glomerulonephritis), human immunodeficiency virus (see Chapter 30, HIV-Associated

Renal Disorders), Epstein-Barr virus, cytomegalovirus, and parvoviruses have been associated with vasculitides and cause medium- or small-vessel vasculitis. Streptococci and staphylococci infections also may cause secondary vasculitis. Infections with methicillin-resistant *Staphylococcus* (MRSA) are associated with vasculitic lesions of lower extremities. Elimination of infection as a cause of vasculitis is critical, because immunosuppressive therapy is the mainstay of treatment for primary forms of vasculitis and could be lethal in a patient with an underlying infection.

4. What is the usual clinical presentation of a patient with vasculitis?
Vasculitis should be considered in a patient who presents with dysfunction of multiple organ systems and with constitutional symptoms such as fever, fatigue, weakness, myalgias, and arthralgias. Various degrees of renal insufficiency are present if the renal parenchyma are involved. The presence of mononeuritis multiplex and palpable purpuric skin lesions are important clues to vasculitis.

5. What are the characteristic urinalysis findings in patients with vasculitis involving the kidney?
The urinalysis generally demonstrates an active sediment with microscopic hematuria and red blood cell casts. However, even with severe vasculitic involvement of the kidney, red blood cell casts can be difficult to identify. Proteinuria is common but usually modest (i.e., less than 3 gm per day).

6. Which of the vasculitides have a predilection for renal involvement?
Kidney involvement in small-vessel vasculitis is quite common. However, polyarteritis nodosa, a medium-size vessel vasculitis, often involves renal arteries. In contrast, Kawasaki syndrome, another vasculitis that affects medium-size vessels, rarely involves renal arteries. Large-vessel vasculitides rarely affect renal blood vessels.

7. Can complement levels be helpful in establishing a diagnosis of vasculitis?
Yes. After exclusion of infectious vasculitic syndromes, low complement levels narrow the differential diagnosis of vasculitis to systemic lupus erythematosus, cryoglobulinemia, and other autoimmune disease–associated vasculitides. Complement levels are generally normal in antineutrophil cytoplasmic antibody (ANCA)–associated small-vessel vasculitides, Henoch-Schönlein purpura, and polyarteritis nodosa. Complement levels also can be depressed in patients with atheroembolic disease, a multisystem disorder that results from dislodged microscopic emboli derived from atherosclerotic plaques (see Chapter 36, Other Vascular Renal Disorders).

8. What are ANCAs?
ANCAs are autoantibodies directed against intracellular neutrophil antigens. These antibodies produce one of two distinct indirect immunofluorescence patterns when serum is incubated with ethanol-fixed neutrophils: cytoplasmic (C-ANCA) or perinuclear staining (P-ANCA). Using specific immunochemical assays, C-ANCAs are directed against a neutrophil and monocyte protease, proteinase 3 (PR3), while P-ANCAs are specific for myeloperoxidase (MPO). ANCAs ares commonly detected in patients with pauci-immune small-vessel vasculitis.

9. What vasculitides cause pulmonary-renal syndrome?
Pulmonary-renal syndrome refers to the constellation of nephritis and hemoptysis or infiltrates on chest x-ray and can be caused by a number of disorders (see Table).

Pulmonary-Renal Vasculitic Syndromes

Microscopic polyangiitis	Goodpasture's syndrome
Wegener's granulomatosis	Henoch-Schönlein purpura
Churg-Strauss syndrome	Behçet's disease
Systemic lupus erythematosus	Rheumatoid vasculitis

Pulmonary-renal syndrome can be caused by both primary and secondary vasculitides. However, other multisystem diseases can present with concurrent pulmonary and renal involvement and need to be considered in the differential diagnosis. These include:
- Congestive heart failure (causing hemoptysis from pulmonary edema) with associated renal failure
- Renal failure complicated by pneumonia (especially *Legionella* infection)
- Nephrotic syndrome with renal vein thrombosis and pulmonary embolism

10. What is pauci-immune glomerulonephritis?

The term *pauci-immune glomerulonephritis* defines a crescentic glomerular disease in which immune deposits are not detected on immunofluorescence microscopy. Eighty percent to 90% of patients with pauci-immune glomerulonephritis are ANCA-positive.

11. How do ANCAs differentiate the etiologies of pauci-immune glomerulonephritides?

Eighty percent to 95% of patients with Wegener's granulomatosis have positive tests for C-ANCA or PR3-ANCA. Five percent to 20% are positive for P-ANCA or MPO-ANCA. Forty percent to 80% of patients with microscopic polyangiitis have positive tests for P-ANCA or MPO-ANCA. Patients with Churg-Strauss syndrome may have positive tests for either C-ANCA or P-ANCA. A number of other diseases, such as rheumatoid arthritis, Behçet's disease, systemic lupus erythematosus, and Sjögren's syndrome, may be associated with a positive P-ANCA on indirect immunofluorescence but will be P-ANCA–negative using the specific enzyme immunoassay for MPO. Differentiating between specific ANCA-associated small-vessel vasculitides in an individual patient is not possible using only ANCA assays, although a positive C- or P-ANCA by indirect immunofluorescence and enzyme immunoassay strongly suggests a diagnosis of small-vessel vasculitis. A tissue biopsy may be needed to differentiate between ANCA-associated small-vessel vasculitides, and biopsy confirmation of vasculitis is also prudent prior to initiation of immunosuppressive therapy.

12. Are there prognostic markers of renal survival in pauci-immune ANCA-related vasculitis?

Yes. The best predictors of renal survival are serum creatinine (high serum creatinine on presentation predicts worse prognosis), race (blacks have a worse prognosis than whites), and presence of arterial sclerosis on kidney biopsy. Age, ANCA pattern, the presence of pulmonary renal involvement, glomerular necrosis, and percent of glomeruli with crescents do not correlate with long-term renal survival.

13. What is the therapy for vasculitis?

Therapy should be guided by the severity of illness. Underlying infection needs to be ruled out before initiating immunosuppressive therapy. Giant cell arteritis and Takayasu's disease are usually treated with high doses of corticosteroids. Steroids are contraindicated in Kawasaki syndrome, which is usually treated with aspirin and high-dose gamma globulin. Henoch-Schönlein purpura is often mild and self-limited and may be treated with supportive care. If intestinal involvement or azotemia complicates Henoch-Schönlein purpura, corticosteroid therapy may be indicated. Patients with ANCA-associated vasculitis (Wegener's granulomatosis and microscopic polyangiitis) usually are treated with a combination of corticosteroids and cytoxic drugs. Plasmapheresis may be beneficial when vasculitis is associated with rapidly progressive glomerulonephritis.

14. Do ANCAs play a pathogenic role or are they an epiphenomenon?

The pathogenic role of ANCAs remains controversial. In support of their pathogenic role, several in vitro studies have demonstrated degranulation of neutrophils and production of oxygen free radicals after incubation with ANCA. These activated neutrophils can then attach to vascular endothelial cells and cause damage. If this theory is correct, circulating (extracellular) ANCAs would need to interact with their target proteins, all of which are intracellular. It has been suggested that these target proteins (e.g., MPO) are translocated to the cytoplasmic membrane through apoptotic or cytokine-primed neutrophils. An alternate hypothesis proposes that release of antigenic proteins from neutrophils at the site of vascular injury occurs secondary to an underlying infection or an immune complex disease in which immune complexes are rapidly cleared from the vascular bed. The latter theory may explain why some patients with mild to moderate Wegener's granulomatosis may respond to antibiotics such as trimethoprim-sulfamethoxazole.

BIBLIOGRAPHY

1. Hagen EC, Daha MR, Hermans J, et al: Diagnostic value of standardized assays for anti-neutrophil cytoplasmic antibodies in idiopathic systemic vasculitis. Kidney Int 53:743–753, 1998.
2. Herbert LA, Cosio FG, Neff JC: Diagnostic significance of hypocomplementemia. Kidney Int 39:811–821, 1991.
3. Hogan SL, Nachman PH, Wilkman S, et al: Prognostic markers in patients with ANCA-associated microscopic polyangiitis and GN. J Am Soc Nephrol 7:23–32, 1996.
4. Jennette JC, Falk RJ: Renal involvement in systemic vasculitis. In Greenberg A (ed): Primer on Kidney Diseases, 2nd ed. San Diego, Academic Press, 1998, pp 200–207.
5. Jennette JC, Falk RJ: Small-vessel vasculitis. N Engl J Med 337:1512–1523, 1997.
6. Johnson RJ: The mystery of the antineutrophil cytoplasmic antibodies. Am J Kidney Dis 26:57–61, 1995.
7. Langford CA, Klippel JH, Balow JE, et al: Use of cytotoxic agents and cyclosporine in the treatment of autoimmune disease. Ann Intern Med 129:49–58, 1998.
8. Rees AJ: Vasculitis and the kidney. Curr Opin Nephrol Hypertension 5:273–281, 1996.
9. Westman KWA, Bygren PG, Olsson H, et al: Relapse rate, renal survival and cancer morbidity in patients with Wegener's granulomatosis or microscopic polyangiitis with renal involvement. J Am Soc Nephrol 9:842–852, 1998.

36. OTHER VASCULAR RENAL DISORDERS

Hany S. Y. Anton, M.D., and Donald E. Hricik, M.D.

1. What are the renal manifestations of scleroderma?
• Hypertension, sometimes malignant (i.e., "scleroderma renal crisis")
• Renal insufficiency
• Varying degrees of proteinuria and hematuria

2. How common is renal disease in patients with scleroderma?
Thirty percent to 50% of patients with scleroderma ultimately develop evidence of renal involvement. Up to 15% of patients develop scleroderma renal crisis.

3. What are risk factors for renal disease in patients with scleroderma?
• Diffuse skin involvement
• African ethnicity
• Female gender (especially in the age range between 20 and 50 years)
• Cold exposure

4. What is the clinical course of patients with scleroderma renal disease?
Renal manifestations typically develop about 4 years following the onset of other systemic manifestations of the disorder. Severe hypertension and abrupt onset of renal failure characterize scleroderma renal crisis. If left untreated, end-stage renal disease usually develops within 1–2 months. Early, aggressive control of hypertension may prevent the development of renal crises and slow the progression of renal insufficiency.

5. What are the pathologic findings in patients with scleroderma renal crisis?
The acute phase comprises fibrinoid necrosis characterized by intravascular deposition of platelet-fibrin thrombi. With healing, there is progressive intimal thickening and concentric hypertrophy of interlobular arteries, leading to an "onion skin" appearance. The histopathology is similar to that seen in patients with other forms of malignant hypertension, thrombotic thrombocytopenic purpura, radiation nephritis, and chronic renal allograft rejection.

6. What is the treatment for renal disease in scleroderma?
The malignant hypertension that occurs in patients with scleroderma is mediated by activation of the renin-angiotensin system resulting from progressive vascular sclerosis. Thus, angiotensin inhibitors are the treatment of choice for both the prevention and treatment of hypertension complicating this disorder.

7. What is atheroembolic renal disease?
Atheroembolic renal disease results from dislodgment of microscopic cholesterol emboli from atherosclerotic plaques leading to occlusion of the lumina of small renal blood vessels, ischemia, and renal dysfunction. The presence of atherosclerotic plaques is obviously the main predisposing factor. Spontaneous atheroembolic disease has been described; however, most cases occur after vascular manipulation (e.g., aortic surgery, arteriography, cardiac catheterization, or angioplasty).

8. What are the clinical features of atheroembolic renal disease?
Renal failure may be the sole manifestation or part of a systemic presentation characterized by ischemia of multiple organs. Renal involvement is characterized by a slow progressive decline

in renal function within days or weeks of vascular manipulation. Beyond the site of plaque dislodgment, bluish discoloration of the extremities, palpable purpura, and livedo reticularis are common. Proteinuria has been reported, and up to 15% of patients exhibit eosinophiluria; however, the urinalysis is more often relatively unremarkable. Peripheral eosinophilia and hypocomplementemia sometimes are observed but are nonspecific findings. In severe cases, signs of ischemia or infarction in other organ systems can be observed (e.g., intestinal infarction). Although the syndrome of atheroembolic renal disease is most often recognized as a catastrophic disorder resulting in irreversible renal failure, it has been recognized recently as a cause of occult and sometimes reversible renal insufficiency.

9. Describe the pathologic findings in atheroembolic renal disease.
    The pathologic hallmark consists of obstruction of small- to medium-sized vessels (ranging from 50 to 900 μm in diameter) with atheromatous debris. During routine fixation of tissues in formalin, cholesterol dissolves, and cholesterol crystals cannot be observed unless special fixatives are used. However, characteristic needle-shaped clefts, previously occupied by the crystals, can be seen within vascular lumina with routine microscopy (see Figure). The deposition of cholesterol crystals leads to vascular and perivascular inflammation that can ultimately result in fibrosis.

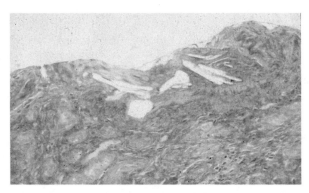

Micrograph showing intravascular needle-shaped clefts in a patient with acute renal failure due to atheroembolic disease.

10. What are the diagnostic and treatment measures in patients with suspected atheroembolic renal disease?
    Most cases diagnosed on clinical grounds. In some cases, biopsies of the kidney, skin, or muscle may be necessary to confirm the diagnosis. There is no specific therapy for this disorder, and management is entirely supportive. Some experts suggest that anticoagulation is contraindicated because it may prevent healing of exposed atherosclerotic plaques.

11. What are the common causes of renal vein thrombosis?
    Renal vein thrombosis can occur in severely dehydrated neonates or children. It also can occur as a complication of trauma or malignancy (especially in cases of renal cell carcinomas that have a proclivity for renal vein invasion). The majority of cases occur in patients with heavy proteinuria and the nephrotic syndrome, usually reflecting a hypercoagulable state (see Chapter 17, Nephrotic Syndrome).

12. What is the clinical presentation of a patient with renal vein thrombosis?
    Most cases are occult and asymptomatic. In severe cases, patients may present with flank pain, microscopic or gross hematuria, high lactate dehydrogenase levels (reflecting renal infarction), or signs of associated pulmonary emboli.

13. What imaging studies are helpful in the diagnosis of renal vein thrombosis?

Computed tomography (CT) scan, magnetic resonance imaging (MRI), and duplex ultrasound have all been used to diagnose renal vein thrombosis noninvasively. However, inferior vena cava venography or the venous phase of arteriography remains the gold standard for diagnosis.

14. What are the clinical characteristics of hemolytic uremic syndrome (HUS) and thrombotic thrombocytopenic purpura (TTP)?

HUS and TTP are disorders characterized by thrombotic microangiopathy. The syndromes differ somewhat with respect to etiology, natural history, and clinical characteristics (see Table).

Clinical Manifestations of Renal Thrombotic Microangiopathies

Hemolytic uremic syndrome	Thrombotic thrombocytopenic purpura
Microangiopathic hemolytic anemia	Microangiopathic hemolytic anemia
Thrombocytopenia	Thrombocytopenia
Renal failure	Renal failure
	Fever
	Neurologic manifestations

15. What are the causes of HUS?

Fifty percent to 90% of cases in children are preceded by diarrhea, often caused by toxigenic *Escherichia coli*. More than half of cases in adults are not associated with diarrheal illness and may be idiopathic, related to nonenteric infections (including pneumonia, meningitis, and human immunodeficiency virus [HIV] infection), or secondary to malignant hypertension, connective tissue disease, or preeclampsia. HUS has been associated with a number of drugs including oral contraceptives, mitomycin C, cyclosporine, and tacrolimus.

16. What therapies are available for patients with HUS and TTP?

HUS is often managed with supportive care, including dialysis when necessary. In contrast, plasma therapies are beneficial in patients with TTP. Plasma exchange using fresh frozen plasma as the initial replacement fluid is associated with a good response in more than 70% of patients. Corticosteroids, vincristine, antiplatelet agents, and splenectomy have each been used in patients with both HUS and TTP, but the absence of controlled trials makes it difficult to ascertain the benefit of these modalities.

BIBLIOGRAPHY

1. Bell WR, Braine HG, Ness PM, Kickler TS: Improved survival in thrombotic thrombocytopenia purpura: Hemolytic uremic syndrome. Clinical experience in 108 patients. N Engl J Med 325:398–403, 1991.
2. Donohoe J: Scleroderma and the kidney. Kidney Int 41:462–477, 1992.
3. Mannesse CK, Blankenstijn PJ, Man int Veld AJ, Schalekamp MADH: Renal failure and cholesterol embolization: A report of 4 surviving cases and a review of the literature. Clin Nephrol 36:240–245, 1991.
4. Rabelink TJ, Zwaginga JJ, Koomans HA, Sixma JJ: Thrombosis and hemostasis in renal disease. Kidney Int 46:287–296, 1994.
5. Remuzzi G, Ruggenenti P: The hemolytic uremic syndrome. Kidney Int 47:2–19, 1995.
6. Steen VD, Costantino JP, Shapiro AP, Medsger TA: Outcome of renal crisis in systemic sclerosis: Relation to availability of angiotensin-converting enzyme (ACE) inhibitors. Ann Intern Med 113:352–357, 1990.
7. Tadhani RI, Carmago CA, Xavier RJ, et al: Atheroembolic renal failure after invasive procedures. Natural history based on 52 histologically proven cases. Medicine 74:350–358, 1995.

37. SICKLE CELL NEPHROPATHY

Chokchai Chareandee, M.D.

1. What renal syndromes occur in sickle cell disease?
- Hematuria
  - Gross
  - Microscopic
- Tubular dysfunction
  - Polyuria (concentrating effect)
  - Renal tubular acidosis
  - Hyperkalemia
- Glomerular disease
  - Focal glomerulosclerosis
  - Membranoproliferative glomerulonephritis
- Chronic renal failure

2. How does sickle cell disease cause kidney damage?
The environment of the renal medulla, characterized by hypoxia, acidosis, and hyperosmolality, predisposes to erythrocyte sickling within medullary capillaries (vasa recta). The sickled erythrocytes reduce blood flow, causing congestion and stasis. If prolonged, interstitial inflammation and papillary infarction occur and eventually result in renal parenchymal fibrosis and tubular atrophy.

3. What is the most common renal abnormality in patients with sickle cell disease?
Hematuria (either microscopic or gross) is the most common abnormality in patients with sickle cell disease and can occur in those who are either homozygous (sickle cell disease) or heterozygous (sickle cell trait) for sickle cell hemoglobin.

4. How should hematuria be treated in patients with sickle cell disease?
Sickle hematuria usually is self-limited. However, persistent hematuria occurs occasionally and can cause a decrease in hematocrit and a worsening of anemia. Conservative therapy to reduce erythrocyte sickling in the renal medulla includes hydration (with hypotonic fluid) and diuretics (either thiazide or loop diuretics) to maintain adequate urine flow. High rates of urine flow not only reduce medullary toxicity but also prevent clot formation in the bladder. Blood transfusion may be required to lower sickle cell hemoglobin concentration. Sodium bicarbonate can reduce the acidity of the renal medulla and, in theory, should reduce sickling by improving hemoglobin oxygen affinity.

Uncontrollable bleeding that is unresponsive to conservative therapy may require other measures. Epsilon-amino caproic acid, an inhibitor of fibrinolysis, has been used successfully, but its use may be complicated by thrombosis in other vascular beds. Arteriographic localization and embolization of the involved renal segment is sometimes necessary to control sickle hematuria.

5. Describe renal papillary necrosis associated with sickle cell disease.
Renal papillary necrosis commonly develops in patients with sickle cell disease or sickle cell trait and frequently is asymptomatic. The lesion results from small, focal infarctions in the renal papillae.

6. What is the earliest evidence of renal dysfunction in the patient with sickle cell disease?

Impairment of urinary concentrating ability occurs early in the course of sickle cell disease and often causes polyuria and nocturia. In children younger than 10–15 years, this defective urinary concentration can often be corrected by blood transfusions that presumably reverse inner medullary congestion. The concentration defect is usually irreversible in older patients. In homozygous patients, maximum urine osmolality after 24 hours of water deprivation is reduced to 400–450 mOsm/kg of water. In heterozygous patients, concentrating ability diminishes with age but usually is less severely compromised than in homozygous patients. In contrast to renal concentrating ability, renal diluting ability remains normal in most sickle cell patients.

7. What are the other clinical manifestations of distal tubular dysfunction in patients with sickle cell disease?

Patients with sickle cell disease often have renal tubular acidosis. Potassium excretion also may be impaired. The defects in excretion of both hydrogen ion and potassium may result from ischemic injury.

8. Is proximal tubular function normal in patients with sickle cell nephropathy?

No. In contrast to the disturbances in medullary tubular function discussed above, both secretory and resorptive function of the proximal tubule is supernormal in patients with early sickle cell nephropathy. The increased secretory capacity results in increased urate clearance that maintains serum urate concentration in the normal range despite overproduction of uric acid resulting from enhanced red cell turnover. Tubular secretion of creatinine also is increased such that creatinine clearances overestimate glomerular filtration rate. Enhanced proximal tubular phosphate resorptive capacity is manifested by increased serum phosphate levels.

9. How common are proteinuria and chronic renal insufficiency in patients with sickle cell disease?

Proteinuria, nephrotic syndrome, and progressive renal failure occur in a minority of patients with sickle cell disease. Approximately 25% of patients with sickle cell disease are proteinuric. Nephrotic syndrome is rare, occurring in 5% of patients. Renal failure develops in 10–25% of patients with sickle cell disease.

10. What is the most common glomerular histopathology in patients with sickle cell disease?

Focal segmental glomerulosclerosis is the most common glomerular lesion identified in renal biopsies of patients with sickle cell disease. Focal segmental glomerulosclerosis occurs in approximately 5% of patients with sickle cell disease. Membranoproliferative glomerulonephritis and minimal change disease also have been described in sickle cell patients.

11. Is therapy available to lessen proteinuria and slow progression of renal insufficiency in sickle cell nephropathy?

No therapy has been shown to prevent glomerular injury in sickle cell disease. However, angiotensin-converting enzyme (ACE) inhibition lowers intraglomerular pressure and probably also improves glomerular permselectivity. Both mechanisms result in diminished proteinuria. Long-term trials are needed to determine whether ACE inhibitor therapy is beneficial in preventing the progression of sickle cell nephropathy to renal failure.

BIBLIOGRAPHY

1. Allon M: Renal abnormalities in sickle cell disease. Arch Intern Med 150:501–504, 1990.
2. Allon M, Lawson L, Eckman JR, et al: Effect of nonsteroidal anti-inflammatory drugs on renal function in sickle cell anemia. Kidney Int 34:500–506, 1988.
3. Bhathena DB, Sondheimer JH: The glomerulopathy of homozygous sickle hemoglobin disease: Morphology and pathogenesis. J Am Soc Nephrol 1:1241–1252, 1991.

4. de Jong PE, Statius van Eps LW: Sickle cell nephropathy: New insights into its pathophysiology. Kidney Int 27:711–717, 1985.
5. Diedrich D: The kidney and sickle cell disease. In Jacobson HR, Striker GE, Klahr S (eds): The Principles and Practice of Nephrology, 2nd ed. St. Louis, Mosby, 1995, pp 246–253.
6. Falk RJ, Scheinman J, Phillips G, et al: Prevalence and pathologic features of sickle cell nephropathy and response to inhibition of angiotensin-converting enzyme. N Engl J Med 326:910–915, 1992.
7. Pariser S, Katz A: Treatment of sickle cell trait hematuria with oral urea. J Urol 151:401–403, 1994.
8. Powars DR, Elliot-Mills DD, Chan L, et al: Chronic renal failure in sickle cell disease: Risk factors, clinical course, and mortality. Ann Intern Med 115:614–620, 1991.
9. Scheinman JI: Sickle cell nephropathy. In Greenberg A (ed): Primer on Kidney Diseases, 2nd ed. San Diego, Academic Press, 1998, pp 309–313.

38. RENAL DISEASE DUE TO DYSPROTEINEMIAS

Edmond Ricanati, M.D.

1. List the different types of dysproteinemias associated with renal disease.

• Multiple myeloma
• Amyloidosis
• Cryoglobulinemia
• Light chain nephropathy
• Waldenström's macroglobulinemia. This produces renal disease only rarely because the monoclonal immunoglobulin M (IgM) paraprotein characteristics of this disorder is generally too large to be trapped by the glomeruli. However, a small percentage of patients with Waldenström's macroglobulinemia (about 20% of cases) have light chains in their urine. These patients are prone to developing renal disease.

2. What is the pathogenesis of renal disease in multiple myeloma?

An estimated 25% of patients with multiple myeloma develop renal failure. The renal injury in multiple myeloma results from overproduction of monoclonal light chains by the rapid proliferation of plasma cells derived from a single clone. These abnormal proteins are freely filtered by the glomerulus and produce extensive renal tubular damage leading to chronic progressive renal disease by:

• Formation of intratubular casts by precipitation of aggregated light chains forming large molecules, which obstruct the tubular lumen. Experimental evidence does show that light chains have an affinity to bind with specific sites on the Tamm-Horsfall glycoprotein, which is locally secreted by the tubular cells of the ascending limb of the loop of Henle. Binding of light chains to this protein causes the formation of intratubular casts.
• Tubular injury due to the reabsorption of the filtered light chains, which are toxic to the tubular cells

3. How are light chains detected in the urine?

The urinary dipstick does not detect light chains; it primarily detects albumin. Sulfosalicylic acid (SSA), which precipitates all proteins in the urine, is the simple test of choice. A positive SSA test with a negative dipstick test is highly suggestive of the presence of light chains. The electrophoretic pattern of urine proteins is characteristic of multiple myeloma and usually shows a sharp monoclonal light chain peak. Patients with multiple myeloma often excrete large quantities of light chains, sometimes exceeding 1 gm per day. Not all light chains are nephrotoxic. Patients excreting lambda chains generally have a more severe form of renal disease than those excreting kappa chains.

4. Patients with multiple myeloma can develop acute renal failure. What predisposing factors can cause this complication?

1. **Hypercalcemia**, which is commonly found in multiple myeloma and is due to increased bone reabsorption (see Chapter 67, Hypocalcemia and Hypercalcemia). This results from the overproduction of cytokines such as interleukin 6, which directly stimulates osteoclasts. Hypercalcemia can precipitate acute renal failure by causing vasoconstriction and by precipitating with light chains in the tubules, causing intratubular obstruction.

2. **Use of radiocontrast agents in the presence of dehydration**. The mechanism for the acute renal failure is not clear; the high concentration of urinary light chains that are excreted

may combine with the contrast agent to produce intratubular obstruction. Hydration is strongly recommended in such patients before use of radiocontrast agents.

3. **Acute urate nephropathy** due to the rapid breakdown of abnormal plasma cells, especially following chemotherapy, with the release of large quantities of uric acid, leading to the formation of intratubular urate casts

5. What are the principal treatments for multiple myeloma with renal failure?

1. **Chemotherapy**
   - In patients with small to moderate tumor burdens, an alkylating agent (e.g., melphalan) and steroids
   - In patients with extensive tumor burdens, treatment regimens include:
     VAD (vincristine, Adriamycin, and dexamethasone)
     ABCM (Adriamycin, carmustine [BCNV], cyclophosphamide, and melphalan)

2. **Plasmapheresis** in combination with chemotherapy to remove more rapidly circulating myeloma proteins. This approach is not very effective in patients with histologic evidence of advanced renal disease (e.g., interstitial fibrosis or amyloidosis). Plasmapheresis is most effective when started early in the course of myeloma kidney disease.

3. **Dialysis** when uremia occurs

6. How does amyloidosis cause renal disease?

Two types of amyloidosis exist: (1) primary amyloidosis (AL amyloidosis) and (2) secondary or reactive amyloidosis (AA amyloidosis). In AL amyloidosis, renal disease results from the deposition of amyloid fibrils, derived from immunoglobulin light chains, in the glomeruli, blood vessels, and tubules. In AA amyloidosis, amyloid fibrils are derived from an acute phase reactant serum protein, amyloid AA, which is a protein produced by the liver in chronic inflammatory conditions. Renal disease due to amyloid AL tends to be more severe than renal disease due to amyloid AA. The amyloid fibrils in AL amyloidosis tend to coalesce and have a characteristic ability to bind to Congo red, producing an intense yellow-green fluorescence under polarized light. It is not clear what stimulates the formation of beta-pleated fibrils from normal plasma proteins.

7. What are the renal manifestations of primary amyloidosis?

The renal manifestations in AL amyloidosis depend on the site of deposition of amyloid fibrils in the kidney. Most commonly, amyloid deposits occur in the glomeruli (both in the mesangium and capillary loops). Such patients usually present with nephrotic-range proteinuria, hypoalbuminemia, and peripheral edema. Initially, plasma creatinine is normal, but with progression of the disease, the plasma creatinine rises and renal failure ensues. In some cases, amyloid fibrils deposit primarily in the blood vessels, leading to progressive renal failure without significant proteinuria. This type of renal disease is apparently more common in secondary amyloidosis (amyloid AA renal disease). Tubular deposits of amyloid fibrils also can occur and may lead to tubular dysfunction such as distal renal tubular acidosis and nephrogenic diabetes insipidus.

8. What is the treatment for amyloidosis?

In secondary amyloidosis, treatment is primarily directed to the underlying inflammatory process (such as osteomyelitis, rheumatoid arthritis, regional enteritis, chronic bronchiectasis with repeated infections), which, if successfully treated, can arrest the progression of the renal disease. In primary amyloidosis, the renal disease progresses relentlessly, and there is no proven effective therapy for this disease. Survival time is short, and death is mostly due to cardiovascular complications resulting from the deposition of amyloid fibrils in the myocardium and blood vessels. Prednisone and melphalan have been used with equivocal results. The addition of colchicine (which has been shown experimentally to decrease amyloid formation) to the prednisone and melphalan regimen has been found to prolong survival in some series.

9. What are cryoglobulins?

Cryoglobulins are immunoglobulins that precipitate when plasma is cooled and redissolve when plasma is warmed. Three types of cryoglobulinemia have been identified. In type I cryoglobulinemia, a single monoclonal immunoglobulin is present. Types II and III cryoglobulinemias are characterized by mixed types of immunoglobulins. In type II cryoglobulinemia, a mixture of polyclonal immunoglobulins and a monoclonal immunoglobulin, usually IgM, is directed against the IgG immunoglobulins. In type III cryoglobulinemia, a mixture of polyclonal antibodies have anti-IgG and anti-IgM (rheumatoid factor) activity.

10. What renal diseases are associated with cryoglobulinemia?

All types of cryoglobulinemias can be associated with glomerular disease. The pattern of glomerular disease depends on the site of immunoglobulin deposition and the types of immunoglobulins involved. The glomerular lesions in type I and III are variable and nonspecific; however, type II cryoglobulinemia results in a well-characterized form of membranoproliferative glomerulonephritis, now recognized to be a manifestation of hepatitis C in most cases (see Chapter 29, Hepatitis-Associated Glomerulonephritis).

11. What is light chain nephropathy?

Light chain nephropathy is a renal disease characterized by the deposition of monoclonal light chains in renal glomeruli or the tubulointerstitium. In contrast to patients with multiple myeloma or amyloidosis, patients with light chain nephropathy exhibit no skeletal evidence of plasma cell overgrowth, and the light chains do not form amyloid fibrils. The characteristic histologic lesion is a nodular glomerulopathy with negative Congo red stains. Patients present either with nephrotic syndrome or with evidence of tubular dysfunction (e.g., Fanconi syndrome). Anecdotal reports have shown improvement following treatment with melphalan and prednisone.

BIBLIOGRAPHY

1. D'Amico G, Fornasieri A: Cryoglobulinemic glomerulonephritis: A membranoproliferative glomerulonephritis induced by hepatitis C virus. Am J Kidney Dis 25:361–369, 1995.
2. Ganeval D, Rabian C, Guérin V, et al: Treatment of multiple myeloma with renal involvement. Adv Nephrol 21:347–370, 1992.
3. Gertz MA, Kyle RA, Greipp PR: Response rates and survival in primary systemic amyloidosis. Blood 77:257–262, 1991.
4. Heilman RL, Velosa JA, Holley KE, et al: Long-term follow-up and response to chemotherapy in patients with light-chain deposition disease. Am J Kidney Dis 20:34–41, 1992.
5. Sanders PW, Herrera GA: Monoclonal immunoglobulin light chain–related renal diseases. Semin Nephrol 13:324–341, 1993.

VI. End-Stage Renal Disease: Causes and Consequences

39. EPIDEMIOLOGY AND OUTCOMES OF END-STAGE RENAL DISEASE

Ashwini R. Sehgal, M.D.

1. What is end-stage renal disease?

End-stage renal disease is irreversible, severe kidney failure for which patients require treatment with dialysis or kidney transplantation in order to survive.

2. How many people have end-stage renal disease?

About 1 of every 1,000 Americans receive treatment for end-stage renal disease, for a total of nearly 300,000 affected individuals. The prevalence of treated end-stage renal disease is increasing at a rate of about 8% per year. It is unclear how many patients with end-stage renal disease are untreated (and die as a result). The prevalence of treated end-stage renal disease in Canada and Western Europe is about half that in the United States.

3. Name the most common causes of end-stage renal disease.

The major causes of end-stage renal disease are diabetes mellitus (one third of patients) and hypertension (one fourth of patients). Other common causes include glomerulonephritis and polycystic kidney disease. In at least 5% of patients, the cause is unknown.

4. What demographic factors are associated with end-stage renal disease?

Advanced age, black race, male sex, and low socioeconomic status are associated with an increased likelihood of end-stage renal disease. For example, blacks account for nearly one third of end-stage renal disease patients but only one eighth of the general population.

5. How is end-stage renal disease treated?

In the United States, end-stage renal disease currently is treated by:
- Hemodialysis (60%)
- Peritoneal dialysis (10%)
- Kidney transplantation (30%)

6. How long do dialysis patients survive?

The death rate among dialysis patients in the United States is approximately 23% per year. A 45-year-old dialysis patient has a life expectancy of about 7 years compared to 35 years for someone from the general population. This marked difference may be due to comorbid conditions, failure of dialysis to completely replace normal kidney function, and/or adverse effects of dialysis treatment.

7. List the factors that influence mortality in dialysis patients.

Demographic factors associated with increased mortality include advanced age, white race, male gender, and low socioeconomic status. Medical factors associated with increased mortality include diabetes mellitus as a cause of renal failure, other comorbid conditions such as cardiovascular disease, and poor nutritional status. A treatment factor associated with increased mortality is inadequate dose of dialysis (see Chapter 45, Hemodialysis: Assessing Adequacy).

8. What are the common causes of death in patients with end-stage renal disease?

The most common causes of death are cardiovascular disease and infection. Withdrawal of dialysis also is a common cause of death, especially among elderly patients. Dialysis most often is withdrawn when new medical complications occur or when patients simply become so tired of treatment that death is preferable to ongoing dialysis.

9. How much does it cost to treat dialysis patients?

Because of congressional legislation, virtually all patients with end-stage renal disease are eligible for Medicare coverage. Total annual Medicare costs for end-stage renal disease are about $10 billion. Outpatient and inpatient Medicare costs per dialysis patient are approximately $50,000 per year. This amount includes care for dialysis-related conditions as well as for other medical conditions.

BIBLIOGRAPHY

1. Alexander GC, Sehgal AR: Barriers to cadaveric renal transplantation among blacks, women, and the poor. J Am Med Assoc 280:1148–1152, 1998.
2. Daugirdas JT, Ing TS: Handbook of Dialysis. Boston, Little, Brown, 1994.
3. Greenberg A: Primer on Kidney Diseases, 2nd ed. San Diego, Academic Press, 1998.
4. Jacobson HR, Striker GE, Klahr S: The Principles and Practice of Nephrology. Philadelphia, Mosby, 1995.
5. Sehgal A, Galbraith A, Chesney M, et al: How strictly do dialysis patients want their advance directives followed? J Am Med Assoc 267:59–63, 1996.
6. U.S. Renal Data Systems: USRDS 1998 Annual Data Report. Bethesda, MD, National Institutes of Health, 1998.

40. RENAL OSTEODYSTROPHY

Lavinia A. Negrea, M.D.

1. What is renal osteodystrophy?
Renal osteodystrophy refers to several bone diseases that occur as a complication of chronic renal insufficiency. In many cases, two or more of these disease processes occur simultaneously.

2. How are renal bone diseases classified?
1. High-turnover bone disease (due to persistently high levels of parathyroid hormone [PTH])
2. Low-turnover bone disease (generally associated with relatively low levels of PTH)

3. Name the factors contributing to sustained increases in PTH secretion, parathyroid hyperplasia, and ultimately high-turnover bone disease.
The factors responsible for secondary hyperparathyroidism associated with renal failure are hyperphosphatemia due to diminished renal phosphorus excretion, hypocalcemia, impaired renal production of active 1,25-dihydroxyvitamin D, alterations in the control of PTH gene transcription, and skeletal resistance to the calcemic action of PTH.

4. What bone lesion is associated with hyperparathyroidism and high turnover of bone?
Osteitis fibrosa cystica.

5. What serum levels of PTH generally are associated with severe hyperparathyroidism and osteitis fibrosa cystica?
Most patients with bone biopsy–proven osteitis fibrosa have serum intact PTH levels above 250–300 pg/ml.

6. Describe the histologic features of osteitis fibrosa cystica.
The histologic features include increased numbers of osteoclasts and osteoblasts, increased amounts of woven osteoid, and peritrabecular fibrosis.

7. What are the radiographic features of osteitis fibrosa cystica?
Typically, these include subperiosteal erosions of the phalanges and erosions at the proximal end of the tibia, the neck of the femur or humerus, and the inferior surface of the distal end of the clavicle. The skull has a mottled and granular "salt-and-pepper" appearance.

8. What bone lesions are classified as low-turnover bone disease?
1. Osteomalacia
2. Adynamic or aplastic bone disease

9. What are the common causes of osteomalacia in dialysis patients?
The most common cause of osteomalacia in patients on dialysis is aluminum intoxication. Abnormalities of vitamin D metabolism and metabolic acidosis may contribute to the development of osteomalacia.

10. What are the "ABCs" of aluminum toxicity?
- Microcytic anemia
- Bone disease
- Central nervous system abnormalities (dialysis encephalopathy)

11. What are the main risk factors for aluminum toxicity?
Diabetes mellitus, prior parathyroidectomy, failed renal transplant, and consumption of aluminum-based phosphate binders over long periods of time are considered the main risks for aluminum toxicity. Citrate markedly enhances intestinal aluminum absorption. Therefore, concomitant use of citrate-containing medications (calcium citrate, Shohl's solution) along with aluminum-containing medications (Amphojel, Carafate) can lead to aluminum accumulation.

12. Why are serum PTH levels generally low in aluminum bone disease?
The low levels of PTH have been attributed to frequent episodes of hypercalcemia (with subsequent suppression of PTH). A direct inhibitory effect of aluminum on the PTH secretion also has been demonstrated.

13. How is aluminum bone disease diagnosed?
The gold standard is the bone biopsy. Alternatively, a basal serum aluminum level of > 100 µg/L plus an increment in aluminum level of > 150 µg/L following deferoxamine administration, in combination with a low PTH level, is highly suggestive of aluminum bone disease.

14. Describe the histologic findings of osteomalacia.
Osteomalacia is characterized by excess of osteoid (unmineralized bone collagen), due to impaired mineralization. Deposits of aluminum can be seen in aluminum-related osteomalacia along trabecular bone surfaces using histochemical staining.

15. Describe the histologic findings of adynamic or aplastic bone disease.
Adynamic bone disease is characterized by decreased bone mineralization but normal amounts of osteoid.

16. What are the risk factors for adynamic bone disease?
Peritoneal dialysis
Diabetes mellitus
Advanced age

17. What serum levels of PTH are generally associated with adynamic bone disease?
Serum levels of intact PTH are, in general, < 100 pg/ml in patients with adynamic bone disease.

18. What is "mixed renal osteodystrophy"?
Mixed renal osteodystrophy entails histologic findings of both osteitis fibrosa cystica and osteomalacia on bone biopsy. It may be seen in patients with established osteitis fibrosa who are developing aluminum-related bone disease.

19. What is dialysis-related amyloidosis?
Dialysis-related amyloidosis refers to the clinical manifestations that result from the deposition of a unique, amyloid fibril protein derived from beta$_2$-microglobulin in bony structures and synovial tissue of patients who have been on dialysis for long periods of time (generally more than 7 years).

20. Name the most common clinical manifestations of dialysis-related amyloidosis.
Carpal tunnel syndrome is the most frequent clinical feature. Scapulohumeral involvement is common and is manifested as shoulder pain. Characteristically, pain is worse at night or at rest and improves with motion. Other affected sites are metacarpophalangeal and interphalangeal joints, shoulders, wrists, and knees. The cervical spine is the most common site of destructive spondyloarthropathy. Bone cysts from amyloid deposition also occur, especially in long bones, and can be associated with pathologic features.

21. Describe the most common radiologic presentation of dialysis-related amyloidosis.
Radiographically, bone cysts occur at the end of long bones, particularly femoral head and proximal humerus. Metacarpal, carpal, and tarsal bones also may be involved. Multiple bone cysts suggest amyloid, whereas brown tumors of osteitis fibrosa are isolated, usually in the rib or jaw.

22. What bone lesion is typical after kidney transplantation?
Osteopenia is common following renal transplantation, with evidence of reduced bone mass found as early as 6 months after transplantation and in nearly all patients within 5 years. The use of corticosteroids for immunosuppression is considered to be the major contributor.

BIBLIOGRAPHY

1. Delmez JA: Renal osteodystrophy and other musculoskeletal complications of chronic renal failure. In Greenberg A (ed): Primer on Kidney Diseases, 2nd ed. San Diego, Academic Press, 1998, pp 448–455.
2. Goodman WG, Coburn JW, Slatopolsky E, Salusky IB: Renal osteodystrophy in adults and children. In Favus MJ (ed): Primer on the Metabolic Bone Diseases and D Disorders of Mineral Metabolism, 3rd ed. Philadelphia, Lippincott-Raven, 1996, pp 341–360.
3. Hruska KA, Teitelbaum SL: Renal osteodystrophy. N Engl J Med 333:166–174, 1995.
4. Pei Y, Hercz G: Low-turnover bone disease in dialysis patients. Semin Dial 9:327–331, 1996.
5. Sprague SM, Moe SM: Clinical manifestations and pathogenesis of dialysis-related amyloidosis. Semin Dial 9:360–369, 1996.

41. UREMIC PERICARDITIS

Marcia R. Silver, M.D.

1. What is uremic pericarditis?

Uremic pericarditis is an inflammation of the pericardium occurring in patients with advanced acute or chronic renal failure. The condition generally is diagnosed by the presence of characteristic chest pain, a pericardial friction rub, typical electrocardiographic changes, and sometimes fever, general malaise, and pericardial effusion. Uremia is probably the most common cause of pericarditis. In 1987, patients with end-stage renal disease were hospitalized for pericarditis at a rate 200 times that of the general population.

2. What is the difference between pericarditis and pericardial effusion?

Pericarditis is inflammation of the pericardium. Pericardial effusion refers to the presence of abnormal amounts of fluid in the pericardial space and may occur without inflammation. Up to 40% of stable dialysis patients studied with echocardiography have pericardial effusions, but most of these patients do not have signs or symptoms of pericarditis.

3. What is pericardial tamponade?

Pericardial tamponade refers to compression of the heart by the pericardium or its contents (fluid or blood) that impedes the inflow of blood into the right and left ventricles. Clinical signs suggesting tamponade include hypotension, tachycardia, jugular venous distention, and pulsus paradoxicus. The electrocardiogram may show decreased voltage and electrical alternans. Echocardiography demonstrates compromise of cardiac filling and the presence of a pericardial effusion. Cardiac catheterization usually shows equalization of pressures in the right and left heart chambers.

4. What is dialysis pericarditis and how does it differ from uremic pericarditis?

Uremic pericarditis usually occurs in patients not yet treated with dialysis and tends to resolve with dialytic therapy, suggesting that uremia per se is important in the pathophysiology. By contrast, dialysis pericarditis most often occurs in patients who have been on dialysis for some time. Although some cases may occur as a consequence of uremia resulting from inadequate dialysis, clusters of dialysis pericarditis suggest that this disorder may sometimes be caused by viral infection. Compared to classic uremic pericarditis, dialysis pericarditis is more often hemorrhagic in character and more often associated with large pericardial effusions and tamponade.

5. What clinical findings suggest uremic pericarditis?

Typically the patient complains of chest pain that is worse in the supine position and that is relieved by sitting up and forward. On physical examination, a two- or three-component pericardial friction rub is characteristic; however, such rubs tend to wax and wane over time. As an effusion increases in size, the rub may disappear because a fluid cushion develops between the walls of the pericardial sac. Precipitous hypotension may be the first sign of pericarditis, usually indicating the presence of tamponade. The electrocardiogram typically reveals widespread ST segment elevations.

The above findings are not specific for *uremic* pericarditis, however. Other causes of pericarditis must be considered, including trauma, infections (viral, bacterial, mycobacterial), malignancies, and myocardial infarction (i.e., Dressler's syndrome). Ultimately, the diagnosis of uremic pericarditis is a diagnosis of exclusion.

6. How common is uremic pericarditis?

Older reports suggest a cumulative incidence of 5–40% in patients with chronic renal failure. However, such data were generated in an era when dialysis was often postponed until patients were severely uremic and when less attention was paid to parameters of dialysis adequacy. In addition, variations in the reported incidence reflect differences in the definition of the disorder— some older studies included all patients with pericardial effusions, even in the absence of other clinical signs and symptoms of pericardial inflammation.

7. What is the treatment for uremic pericarditis?

While patients with pericardial tamponade clearly require urgent therapy that may include either pericardiocentesis or surgery for creation of a "pericardial window," the management of patients with uremic or dialysis pericarditis in the absence of tamponade is less certain. Uremic pericarditis is treated promptly with dialytic therapy performed on a daily basis until there is clear resolution of pericarditis. Heparin use is kept to a minimum in order to minimize the risk of bleeding into the pericardial space. Dialysis pericarditis is treated similarly, with institution of daily dialysis without heparin and careful examination of all aspects of the dialysis procedure looking for problems leading to underdialysis. Volume removal should be attempted if there is evidence of fluid overload. Improvement is usually seen in 1–2 weeks. If there is no evidence of underdialysis, and other causes have been excluded, a viral etiology may be presumed and the dialysis schedule may not need to be altered. Persistent chest pain may be treated with nonsteroidal anti-inflammatory drugs, although these agents may increase the risk of pericardial hemorrhage and should be used cautiously. Patients with slowly evolving tamponade physiology or persistent, large pericardial effusion despite weeks of daily dialysis may require either simple pericardiocentesis or a few days of continuous catheter drainage with instillation of nonabsorbable steroids into the pericardial space. Rarely, pericardial window or even pericardiectomy may be required.

8. What is the prognosis of patients with uremic or dialysis-related pericarditis?

In the setting of acute renal failure, complete resolution of pericarditis is the rule in patients who recover from the underlying renal failure. Mortality rates of up to 5% have been reported in patients with dialysis-associated pericarditis. However, data from serial reports of the United States Renal Data System suggest that mortality rates from this complication of end-stage renal disease have decreased with time (see Table).

Death Rates (from Pericarditis) per 1000 Patient Years

TIME PERIOD	DEATH RATE
1987–1989	1.6
1988–1990	1.4
1989–1991	1.0
1991–1993	< 1
1994–1996	0.3

BIBLIOGRAPHY

1. Comty CM, Cohen SL, Shapiro FL: Pericarditis in chronic uremia and its sequels. Ann Intern Med 75:173–183, 1971.
2. DePace NL, Nestico PF, Schwartz AB, et al: Predicting success of intensive dialysis in the treatment of uremic pericarditis. Am J Med 76:38–46, 1984.
3. Silverberg S, Oreopoulos DG, Wise DJ, et al: Pericarditis in patients undergoing long-term hemodialysis and peritoneal dialysis. Am J Med 63:874–880, 1977.
4. Silver MR, Logue E, McCord G: Rates of pericarditis associated with various treatment modalities for end-stage renal disease [abstract]. J Am Soc Nephrol 3:394, 1992.
5. Wray TM, Stone WJ: Uremic pericarditis: A prospective echocardiographic and clinical study. Clin Nephrol 6:295–301, 1976.

42. ANEMIA ASSOCIATED WITH RENAL FAILURE

Jay B. Wish, M.D.

1. What causes the anemia in patients with renal disease?

The anemia of chronic renal disease is caused primarily by deficiency of erythropoietin. The kidneys are the major source of erythropoietin and, as renal function declines, production of erythropoietin declines proportionately. As a result, there tends to be a linear relationship between hematocrit and creatinine clearance in patients with renal insufficiency, although a wide range of hematocrit levels may be observed for any degree of renal disease.

A number of other factors tend to decrease red cell life span from the normal of 120 days to approximately 70–80 days in patients with chronic renal failure. These include red cell trauma due to microvascular disease from diabetes or hypertension, blood loss due to the hemodialysis procedure, an increased incidence of gastrointestinal bleeding due to peptic ulcer disease and angiodysplasia of the bowel, and increased oxidative stress leading to shortened red cell survival.

2. How does one evaluate anemia in a patient with chronic renal disease?

Erythropoietin deficiency is a diagnosis of exclusion, and determination of erythropoietin levels in patients with chronic renal disease is generally not indicated. The routine evaluation of such patients should include measurement of red blood cell indices, reticulocyte count, transferrin saturation, serum ferritin, and a test for occult blood in the stool. If these tests reveal no easily correctable cause of anemia, such as gastrointestinal bleeding or iron deficiency, it can be presumed that the anemia is due primarily to erythropoietin deficiency.

3. How are the tests of iron status in patients with chronic renal disease interpreted?

The two most commonly used tests of iron status are transferrin saturation and serum ferritin. Transferrin saturation is computed by dividing the serum iron level by the total iron-binding capacity. The total iron-binding capacity correlates with circulating transferrin, which is the major iron-binding protein in plasma. Transferrin saturation correlates with the amount of iron available for erythropoiesis because only circulating iron is available to the bone marrow for incorporation into newly synthesized red blood cells. The serum ferritin level correlates with storage iron located primarily in the reticuloendothelial system. Interpretation of serum ferritin levels is confounded by the fact that ferritin will rise as an acute phase reactant in the setting of acute or chronic inflammation. In patients with chronic renal disease, a serum ferritin less than 100 ng/ml correlates with the deficiency in storage iron; such patients will almost invariably respond to supplemental iron therapy. Patients with a transferrin saturation of less than 20% have decreased iron delivery to the erythroid marrow, but supplemental iron may or may not correct this problem, depending on whether storage iron can effectively be released to the transferrin carrier protein.

4. What is functional iron deficiency?

Functional iron deficiency is a phenomenon that occurs in patients treated with pharmacologic doses of erythropoietin when the bone marrow is stimulated to produce red blood cells faster than the transferrin carrier protein can deliver adequate iron substrate. In such patients, the transferrin saturation tends to be low or low-normal, while the serum ferritin level may be normal or even high. The operative definition of functional iron deficiency is based on a response to intravenous iron supplementation characterized by either an increase in hematocrit or a decrease in erythropoietin requirements to achieve the same hematocrit. Studies have demonstrated that functional iron deficiency is common in patients with end-stage renal disease who are treated with erythropoietin and that intravenous iron supplementation will decrease erythropoietin requirements by approximately 30–35%.

5. Why are oral iron supplements often ineffective in treating the iron deficiency in patients on chronic hemodialysis?

Oral iron absorption tends to be inversely proportional to serum ferritin levels. In patients with a serum ferritin of 100 ng/ml or higher, oral iron absorption is approximately 1–2% of the administered load. A patient taking ferrous sulfate, 325 mg three times daily, will consume 200 mg of elemental iron, of which 2–4 mg will be absorbed daily. The iron requirements in anemic patients undergoing hemodialysis are often enormous. To increase the hematocrit from 25% to 35% in a 70-kg patient requires the incorporation of 600 mg of elemental iron into the newly synthesized red blood cells. In addition, the estimated daily iron losses in hemodialysis patients are approximately 4–7 mg. Thus, the 2–4 mg of oral iron absorbed daily would barely keep pace with ongoing iron losses let alone repair the accumulated iron deficit. Compounding this problem is the phenomenon of functional iron deficiency, which often results in the need for high levels of storage iron to facilitate release of iron to transferrin and delivery of that iron to the erythroid marrow. As a result, the majority of hemodialysis patients receiving erythropoietin require intravenous iron supplements.

6. How is erythropoietin administered?

Human recombinant erythropoietin is a polypeptide hormone that, like insulin, must be given parenterally through a subcutaneous or intravenous route. A number of studies have demonstrated that subcutaneously administered erythropoietin, because of its slower absorption and longer half-life, is more effective than a comparable dose administered intravenously. Several studies have demonstrated a 30–35% reduction in the erythropoietin dose required to achieve the same hematocrit when patients are switched from the intravenous to the subcutaneous route of administration.

For patients receiving erythropoietin intravenously on hemodialysis, the recommended starting dose is 50 U/kg of body weight three times weekly, with the dose titrated at monthly intervals depending on the hematocrit response. For patients receiving erythropoietin therapy subcutaneously, the recommended starting dose is 30 U/kg administered three times weekly (as is typically done in hemodialysis facilities) or 50 U/kg administered twice weekly (which is typical for predialysis and peritoneal dialysis patients). Again, the dose would be titrated at monthly intervals depending on the hematocrit response.

7. What is the target hematocrit or hemoglobin for patients receiving erythropoietin therapy?

The practice guidelines prepared by the National Kidney Foundation's Dialysis Outcomes Quality Initiative (DOQI) recommend a target hematocrit of 33–36% or a target hemoglobin of 11–12 gm/dl. This is supported by a number of studies that demonstrate that this hematocrit and hemoglobin level is associated with improved functional and cognitive status, improved quality of life, regression of left ventricular hypertrophy, and decreased morbidity and mortality when compared to patients with chronic renal failure and lower hematocrit and hemoglobin levels. Whether patients with chronic renal failure would benefit from having hematocrit and hemoglobin levels closer to those of the normal population remains a subject of some controversy. As of 1999, medical justification is required for reimbursement from Medicare or Medicaid for erythropoietin administered to patients with a 3-month rolling average hematocrit greater than 37.5.

BIBLIOGRAPHY

1. Eschbach JW: The anemia of chronic renal failure: Pathophysiology and the effects of recombinant erythropoietin. Kidney Int 35:134–148, 1989.
2. Fishbane S, Frei GL, Maesaka J: Reduction in recombinant human erythropoietin doses by the use of chronic intravenous iron supplementation. Am J Kidney Dis 26:41–46, 1995.
3. Foley RN, Parfrey PS, Harnett JD, et al: The impact of anemia on cardiomyopathy, morbidity, and mortality in end-stage renal disease. Am J Kidney Dis 28:53–61, 1996.
4. Horl WH, Dreyling K, Steinhauer HB, et al: Iron status of dialysis patients under r-HuEPO therapy. Contrib Nephrol 87:78–86, 1990.
5. Taylor JE, Belch JJF, Fleming LW, et al: Erythropoietin response and route of administration. Clin Nephrol 41:297–302, 1994.
6. Wingard RL, Parker RA, Ismail N, Hakim RM: Efficacy of oral iron therapy in patients receiving recombinant human erythropoietin. Am J Kidney Dis 25:433–439, 1995.

43. OTHER MANIFESTATIONS OF UREMIA

Donald E. Hricik, M.D.

1. What is the cause of and treatment for uremic pruritis?

The cause is unknown. Some, but certainly not all, cases are associated with secondary hyperparathyroidism or a high calcium × phosphorus product and respond to appropriate measures (see Chapter 40, Renal Osteodystrophy). Itching often persists despite otherwise adequate dialysis. Antihistamines constitute the mainstay of therapy. In severe cases, ultraviolet phototherapy can be helpful.

2. What are the neurologic effects of uremia?

Central nervous system	Peripheral nervous system
Lethargy	Symmetric sensorimotor polyneuropathy
Irritability	"Restless leg syndrome"
Alterations in memory	
Coma (severe cases)	
Seizures (rare)	
Myoclonus or asterixis	

3. How does uremia affect sexual function?

In men, erectile dysfunction and decreased libido are common and related, in part, to hypogonadism and low testosterone levels. Women may exhibit signs and symptoms of hyperprolactinemia but generally show signs of hypogonadism manifested either by dysfunctional uterine bleeding or amenorrhea. Fertility is not always impaired, but term pregnancy is rare in women with end-stage renal disease. Spontaneous abortion is the rule in women who become pregnant. Fertility can be fully restored after successful kidney transplantation.

4. What is the nature of the bleeding diathesis in patients with uremia?

Uremic patients commonly exhibit platelet dysfunction best assessed by measurement of a bleeding time. At best, only a crude correlation exists between the degree of azotemia and the degree of platelet dysfunction.

5. What is the clinical significance of uremic platelet dysfunction?

Spontaneous or surgically induced bleeding is common in patients with uremia. In the absence of risk factors such as heart failure, obesity, and immobilization, thromboembolic events are less common in patients with renal failure than in the general population.

6. What pharmacologic agents have been used to prevent or treat uremic bleeding?

1. Desmopressin (DDAVP)
2. Cryoprecipitate
3. Conjugated estrogens (particularly for chronic gastrointestinal bleeding)

7. What is uremic serositis?

Akin to uremic pericarditis, uremia can be associated with inflammation of other serous membranes leading, for example, to noninfectious pleuritis or peritonitis. In addition, uremia has been named as an occasional cause of gastritis, enteritis, and even pancreatitis.

8. What is uremic cardiomyopathy?

It remains unclear whether uremia per se can suppress myocardial function. However, successful renal transplantation is sometimes associated with improved myocardial performance in patients previously deemed to have heart failure, suggesting that uremic cardiomyopathy probably occurs in some patients.

9. How does uremia affect glucose tolerance?

Most nondiabetic patients with uremia exhibit mild glucose intolerance that is rarely of clinical significance. Because the kidney is involved in the metabolism of insulin, patients with type II diabetes mellitus often exhibit reduced insulin requirements as renal failure progresses to end stage. A poorly understood syndrome of spontaneous hypoglycemia has been observed in some dialysis patients. It appears to be associated with defects in gluconeogenesis and generally is associated with a poor prognosis.

10. Name some other metabolic abnormalities associated with uremia.

Hypertriglyceridemia is common and related both to overproduction and decreased clearance of very low density lipoproteins. Recent studies suggest that advanced glycation end products accumulate in patients with renal failure, even in the absence of diabetes. The mechanism is unclear, but these compounds may contribute to cardiovascular disease. Abnormal glycation of $beta_2$-microglobulin is now known to cause a secondary form of amyloidosis associated with arthropathy in dialysis patients.

BIBLIOGRAPHY

1. Bagdade JD, Porte D, Bierman EL: Hypertriglyceridemia: A metabolic consequence of chronic renal failure. N Engl J Med 279:181–186, 1968.
2. DeFronzo RA, Alvestrand A: Glucose intolerance in uremia: Site and mechanisms. Am J Clin Nutr 33:1438–1444, 1980.
3. Lim VS, Henriquez C, Sievertsen G, et al: Ovarian function in chronic renal failure: Evidence suggesting hypothalamic anovulation. Ann Intern Med 93:21–27, 1980.
4. Manucci PM, Remuzzi G, Pusineri F, et al: Deamino-8-D-arginine vasopressin shortens the bleeding time in uremia. N Engl J Med 308:8–12, 1983.
5. Miyata T, Wada Y, Jida Y, et al: Implications of an increased oxidative stress in the formation of advanced glycation end products in patients with end-stage renal failure. Kidney Int 51:1170–1181, 1997.
6. Procci SR, Goldstein DA, Adelstein J, et al: Sexual dysfunction in the male patient with uremia. A reappraisal. Kidney Int 19:317–323, 1981.
7. Shemin D, Elnour M, Amarantes B, et al: Oral estrogens decrease bleeding time and improve clinical bleeding in patients with renal failure. Am J Med 89:436–440, 1990.

VII. End-Stage Renal Disease: Management

44. TECHNICAL ASPECTS OF HEMODIALYSIS

Jay B. Wish, M.D.

1. What is the technical basis for dialysis?

Dialysis refers to the diffusion of small molecules down their concentration gradient across a semipermeable membrane. In hemodialysis, blood is withdrawn from the patient's body and passed by a membrane that separates the blood from a dialysate solution on the other side. The dialysate solution contains electrolytes and glucose. Small molecules such as urea, potassium, and phosphorus diffuse down their concentration gradients from the blood into dialysate solution. Small molecules such as calcium and bicarbonate move down their concentration gradients from the dialysate solution into the blood. The effect is to remove low–molecular-weight toxins from the blood while, at the same time, increasing the plasma concentration of molecules that may be deficient in the patient with renal failure.

2. What are the two components of hemodialysis?

Hemodialysis is a process that consists of **diffusion** and **ultrafiltration**. Diffusion refers to the movement of small molecules down their concentration gradients. Urea is most commonly chosen as the marker for small molecule diffusion during dialysis. Urea itself is not a uremic toxin, but its blood level and clearance by dialysis seem to correlate with that of other uremic toxins. Diffusive clearance of urea by hemodialysis is a function of three factors:

1. **Blood flow rate:** More urea diffusion will occur if more blood is exposed to the dialysis membrane per unit of time.

2. **Membrane surface area:** The larger the surface area of the membrane, the more urea diffusion can occur per unit of time.

3. **Time:** The longer the dialysis treatment, the more urea diffusion will occur.

Ultrafiltration refers to the removal of water from the patient's circulation during the dialysis treatment. In peritoneal dialysis, the movement of water from the patient's circulation into the dialysate is propelled by an osmotic radiant caused by the high concentration of glucose in the dialysate (see Chapter 47, Technical Aspects of Peritoneal Dialysis). In hemodialysis, the movement of water from the patient's circulation to the dialysate is propelled by a transmembrane hydrostatic pressure gradient. The blood compartment is under positive pressure because the blood is being pushed by a pump through the extracorporeal circuit. Dialysate is under negative pressure, because the dialysate fluid is being pulled by a pump through the circuit. The sum of the positive pressure in the blood compartment and the negative pressure in the dialysate compartment equals the transmembrane pressure. Removal of water during the dialysis treatment is a function of three factors:

1. The transmembrane hydrostatic pressure

2. The ultrafiltration coefficient of the dialysis membrane, which is a function of its surface area, composition, thickness, and porosity

3. The duration of the dialysis treatment

3. What is the composition of the dialysate solution used for hemodialysis?

The dialysate solution consists of sodium, chloride, bicarbonate, calcium, magnesium, potassium, and dextrose. The concentrations of sodium and chloride approximate those in plasma.

Because the concentration of bicarbonate generally exceeds that of plasma in patients with renal failure, there is net diffusion of bicarbonate from the dialysate into the plasma. Concentration of magnesium in the dialysate is generally less than that of plasma, so that removal of magnesium usually occurs during the dialysis treatment. Concentration of potassium in the dialysate is variable and can be adjusted depending on the patient's serum potassium level. Concentration of calcium in the dialysate is also variable, so that net removal or delivery of calcium can occur during the dialysis, depending on the clinical indications. Concentration of glucose in dialysate is generally around 200 mg/dl, so that net diffusion of glucose into the patient occurs during the hemodialysis treatment.

4. What is the composition of the dialysis membrane?

Most dialysis membranes used in the United States are of a hollow fiber design. A typical hollow fiber artificial kidney is composed of approximately 10,000 capillary tubes arranged in parallel. The blood circulates through the lumen of the capillary tubes, and dialysate solution bathes the capillary tubes from the outside, moving in the opposite direction. A small minority of dialysis procedures in the United States are performed using parallel plate membranes, which are a stacked array of flat membrane envelopes. Blood circulates through the inside of the envelope, and the dialysate solution bathes the envelope from the outside.

Dialysis membranes are either cellulose-based or polymer-based. Cellulosic membranes cost less because of the abundance of raw cellulose in the environment. They tend to have a low ultrafiltration coefficient, can be reused frequently, and can be used with less technically sophisticated dialysis machines. A major disadvantage of cellulosic membranes is their "bioincompatibility." Some types of cellulosic membranes activate complement through the alternative pathway, leading to agglutination of white blood cells in the lungs and transient hypoxemia during dialysis. Chronic complement activation may contribute to the amyloidosis that may develop in patients who have been dialyzed for many years. Some studies suggest that the use of cellulosic membranes may be associated with higher rates of morbidity and mortality among patients with acute renal failure than those observed with the use of polymer membranes.

Polymer membranes cost more and must be used with more expensive dialysis machines that tightly control ultrafiltration. However, they are more biocompatible than cellulosic membranes and do not cause any complement activation. Furthermore, the high porosity of some of these membranes (termed *high-flux*) may augment the convective removal of uremic toxins through increased "solvent drag." Water purification standards for dialysate used with high-flux membranes must be extremely rigorous because of the potential for back filtration of contaminants (such as endotoxins) through the large pores in such membranes.

5. How is blood removed from the patient's body during hemodialysis?

Patients undergoing hemodialysis must have adequate access to their circulation to sustain extracorporeal blood flow rates of 300–400 ml/min. The superficial venous circulation is inadequate for this purpose. Most chronic hemodialysis patients have an arteriovenous fistula or an arteriovenous graft. An arteriovenous fistula is a direct surgical anastomosis between an artery and a superficial vein that causes the vein to dilate and develop a thickened wall. A well-developed arteriovenous fistula is the most desirable permanent hemodialysis access because it involves no foreign body and is able to sustain the greatest extracorporeal blood flow rates. An arteriovenous graft involves the surgical interposition of a synthetic blood vessel between an artery and a vein. This artificial vessel is placed below the skin such that it can be repeatedly cannulated with a large-bore needle as necessary to sustain adequate extracorporeal blood flow rate. The major complications associated with arteriovenous grafts or fistulas are thrombosis and infection.

When hemodialysis is required in patients who do not have a functioning arteriovenous fistula or graft, temporary or semipermanent vascular access is achieved by the use of a central venous catheter with two large-bore lumens; blood is removed from the patient through one lumen and blood is returned to the patient through the other lumen. Such catheters are generally placed into the superior vena cava through the internal jugular veins or into the interior vena cava through the femoral veins. If catheter access for hemodialysis is required for a long period of time, the catheter often is placed using a cuffed subcutaneous tunnel to decrease the incidence of infection. Such catheters generally are discouraged as long-term vascular access for hemodialysis patients because of their significantly higher rate of infectious complications when compared to arteriovenous fistulas and grafts. Subclavian vein dialysis catheters are discouraged because of a high rate of subsequent subclavian vein stenosis that may impede the ability to successfully construct a fistula or graft in the affected extremity.

6. What prevents the patient's blood from clotting while it is in the extracorporeal hemodialysis circuit?

Hemodialysis patients are routinely given heparin during the hemodialysis treatment to prevent thrombosis in the extracorporeal circuit. Although the dose of heparin required generally correlates with the weight of the patient and the duration of the hemodialysis treatment, the heparin dose must be individualized for each dialysis patient to prevent complications. Some dialysis facilities give an initial bolus of heparin followed by an infusion of heparin administered up to the last hour of the dialysis treatment. Other facilities administer heparin in 2 boluses, with approximately two thirds of the total dose given at the initiation of the dialysis treatment and approximately one third of the heparin dose given about 2 hours into the dialysis treatment. The appropriate dose of heparin is generally that which prevents clotting in the extracorporeal circuit and, at the same time, does not lead to bleeding from the needle puncture sites for more than 10 minutes after the needles are removed at the end of the hemodialysis treatment.

BIBLIOGRAPHY

1. Cimochaowski GE, Worley E, Rutherford WE, et al: Superiority of the internal jugular over the subclavian access for temporary dialysis. Nephron 54:151–161, 1990.
2. Dobkin JF, Miller MH, Steigbigel NH: Septicemia in patients on chronic hemodialysis. Ann Intern Med 88:28–33, 1987
3. Hakim RM: Clinical implications of hemodialysis membrane biocompatibility. Kidney Int 44:484–494, 1993.
4. Jannett TC, Wise MG, Shanklin NH, Sanders PW: Adaptive control of anticoagulation during hemodialysis. Kidney Int 45:912–915, 1994.
5. Ketchersid TL, van Stone JC: Dialysate potassium. Semin Dial 4:46–51, 1991.
6. Palmer BF: The effect of dialysate composition on systemic hemodynamics. Semin Dial 5:54–60, 1992.
7. Shusterman NH, Feldman HI, Wasserstein A, Strom BL: Reprocessing of hemodialyzers: A critical appraisal. Am J Kidney Dis 14:81–91, 1989.

45. HEMODIALYSIS: ASSESSING ADEQUACY

Eduardo Lacson, Jr., M.D.

1. What is adequate hemodialysis?

Adequate hemodialysis can be defined as the amount of dialysis required for optimal patient survival. Patient survival, morbidity, and quality of life all have been linked to measures of hemodialysis adequacy. Thus, it is important to know what adequate hemodialysis means and to be able to prescribe it, deliver it, and monitor its influence on the dialysis patient population.

2. How is the dose of dialysis measured?

In hemodialysis, an artificial kidney is used to replace the natural kidney's function to eliminate waste products and endogenous toxins. The dose of dialysis can therefore be measured by the clearance of these waste products. Like any drug clearance, this can be measured as:

$$\text{Clearance} = \log (C_t/C_o)^{Kt/V}$$

where C_t = concentration of the drug (toxin) at time point t, C_o = initial concentration prior to clearance, K = constant (value for rate of diffusion), t = time elapsed, and V = volume of distribution of the substance. Although many waste products accumulate in renal failure, by convention, clearance of urea has been used as a surrogate for clearance of "uremic" toxins.

3. Is urea the primary toxin that causes the signs and symptoms of uremia?

No. This is a common misconception. Urea per se is not inherently toxic and is not responsible for most of the signs and symptoms associated with uremia. It was chosen as a marker because it is easily measurable, well distributed in body tissues, elevated in renal failure, and dialyzable. The clearance of urea forms the cornerstone of measuring the efficacy, and by inference, the adequacy of dialysis therapy.

4. How do urea levels translate into practical and useful parameters to measure dialysis dose?

The serum urea levels before and after hemodialysis therapy are the main values considered when assessing the adequacy of treatment. Urea levels in dialysate also can be used but are not widely available. The Clinical Practice Guidelines Committee of the National Kidney Foundation's Dialysis Outcomes Quality Initiative (DOQI) recommends using serum levels to assess dialysis adequacy in conjunction with formal urea kinetic modeling, which uses complicated calculations to plot urea removal, urea generation, and volume of distribution. Recognizing that the parameter Kt/V is an exponent in the formula in question 2, the equation can be rearranged:

$$Kt/V = -Ln(C_t/C_o)$$

where C_t = postdialysis serum urea nitrogen and C_o = predialysis serum urea nitrogen level. In essence, Kt/V describes the fractional clearance of urea in relation to its distribution volume. The DOQI guidelines recommend the use of formal kinetic modeling, the natural logarithm formula, or the urea reduction ratio (see question 5) for assessment of dialysis adequacy.

5. How can Kt/V be measured if the tools for formal kinetic modeling are unavailable?

To further define Kt/V, one must understand that K ultimately represents the clearance coefficient of the dialyzer, t is the time on dialysis, and V is the volume of distribution of urea. Thus, Kt actually represents the volume of blood cleared of urea as it passes through the dialyzer. Because urea is also distributed in tissues, it must equilibrate with blood during dialysis so that only a certain portion of the total body urea can be cleared at any given time. Thus, the initial natural logarithm formula for Kt/V in question 4 was further refined by Daugirdas into:

$$Kt/V = -\text{Ln} (R - 0.008 \times t) + (4 - 3.5 R) (UF/W)$$

where R is the postdialysis over predialysis serum urea level (C_t/C_o), t = time of dialysis (in hours), UF = ultrafiltration volume in liters (amount of fluid removed by dialysis), and W = patient's postdialysis weight in kilograms. The first part of the equation represents the effects of urea generation during dialysis, and the second part represents the additional urea removed with the fluid during dialysis. Thus, even with a simple scientific calculator, one can calculate the Kt/V if one knows the predialysis serum urea level, the postdialysis serum urea level, the patient's predialysis weight, the postdialysis weight, and the duration of dialysis therapy.

6. What about the urea reduction ratio (URR)?

This even simpler calculation represents the drop in urea levels after dialysis in the form of a percentage. It is calculated as follows:

$$URR = 100\%[1 - (C_t/C_o)]$$

where C_t and C_o represent postdialysis and predialysis serum urea levels. However, the URR does not account for the contribution of ultrafiltration to the final delivered dose of dialysis. The inaccuracy makes it unreliable as the sole measure of the delivered dose of dialysis in individual patients. It remains a useful epidemiological tool, however.

7. Is Kt/V related to patient outcome?

Yes. Results of the National Cooperative Dialysis Study (NCDS) indicated high rates of morbidity in patients with a Kt/V < 1. Subsequent studies have correlated low Kt/V with mortality.

8. What is the target Kt/V for adequate hemodialysis?

The target delivered Kt/V has been subject to debate, and the DOQI Committee has stated after a thorough review of the literature that there is insufficient evidence to set an optimal value. However, with the support of data from the NCDS and other studies, the minimum delivered Kt/V recommended for all patients is set at 1.2 (this would roughly correlate to an average URR of > 65%). Some centers advocate higher Kt/V values of 1.4–1.6.

9. What is the difference between the prescribed dose and the delivered dose of hemodialysis?

Delivered Kt/V reflects the amount of dialysis the patient is actually getting. When starting a patient on dialysis, an estimate of the Kt/V prescription can be made by establishing values for K, t, and V. Most dialyzers will have a K value written on them as tested in vitro in ml/min that indicates the volume cleared of urea; t is the time (duration) of dialysis that is prescribed by the physician and is thus the variable under our control. V is the calculated volume of distribution of urea, which roughly corresponds to 0.6 ml/gm × body weight in grams. Therefore, a 60-kg man with a time of 3 hours on a polysulfone F8 dialyzer (K = 240 ml/min at a blood flow of 300 ml/min) will have a prescribed Kt/V of:

$$(240 \text{ ml/min}) \cdot (240 \text{ min})/(0.6) \cdot (60,000) = 57,600 \text{ ml}/36,000 \text{ ml} - Kt/V = 1.6$$

10. What Kt/V should be prescribed?

To prevent the delivered dose of hemodialysis from falling below the recommended minimum dose, the DOQI guidelines recommend a minimum prescribed Kt/V of 1.3. After all, in a random distribution falling on a bell-shaped curve, if the median is 1.2, half of the Kt/V will be less than 1.2 if it is the target. Thus, to increase the chances of most people having a delivered Kt/V of 1.2, the prescribed Kt/V should be at least 1.3.

11. What factors account for differences between prescribed and delivered Kt/V?

The many factors that can cause a discrepancy between the prescribed and delivered dose of dialysis can be grouped under (1) compromised urea clearance and (2) reductions in treatment time (see Tables).

Reasons for Compromised Urea Clearance

PATIENT-RELATED REASONS	STAFF-RELATED REASONS	MECHANICAL PROBLEMS
Decreased effective time on dialysis	Decreased effective time	Dialyzer clotting during
Decreased blood flow rates (BFR)	Decreased blood flow rate	reuse
Access clotting	Less than prescribed	Blood pump calibration
Use of intravenous catheters (instead	Difficult cannulation	error
of an arteriovenous graft or fistula)	Decreased dialysate flow rate	Dialysate pump
Inadequate flow through vascular	Less than prescribed	calibration error
access	Inappropriately set	Inaccurate estimation of
Recirculation	Dialyzer	dialyzer performance
Use of catheters	Inadequate quality control	by the manufacturer
Inadequate access for prescribed	of "reuse"	Variability in blood
BFR		tubing
Stenosis, clotting of access		

Adapted from Parker TF: Trends and concepts in the prescription and delivery of dialysis in the United States. Semin Nephrol 12:267–275, 1992.

Reasons for Decreased Effective Time on Dialysis

PATIENT-RELATED REASONS	STAFF-RELATED REASONS	MECHANICAL REASONS
Late start (patient tardy)	Late start (staff tardy)	Clotting of dialyzer
Early sign-off	Wrong patient taken off	Dialyzer leaks
With consent (i.e., symptoms)	Time calculated incorrectly	Machine malfunction
Against advice (i.e., social)	Time on/off read incorrectly	
Medical complications (e.g., hypo-	Clinical deficiencies (e.g.,	
tension)	no time registered)	
"No show"	Premature discontinuation	
	for unit convenience	
	Scheduling conflicts	
	Emergencies	
	Incorrect assumptions of	
	continuous treatment time	
	(e.g., failure to account	
	for interruptions of treat-	
	ment such as repositioning	
	needles or accidental	
	removal)	
	Inaccurate assessment of ef-	
	fective time by using	
	variable time pieces	

Adapted from Parker TF: Trends and concepts in the prescription and delivery of dialysis in the United States. Semin Nephrol 12:267–275, 1992.

12. How often should adequacy of hemodialysis be measured?

Because clinical signs and symptoms alone are not reliable indicators of dialysis adequacy, it is recommended that adequacy be measured using Kt/V for the delivered dose of dialysis. By convention, dialysis lab tests are drawn monthly, and it is pragmatic to do Kt/V measurements at the same time.

13. What are middle molecules?

There are hypothetical substances, theorized to be 500–2,000 daltons in molecular weight, that were historically thought to affect patient outcome as they accumulated in renal failure. No middle molecular toxins have ever been specifically identified. However, the benefits of longer dialysis time on patient survival theoretically could reflect clearance of middle molecules. The newer high-flux membranes with larger pores are theoretically able to clear middle molecules better than regular high-efficiency or cellulosic dialysis membranes. The benefit of high-flux dialysis will need to be proven in future clinical trials.

14. What lies ahead for optimizing dialysis therapy?

The National Institutes of Health (NIH) are currently conducting a multicenter trial called the Hemo Study, which is a prospective, randomized trial designed to assess the effect of hemodialysis dose (small molecule clearance) and flux (middle molecule clearance) on morbidity and mortality. Results of this trial may establish new goals and guidelines that may strengthen or revise current standards for adequate hemodialysis. Many researchers are also trying to find novel measures of and correlations with outcome and to improve the current methods by incorporating factors such as urea rebound.

BIBLIOGRAPHY

1. Collins AJ, Ma JZ, Umen A, Keshaviah P: Urea index and other predictors of hemodialysis patient survival. Am J Kidney Dis 23:272–282, 1994.
2. Consensus Conference Development Panel: Morbidity and mortality of renal dialysis: An NIH consensus conference statement. Ann Intern Med 121:62–70, 1994.
3. Daugirdas JT: Second generation logarithmic estimates of single-pool variable volume Kt/V: An analysis of error. J Am Soc Nephrol 4:1205–1213, 1992.
4. Gotch FA, Sargent JA: A mechanistic analysis of the National Cooperative Dialysis Study (NCDS). Kidney Int 28:526–534, 1985.
5. Hakim RM: Assessing the adequacy of dialysis. Kidney Int 37:822–832, 1990.
6. Held PJ, Levin NW, Randall R, et al: Mortality and duration of hemodialysis treatment. JAMA 265:871–875, 1991.
7. Lacson E, Wish JB: Hemodialysis adequacy. In Henrich W (ed): Principles and Practice of Dialysis, 2nd ed. Baltimore, Williams & Wilkins, 1998.
8. NKF-DOQI: Clinical practice guidelines for hemodialysis adequacy. Am J Kidney Dis 50(suppl 2):S15–S66, 1997.
9. Parker TF: Trends and concepts in the prescription and delivery of dialysis in the United States. Semin Nephrol 12:267–275, 1992.
10. Sehgal AR, Snow RJ, Singer ME, et al: Barriers to adequate delivery of hemodialysis. Am J Kidney Dis 31:593–601, 1998.

46. COMPLICATIONS OF HEMODIALYSIS

Lavinia A. Negrea, M.D.

1. What is the most common intradialytic complication?

Hypotension occurs in 10–30% of hemodialysis treatments. It is more frequent in the elderly and in women.

2. Name the most common causes of intradialytic hypotension.

Factors related to **decreases in blood volume** include:
• Target "dry" weight set too low
• Too rapid removal of water (high ultrafiltration rate)
• Low dialysate sodium concentration
Cardiovascular factors include:
• Dialysate that is relatively too warm
• Food ingestion during dialysis (splanchnic vasodilatation)
• Administration of short-acting antihypertensive medications prior to dialysis
• Lack of peripheral vasoconstriction due to autonomic neuropathy
• Congestive heart failure
• Acetate-containing dialysate

3. What life-threatening disorders should be considered in the differential diagnosis of hypotension during dialysis?

Myocardial infarction
Pericardial tamponade
Arrhythmia
Internal hemorrhage
Sepsis
Air embolism

4. What approaches will prevent hypotension during dialysis?

Prevention of hypotension can be achieved by frequent determinations of the "dry weight" (the weight below which the chronic hemodialysis patient has orthostatic hypotension), avoiding large interdialytic fluid gains, and holding short-acting antihypertensive medications until immediately prior to dialysis.

5. Describe the clinical manifestations of dialysis dysequilibrium syndrome.

Clinical manifestations occur during or immediately after dialysis and include headache, lethargy, nausea, muscular twitching, and malaise. Symptoms can progress to obtundation, seizures, or coma. The syndrome occurs most commonly after the first few dialysis treatments in patients with chronic renal failure and long-standing uremia.

6. What causes dialysis dysequilibrium, and how can it be prevented?

The syndrome occurs when the plasma solute level is rapidly lowered during dialysis. Plasma becomes hypotonic with respect to the brain tissue and water shifts in the brain, leading to cerebral edema. Acute changes in cerebrospinal fluid pH also have been incriminated. Dysequilibrium is best prevented by deliberately limiting solute removal during the first treatment session and by stepwise increases in the subsequent sessions. Administration of mannitol also may prevent shifts of water into the brain.

7. What are dialyzer reactions?

There are two main types of dialyzer reactions:

1. **Type A, or anaphylactic reaction**. The symptoms occur during the first few minutes of dialysis and include anxiety, dyspnea, urticaria, and pruritus. These reactions are thought to be due to residual amounts of ethylene oxide, used for sterilization of dialyzers, and can range from mild discomfort to true anaphylaxis.

2. **Type B, or nonspecific dialyzer reaction**. Symptoms occur within the first 30 minutes of dialysis and are less severe, much more common, and include chest pain, back pain, varying degrees of nausea, and pruritus. Use of unsubstituted cellulose membranes and activation of complement are the implicated etiologies.

8. Which processes are responsible for dialysis-associated hypoxemia?

Hypoxemia occurs commonly during hemodialysis. With acetate dialysis, the primary mechanism is the loss of bicarbonate and carbon dioxide by diffusion into the dialysate, with subsequent hypoventilation. Unsubstituted cellulose dialysis membranes can impair intrapulmonary oxygen diffusion through complement activation and sequestration of neutrophils within pulmonary capillaries.

9. Name the most important factors contributing to arrhythmias during dialysis.

The hemodialysis procedure does not increase the likelihood of arrhythmias in all patients. In patients with ischemic heart disease and those receiving cardiac glycosides, factors contributing to arrhythmias are acidosis, hypoxemia, hypotension, removal of certain antiarrhythmic agents during dialysis, hypokalemia, and hypomagnesemia.

10. What accounts for increased bleeding tendencies in hemodialysis patients?

Uremic bleeding (see Chapter 43, Other Manifestations of Uremia) can persist in some patients after initiation of dialysis. This can be aggravated by intradialytic administration of heparin.

11. What causes chest pain during hemodialysis?

Chest pain occurs in 1–4% of dialysis treatments. It is often associated with back pain when due to "dialyzer reaction" (see question 7). It should be differentiated from other causes such as angina or hemolytic reactions.

12. What factors are responsible for headaches during dialysis?

Headaches can be a subtle manifestation of dysequilibrium syndrome. In patients who are coffee drinkers, headache can be a manifestation of caffeine withdrawal as the blood caffeine concentration is acutely reduced during dialysis.

13. What causes nausea and vomiting during dialysis?

Nausea and vomiting occur in up to 10% of dialysis treatments. Most episodes are related to hypotension. Nausea can also be an early manifestation of dysequilibrium syndrome.

14. What causes pruritus during dialysis?

Pruritus is experienced by many dialysis patients, sometimes with exacerbation during or immediately after dialysis. Proposed causes are dryness of the skin, secondary hyperparathyroidism, abnormal calcium-phosphorus product, and elevated plasma histamine concentration.

15. Are fever and chills during hemodialysis always caused by infection?

Febrile episodes in dialysis should always be aggressively evaluated, with infection-induced fevers representing the main concern. The vascular access site is the source of 50–80% of bacteremic episodes in hemodialysis patients, most often associated with temporary catheters, least often with native arteriovenous fistulas. Febrile reactions during hemodialysis also can be related to exposure to endotoxins originating from the dialyzer or dialysate. These "pyrogenic reactions" are manifested by fever, chills, nausea, and hypotension. Patients with pyrogen-related fever are afebrile prior to dialysis, and no bacteremia can be demonstrated in blood cultures.

16. What causes hemolysis during dialysis?

Hemolysis can be a medical emergency, presenting with chest tightness, back pain, shortness of breath, fall in hematocrit, and hyperkalemia. Acute hemolysis almost always is due to a technical problem (chloramine-T or nitrates contamination, overheated or hypotonic dialysis solutions).

17. What is the cause of muscle cramps during dialysis?

Muscle cramps occur in up to 20% of hemodialysis treatments and appear to be related to rapid ultrafiltration. Preventive measures include avoidance of large fluid gains between treatments and administration of quinine sulfate prior to dialysis.

BIBLIOGRAPHY

1. Bregman H, Daugirdas JT, Ing TS: Complications during hemodialysis. In Daugirdas JT, Ing TS (eds): Handbook of Dialysis, 2nd ed. Boston, Little, Brown, 1994, pp 149–168.
2. Jameson MD, Wiegmann TB: Principles, uses and complications of hemodialysis. Med Clin North Am 74:945–960, 1990.
3. Kaufman AM, Polaschegg H, Levin NW: Complications during hemodialysis. In Nissenson AR, Fine RN (eds): Dialysis Therapy, 2nd ed. St. Louis, Mosby, 1993, pp 109–132.
4. Schulman G, Hakim RM: Complications of hemodialysis. In Jacobson HR, Striker GE, Klahr S (eds): The Principles and Practice of Nephrology, 2nd ed. St. Louis, Mosby, 1995, pp 673–683.

47. TECHNICAL ASPECTS OF PERITONEAL DIALYSIS

Miriam F. Weiss, M.D.

1. How is a peritoneal dialysis patient like a salmon?

A canal that passes from the peritoneal cavity through the body wall to a pore on the surface of the abdomen has been identified in salmonids (*Salmo giardneri, Salmo salar, Coregonus arte-dii*). Peritoneal fluid, cells, and injected particles or bacteria are actually "voided" from the pore enabling the peritoneum to function like an excretory organ. By creating an artificial abdominal pore (peritoneal dialysis catheter), the inherent "excretory" capacity of the peritoneum is made available to sustain life in patients with kidney failure.

2. How does peritoneal dialysis work?

Dialysate solution (containing balanced electrolytes and high concentrations of dextrose) is introduced into the peritoneal cavity. Uremic toxins diffuse across peritoneal capillaries, through the interstitium, across the peritoneal mesothelial layer, and into the peritoneal cavity. Fluid is removed by ultrafiltration when water in the blood moves across these peritoneal layers into the hypertonic dialysate along an osmotic gradient. Toxins and ultrafiltered water are removed when the dialysate is drained from the peritoneal cavity.

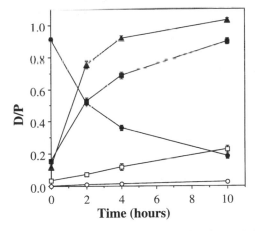

Increasing dialysate levels of urea (*closed triangle*), creatinine (*closed square*), beta$_2$-microglobulin (*open square*), and protein (*open circle*) over the course of a long dwell. Results are expressed as the ratio of the level in dialysate (D) to the level in plasma (P). The decrease in the ratio of initial dialysate glucose to dialysate glucose (*closed circle*) is also shown (D/D0). The data represent the mean ± standard error of 38 peritoneal equilibration tests.

3. What is the peritoneum?

The peritoneum is a membrane lining the surface of the abdominal cavity and its organs. It includes the visceral peritoneum, lining the abdominal and pelvic walls and the diaphragm, and the parietal peritoneum, covering the stomach, intestines, and surface of the liver and spleen. In the supine position, most of the dialysate in the peritoneal cavity is distributed near the liver and spleen and between the small intestines. The peritoneum forms a closed sac in men. In women, the fallopian tubes open into the peritoneum.

4. Why doesn't dialysis fluid drain through the fallopian tubes and leak from the uterus in women treated by peritoneal dialysis?

The tubes are usually collapsed, so there is no free communication between the peritoneum and the exterior. On the other hand, female patients occasionally report blood in their dialysate during ovulation. In patients with endometriosis, intraperitoneal bleeding may be seen as blood-tinged dialysate during the menstrual period.

5. How big is the peritoneum?

The surface area of the peritoneum is equivalent to that of the skin, approximately 1.73 m^2 in an average-sized adult male. Peritoneal blood flow is between 75 and 200 ml/minute, compared with normal renal blood flow of ~400 ml/minute. The hypertonic dialysate instilled into the peritoneal cavity causes vasodilation, thus increasing blood flow.

6. What are the indications for peritoneal dialysis?

Peritoneal dialysis is a long-term treatment alternative for *any* patient with end-stage renal disease. Peritoneal dialysis has medical advantages over hemodialysis in some circumstances. It has been a successful adjuvant to the management of congestive heart failure refractory to conventional medical treatment, even in patients who do not have renal failure.

7. What are the contraindications to peritoneal dialysis?

There are few absolute contraindications to peritoneal dialysis. A patient or caregiver must be able to master the concepts and procedures necessary to perform dialysis in a safe way. Relative but major contraindications to peritoneal dialysis include (1) inguinal, umbilical, or diaphragmatic hernias, particularly if pleuroperitoneal leak and hydrothorax develop; (2) ostomies (colostomy or nephrostomy); (3) recent aortic valve prosthesis; and (4) abdominal wall abscess. Minor contraindications include morbid obesity (may necessitate omentectomy at the time of catheter placement), polycystic kidneys (increased intra-abdominal pressure), and diverticulosis.

8. What are the unique design features of a chronic peritoneal dialysis catheter?

In 1968, Tenckhoff developed a silicone catheter with two Dacron cuffs. The cuffs are positioned within the abdominal wall just above the peritoneum and just below the skin (see Figure). The Dacron cuffs heal with the formation of fibrosis, preventing bacteria from moving from the skin into the tunnel (which bridges the distance between the two cuffs) and the peritoneum. A patient with a well-healed peritoneal catheter is free to shower or swim without danger of bacteria entering the peritoneum around the catheter.

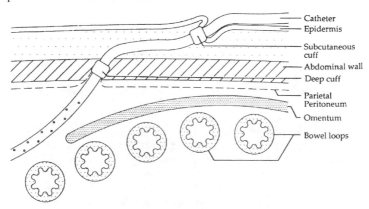

Cross section of the proper position of a double-cuffed Tenckhoff catheter as it crosses the abdominal wall. (From Ash SR, Carr DJ, Diaz-Buxo JA: Peritoneal access devices. In Nissenson AR, Fine RN, Gentile DE (eds): Clinical Dialysis, 2nd ed. Norwalk, CT, Appleton & Lange, 1990, pp 212–239, with permission.)

9. Compare peritoneoscopic to surgical placement of chronic peritoneal dialysis catheters.

	Advantages	*Disadvantages*
Peritoneoscopy	Outpatient procedure, local anesthesia and analgesia Smaller exit-site incision	Requires specialized equipment Greater risk of subcutaneous leak of dialysate, if catheter is used early Greater likelihood of developing late pericatheter hernia
Surgical Placement	Direct visualization of placement for both external and internal cuffs Reduced risk of subcutaneous leak of dialysate, if catheter used early	Surgical procedure, requiring general anesthesia Larger exit-site incision

10. How long is the healing period after catheter placement?

Catheter break-in periods of 10 days to 2 weeks are recommended to allow the cuffs to seal. To prevent increased intra-abdominal pressure that may disrupt fibroblast ingrowth into the cuffs, patients should avoid strenuous activity or heavy lifting. Physicians should avoid infusing full volumes of dialysate into the peritoneal cavity. Fluid leakage around the cuffs inhibits fibroblasts from growing into the cuffs and encourages the development of infection along the catheter tract, or peritonitis. When the need to treat uremia is urgent, patients can be started on hemodialysis through a temporary catheter. Alternatively, they can be hospitalized for low-volume exchanges while on bed rest.

11. What is an "exchange"?

An exchange consists of draining out dialysate that has been dwelling in the peritoneum and infusing a fresh volume of dialysate. Commercial dialysate comes in flexible plastic bags. The standard size is 2–3 L per exchange. An array of devices and systems are available to enable patients to perform sterile connection and disconnection procedures during the exchange.

12. What do CAPD, CCPD, and NIPD stand for?

- Chronic ambulatory peritoneal dialysis (CAPD) consists of 4–5 exchanges using 2–3 L of dialysate with each exchange. The patient carries fluid in the abdomen 24 hours per day. Exchanges are spaced out throughout the day, usually upon awakening, at lunchtime, at dinnertime, and before bed.
- In continuous cycler-assisted peritoneal dialysis (CCPD), an automated cycler machine performs some of the dialysis exchanges (usually at night while the patient is asleep). When the patient is not connected to the cycler machine, the peritoneal cavity is filled with a volume of dialysate that is either drained by hand or drained when the patient connects back to the machine for another set of exchanges.
- Nocturnal intermittent peritoneal dialysis (NIPD) is like CCPD, except the peritoneal cavity is empty of fluid when the patient is not using the cycler machine.

13. What is the composition of peritoneal dialysate?

Current commercially available dialysate solutions contain dextrose, in concentrations of 1.5%, 2.5%, or 4.25%, as the main osmotic solute. Maximal ultrafiltration occurs by 3–4 hours using 1.5% dextrose (see Figure). By 8–10 hours, most patients will have absorbed a significant amount of dextrose or diluted the dextrose content with ultrafiltrate. As a result, the osmotic gradient will be dissipated. At this point, dialysate can be absorbed, resulting in a net positive fluid balance. Using 4.25% dextrose dialysate, maximal ultrafiltration occurs about 5 hours after infusion, and net positive ultrafiltration is not dissipated for 12–15 hours. Therefore, higher concentrations of dialysate glucose are useful in CAPD for the overnight dialysis exchange and in CCPD for the long diurnal dwell. Polyglucose solutions that are not absorbed are currently undergoing testing as alternative osmotic agents. These solutions will have the advantage of providing continuous ultrafiltration without dissipation of the osmotic gradient.

The major bicarbonate-generating base used in peritoneal dialysate is lactate (35–40 mEq/L). Although only L-lactate is normally present in the body, DL-lactate is used. The liver can generate bicarbonate from both isomers. Some loss of bicarbonate into the dialysate occurs early in the exchange but is compensated by the metabolism of the administered lactate.

The sodium concentration of the dialysate, 132 mEq/L, is slightly lower than serum (135–142 mEq/L) to allow net removal of Na^+ and Cl^- to take place across the dialysate. Commercial dialysate contains no potassium. Peritoneal dialysis is effective at controlling hyperkalemia in most patients treated with peritoneal dialysis, in part, through constant removal of K^+ across the peritoneum.

Standard dialysate solutions contain 3.5 mEq/L of calcium. Thus, the ionized calcium concentration is much higher than normal blood ionized calcium, causing a net positive calcium balance. Over time, the increased absorption of calcium from dialysate, concurrent with the routine use of calcium-containing phosphate binders, can result in excessive suppression of hyperparathyroidism, a form of renal osteodystrophy called *hypoplastic bone disease*, and hypercalcemia. Dialysate solutions containing 2.5 mEq/L of calcium are also available and may mitigate this problem.

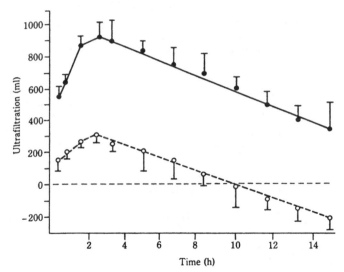

Net ultrafiltration (volume drained versus volume instilled) as a function of time after infusion of dialysate. The figure compares 1.5% dextrose (open circles) with 4.25% dextrose (closed circles). (From Sorkin MI, Diaz-Buxo JA: Physiology of peritoneal dialysis. In Daugirdas JJ, Ing TS (eds): Handbook of Dialysis, 2nd ed. Boston, Little, Brown, 1994, pp 245–261, with permission.)

14. What is a peritoneal dialysis prescription, and how is it determined?

The dialysis prescription encompasses the volume of dialysate, the osmolality of the dialysate, and the frequency of exchanges—three factors that determine solute clearance in peritoneal dialysis. Peritoneal permeability is a major factor in determining the rate of fluid and solute removal during peritoneal dialysis. Norms have been established that enable the nephrologist to categorize patients' permeability patterns (see question 15). Patients with high peritoneal permeability (rapid transporters) have an early loss of osmotic gradient because glucose is quickly absorbed across the peritoneum. To prevent fluid overload, such patients must have decreased dwell time in order to drain dialysate when the osmolality of the fluid is still high. These patients respond best when treated with CCPD or NIPD.

15. What is the peritoneal equilibration test?

Although several standardized tests to determine the function of the peritoneal membrane have been developed, the fast peritoneal equilibration test is most widely used. This test is reproducible and accurate. The test starts with drainage of the previous night's dialysis bag. A fresh bag of 2.5% dextrose is infused over 10 minutes. A blood sample is taken during the equilibration period. After 4 hours, the dialysate is drained, and a sample is taken. The volume of the drained dialysate is ascertained. Both dialysate and blood are assayed for creatinine. The 4-hour dialysate/plasma ratio (D/P creatinine) and the net ultrafiltration (volume drained minus volume exchanged) are compared to standards that allow the nephrologist to classify the patient's peritoneal function as low, low-average, high-average, or high in its transport characteristics. Patients with high transport characteristics do better with relatively short dwells. These rapid transporters will have optimal clearance of uremic toxins and removal of fluid with frequent short exchanges, such as can be provided by an automatic cycling device. Patients with low transport characteristics need to allow the dialysate to dwell for longer periods of time to optimize removal of uremic toxins and excess water.

16. How is adequacy of treatment determined in patients on peritoneal dialysis?

In contrast to the experience with hemodialysis (see Chapter 45, Hemodialysis: Assessing Adequacy), no large, multicenter study has been performed to determine the optimal amount of peritoneal dialysis. It is difficult to compare peritoneal dialysis and hemodialysis, because one is a continuous therapy and the other intermittent. Peritoneal dialysis patients seem to get by on about half the urea clearance of hemodialysis patients. This may be because the peritoneum is removing more large uremic toxins than the hemodialysis membrane. Alternatively, patients treated by peritoneal dialysis may tolerate a constant level of uremic toxins better than the peaks and valleys experienced by patients treated by hemodialysis.

Whereas the formula Kt/V (K − clearance coefficient of the dialyzer, t = time on dialysis, and V = volume of distribution of urea) is a very good way of assessing if adequate hemodialysis is being given to a patient, the best method for assessing adequacy for peritoneal dialysis has not been determined. Many centers ask patients to collect all of their dialysate (and any urine they have made) for a 24-hour period and to bring these volumes of fluid for testing every 6 months. The volume of urine and dialysate and the urea and creatinine concentrations are then measured, along with blood levels of these solutes, and total clearance of urea and creatinine are calculated by standard formulas. Mathematical approximations of Kt/V in peritoneal dialysis may be particularly inaccurate because they are based on assumptions about the patient's weight and the volume of distribution of urea that are probably incorrect. Nonetheless, it is recommended that patients on peritoneal dialysis reach an average weekly Kt/V target of 1.7–2.2. The total weekly creatinine clearance should be greater than 60 L/week, corrected for body surface area.

17. Why do patients treated with peritoneal dialysis require a high-protein diet?

Patients treated by hemodialysis are given a low-protein diet to reduce the intake of urea precursors. By contrast, patients treated by peritoneal dialysis lose between 10 and 40 gm of protein across the peritoneal membrane each day. As a result, high-protein diets (1.8–2.5 gm/kg body weight/day) are prescribed to replace these losses. Amino acid dialysate solutions are also available to malnourished patients treated by peritoneal dialysis. Amino acids contribute to the hypertonicity of the dialysate but also are absorbed across the peritoneal membrane and through the peritoneal lymphatics.

18. How does peritoneal dialysis compare to hemodialysis?

The usual peritoneal dialysis prescription does not provide as much clearance of low–molecular-weight solutes as does the usual hemodialysis regimen. However, peritoneal dialysis removes high–molecular-weight substances better than hemodialysis. In theory, increased clearance of high–molecular-weight solutes may improve long-term control of the uremic syndrome. However, recent studies have raised the concern that patients treated by peritoneal dialysis may not exhibit adequate clearance of uremic toxins over long periods of time. Current standard of care is to increase clearance by using the maximum volume of dialysate tolerated by patients and by increasing the frequency of dialysis exchanges consistent with the patient's underlying transport characteristics, as determined by the peritoneal equilibration test (see Chapter 48, Complications of Peritoneal Dialysis).

BIBLIOGRAPHY

1. Ash SR, Carr DJ, Diaz-Buxo JA: Peritoneal access devices. In Nissenson AR, Fine RN, Gentile DE (eds): Clinical Dialysis, 2nd ed. Norwalk, CT, Appleton & Lange, 1990, pp 212–239.
2. Blake PG: A review of the DOQI recommendations for peritoneal dialysis. Perit Dial Int 18:247–251, 1998.
3. Dobbie JW: From philosopher to fish: The comparative anatomy of the peritoneal cavity as an excretory organ and its significance for peritoneal dialysis in man. Perit Dial Int 8:1–3, 1988.
4. Keshaviah PR: Adequacy of CAPD: A quantitative approach. Kidney Int 42(Suppl 38):S160–S164, 1992.
5. Kopple JD, Gao XL, Qing DP: Dietary protein, urea nitrogen appearance, and total nitrogen appearance in chronic renal failure and CAPD patients. Kidney Int 52:486–494, 1997.
6. Nolph JD, Lindblat AS, Navak JW: Current concepts: Continuous ambulatory peritoneal dialysis. N Engl J Med 318:1595–1600, 1988.
7. Pastan S, Bailey J: Dialysis therapy. N Engl J Med 338:1428–1437, 1998.
8. Sorkin MI, Diaz-Buxo JA: Physiology of peritoneal dialysis. In Daugirdas JT, Ing TS (eds): Handbook of Dialysis, 2nd ed. Boston, Little, Brown, 1994, pp 245–261.
9. Twardowski ZJ, Nolph KD, Khanna R: Peritoneal equilibration test. Perit Dial Bull 7:138–147, 1987.
10. Tzamaloukas AH, Murata GH, Piraino B, et al: Peritoneal urea and creatinine clearances in continuous peritoneal dialysis patients with different types of peritoneal solute transport. Kidney Int 53:1405–1411, 1998.

48. COMPLICATIONS OF PERITONEAL DIALYSIS

Carolyn P. Cacho, M.D.

1. What is peritonitis?

The presence of more than 100 white blood cells per cubic millimeter in the peritoneal fluid and greater than 50% polymorphonuclear neutrophils defines peritonitis in the peritoneal dialysis patient. Visibly cloudy effluent and abdominal pain usually herald the onset of the illness. Fever, nausea, and diarrhea are less consistently present. On examination, abdominal pain, decreased bowel sounds, guarding, and rebound tenderness are all typical findings.

2. What is the cause of peritonitis in patients treated with peritoneal dialysis?

About 95% of cases are caused by bacterial infection. Historically, *Staphylococcus epidermidis* infections due to touch contamination were the most common causative agents. However, with the introduction of the Y-set and double-bag peritoneal dialysis systems, touch contamination has declined as the cause of peritonitis. Currently, gram-positive infections account for 50–80% of all episodes of peritonitis in peritoneal dialysis patients. Gram-negative organisms account for 20–30% of all episodes. Unlike infections caused by gram-positive organisms, which usually result from touch contamination, gram negative infections derive from a variety of sources including the skin, bowel, urinary tract, and contaminated water. Less than 5% of cases are caused by fungi, usually *Candida* species. While the number of cases is relatively small, fungal peritonitis often follows repeated episodes of bacterial peritonitis and invariably necessitates removal of the peritoneal dialysis catheter. Rare cases of peritonitis are caused by anaerobic bacteria or mycobacteria. Finally, peritonitis may be caused by hypersensitivity to intraperitoneally administered drugs (e.g., vancomycin), a phenomenon characterized by a high number of eosinophils in the dialysis effluent.

3. What is the appropriate diagnostic work-up of peritonitis in a peritoneal dialysis patient?

The appearance of cloudy dialysis effluent should prompt the simultaneous initiation of the diagnostic evaluation and treatment of peritonitis. A dialysate cell count and differential are obtained to provide quick confirmation of the diagnosis. The Gram stain is often negative early in the course of infection. However, when organisms are seen, the results can be used to tailor therapy. Bacterial, fungal, and mycobacterial cultures should be obtained and are positive in more than 80% of cases. Because it is unusual for peritonitis to cause systemic illness in this setting, blood cultures are indicated only when signs of bowel perforation or sepsis are present.

4. How should peritonitis be treated?

Initiation of therapy need not be delayed until results of the diagnostic work-up are available. Initial therapy should cover both gram-positive and gram-negative organisms. The emergence of vancomycin-resistant organisms and concern over the adverse effect of aminoglycosides on residual renal function has increased the controversy regarding the choice of antibiotics. A first-generation cephalosporin can be administered intraperitoneally for initial gram-positive coverage instead of vancomycin. However, this choice requires careful follow-up of culture results because gram-positive infecting agents are more likely to be resistant to a cephalosporin than to vancomycin. An alternative protocol may use vancomycin initially with a change to a second agent when culture results are available. Intraperitoneal aminoglycosides remain the first choice for gram-negative coverage; however, recent guidelines recommend omitting a loading dose. This empiric regimen should be modified based on culture and sensitivity results. Treatment typically is continued for a total of 10–14 days.

Peritonitis in the peritoneal dialysis patient is usually a benign disease, and a response to treatment, indicated by a normalization of the cell count, clearing of the dialysate, and improvement of clinical symptoms, should occur within 48 hours. Persistent elevation of the white cell count or predominance of neutrophils, cloudy dialysate, or continued abdominal pain should increase concern about infections with *Staphylococcus aureus, Pseudomonas,* or fungal species. In comparison to patients with other gram-positive infections, those with *Staphylococcus aureus* infections generally have more severe disease and may even present with toxic shock–type illness. For this reason, a longer treatment course of 21 days is recommended. Pseudomonal infections are particularly difficult to eradicate and should be treated with two antibiotics for at least 21 days. Frequently, this regimen fails, and the catheter must be removed. The diagnosis of a fungal peritonitis must be considered if the dialysate is slow to clear. On occasion, fungal elements can be seen on the Gram stain, and the organisms will grow when the peritoneal fluid is sent for fungal culture. Recent recommendations for the treatment of fungal peritonitis suggest a trial of intraperitoneal fluconazole and oral flucytosine without the removal of the catheter. A more conservative alternative is to remove the catheter and administer a prolonged course of amphotericin B (total dose of about 1 gm) on hemodialysis. Once the infection has cleared, the peritoneal dialysis catheter can be reinserted. As is often the case after severe or repeated episodes of peritonitis, peritoneal scarring may prevent successful resumption of peritoneal dialysis.

Treatment of peritonitis often fails when the disease is caused by an abdominal catastrophe such as bowel perforation. The mortality rate in such cases is as high as 50%. Diagnostic studies such as computed tomography (CT) scans or contrast enemas are helpful when they confirm the presence of a perforated viscus or bowel interruption. However, a negative study does not rule out the presence of an abdominal catastrophe. The approach to such cases includes broadening of antibiotic coverage to include gram-negative organisms and antianaerobic coverage, consideration of empiric antifungal therapy, and early exploratory laparotomy. At least one study has found a correlation between mortality and time to surgical intervention.

5. What is an exit site infection?

Unlike peritonitis, which has a well-established and accepted definition, criteria for establishing diagnosis of an exit site infection are somewhat unsettled. Bacteria colonize most healed exit sites. These bacteria can cause infection if the exit site is traumatized, improperly anchored, or subjected to prolonged soaking. An infected exit site is often erythematous, indurated, and tender. It may bleed or exude pus. In most cases the infecting organism can be determined from a swab culture. If left untreated, the infection may extend into the tunnel and eventually cause peritonitis.

6. How is an exit site infection treated?

The treatment of exit site infection ranges from the use of astringent soaks to the administration of parenteral antibiotics. In cases of mild erythema and a negative bacterial culture, hypertonic saline or dilute solutions of bleach and hydrogen peroxide may reverse the condition. Induration, tenderness, or a positive culture warrants the use of antibiotics. Topical vancomycin, tobramycin, or gentamicin, in combination with an astringent soak, often will cure exit site infections. When topical treatment fails or in the case of *Pseudomonas* exit site infection, parenteral antibiotics should be used. For gram-positive infections, vancomycin may be given intraperitoneally. For persistent infections, the addition of oral rifampin is helpful. Gram-negative infections usually respond to the intraperitoneal administration of an aminoglycoside or a third-generation cephalosporin. Infections due to *Pseudomonas* also should be treated with a second agent such as ciprofloxacin. Failure to respond to parenteral antibiotics or the occurrence of relapsing exit site infections should prompt catheter replacement.

7. How can exit site infections be prevented?

The most important step in the prevention of exit site infection occurs at the time of catheter implantation. The use of a catheter with a swan-neck, which drains downward, and two cuffs, which serve as barriers to bacteria, has been shown to decrease the rate of exit site infection. Perioperative antibiotics, catheter immobilization, and perioperative eradication of nasal

Staphylococcus aureus are additional helpful measures. Long-term strategies for prevention of exit site infection include daily care with a nonirritating cleansing agent.

8. What is the approach to inflow and outflow pain?

Pain with instillation of dialysate occasionally occurs, especially in patients who have recently started peritoneal dialysis. The pain is caused by the jet of fluid striking the viscera. Catheters with a curled intraperitoneal segment distribute the fluid over a wider area and therefore are less likely to cause this problem. However, these catheters may be more prone to kinking. Lowering the bag of dialysate decreases the rate of flow and is usually enough to stop the pain. Laparoscopic manipulation and laxation may also allow the catheter to migrate to a more comfortable position.

Outflow pain most commonly occurs at the end of drain when the abdomen is empty. It is caused by the tip of the catheter irritating the bladder or intestine. Like inflow pain, it is observed less often with curled catheters. The problem can be improved by instructing the patient to start filling with the onset of the pain and to avoid an empty peritoneum. A tidal program that leaves a small (200 ml) volume of dialysate in the peritoneum with each drain may relieve symptoms in patients who experience pain during cycling.

9. What causes poor dialysate drainage?

Poor outflow is one of the most common problems encountered in a peritoneal dialysis practice. Recall that net ultrafiltration is determined by the osmotic tonicity of the dialysate, the length of the dwell time, the peritoneal kinetics of the patient, and any internal or external impediments to outflow. All of these factors should be considered when presented with a patient whose inflow volume is greater than outflow volume. In general, hypotonic dialysate, long dwell times, or rapid kinetics result in small net negative balances that can slowly lead to fluid overload. By comparison, mechanical impediments lead to fluid overload more rapidly.

If maneuvers such as increasing the tonicity of the dialysate, shortening the dwell time, checking for kinked tubing, and changing positions with draining have failed to solve the problem, the most likely cause of the outflow failure is an internal impediment to flow. The most common internal cause of decreased flow is constipation, which decreases the effective area available for ultrafiltration and can mimic external compression on the catheter. A fibrin clot may obstruct inflow or outflow and usually responds to the instillation of heparin in the dialysate. Rarely, dissolution of the clot with streptokinase may be necessary.

Outflow failure may also occur when the catheter becomes encased in omentum. Fortunately, this problem can be recognized by the ease of inflow and normal initial rate of outflow, which, after a few hundred milliliters of drainage, abruptly stops. Partial omentectomy through a small midline incision with catheter repositioning solves the problem. Catheter malposition is another cause of outflow failure that often occurs shortly after catheter placement. This can avoided by testing inflow and outflow at the time of catheter implantation and by checking the catheter position on plain films of the abdomen. Poor outflow also may be seen when the dialysate becomes loculated, as in cases of leaks into the abdominal or pleural cavity (see question 11).

10. What is the approach to the peritoneal dialysis patient with a hernia?

Hernias occur in about 10% of peritoneal dialysis patients. The prevalence of this complication appears to be related to the increase in intra-abdominal pressure, which rises with increasing volume of dialysate instilled in the abdomen. The intra-abdominal pressure may increase four- to sixfold with the instillation of standard dialysate volumes. With cough and straining at stool, these pressures may increase 100 times above normal. Hernias occur most commonly in the umbilical, inguinal, and pericatheter regions and at sites of earlier surgical incisions.

The best approach to pericatheter hernias in the peritoneal dialysis patient is to prevent formation by allowing the catheter to mature for 10–14 days prior to instilling full volumes in the peritoneal cavity. If the patient must undergo peritoneal dialysis during this break-in period, keeping the patient in a supine position keeps the intra-abdominal pressure as low as possible. Depending on the location of the hernia, the patient may present with swelling at the hernia site, genital edema, intestinal obstruction, and, in the most severe cases, strangulation with peritonitis due to bowel infarction. Because of the high intra-abdominal pressure, hernias in this patient population tend to enlarge over time and so should be repaired when they become clinically significant. Following hernia repair, it is advisable to resume peritoneal dialysis with smaller volumes of dialysate in the first 7 days after surgery.

11. Can peritoneal dialysis patients develop leaks?

Yes. Sometimes peritoneal dialysis patients present with abdominal or genital edema of unclear origin. This complication likely is due to dialysate seeping through the peritoneal dialysis membrane into the adjacent tissues under the influence of increased intra-abdominal pressure. If a hernia cannot be palpated, a CT scan with intraperitoneal injection of contrast dye may pinpoint the source of the leak. An alternative course is to temporarily reduce daytime volumes. If that is not successful, temporary discontinuation of peritoneal dialysis may allow the path of the leak to heal. Recurrent leaks should probably be surgically explored to find and repair the breach.

12. Is a pleural effusion in a peritoneal dialysis patient cause for concern?

A pleural effusion in a peritoneal dialysis patient usually is due to fluid overload and can be treated by increasing ultrafiltration through use of dialysate with higher tonicity. Occasionally, however, fluid in the pleural cavity is due to leaking of dialysate from the peritoneal space. This problem can occur at any time and may develop either rapidly and dramatically or so slowly that it is discovered only on routine x-ray examination. It is more common in females and more frequently involves the right side. The finding of a high glucose concentration in the pleural fluid is diagnostic. In equivocal cases, demonstration of contrast dye in the pleural space following injection into the peritoneum confirms the diagnosis. Treatment of this condition begins with temporary transfer to hemodialysis because cases of spontaneous remission have been reported. Unfortunately, reinitiation of peritoneal dialysis often leads to reaccumulation of dialysate in the pleural cavity. In this situation, stimulation of adhesion formation with irritants such as talc, tetracycline, and autologous blood or surgical closure of the pleural space have at times been successful.

13. What are the other mechanical complications of peritoneal dialysis?

Peritoneal dialysis patients may suffer from compromised respiratory function, back pain, dyspepsia, and early satiety as a direct result of the dialytic method. The large amount of instilled fluid may cause impairment of respiratory function similar to that seen in obese or pregnant patients. Symptoms are worse in the supine position, and, therefore, patients with this difficulty should carry larger volumes when ambulatory. The dialysate volume and the increased intra-abdominal pressure also can precipitate or exacerbate back pain syndromes. Patients with back pain usually are more symptomatic with large volumes while ambulatory and therefore are best treated with large volume cycling at night and smaller daytime volumes. Peritoneal dialysis can result in early satiety and even dyspepsia due to large volume dialysis and increased intra-abdominal pressure. Strategies to ameliorate this problem include eating while empty or at the beginning of a dwell, decreasing the volume of daytime dwells, and using intestinal propulsants and antireflux medications.

14. What are the indications for catheter removal?

The three major indications for removal of a peritoneal dialysis catheter are intractable infection of the exit site, tunnel, or peritoneum; failure to effect adequate fluid removal; and failure to support adequate clearance. Persistent leaks or inflow pain also may prompt catheter removal. In the past, removal of the catheter has usually meant at least transient transfer to hemodialysis. More recently, simultaneous removal and replacement has been shown to be successful in noninfectious indications for catheter removal such as leaks and inflow pain and in infectious cases such as nonpseudomonal exit site and tunnel infections. Furthermore, repositioning of the catheter and partial omentectomy through a midline minilaparotomy incision now treat outflow obstruction, which used to be treated with catheter removal. Peritoneal dialysis can be restarted with low fill volumes after 48 hours. If the catheter was removed for *Pseudomonas* exit site or tunnel infection or for persistent peritonitis, catheter should be replaced after the infection has been completely eradicated. Patients with ultrafiltration failure and inadequate dialysis are transferred permanently to hemodialysis.

BIBLIOGRAPHY

1. Burkhart J, Nolph K: Peritoneal dialysis. In Brenner B (ed): The Kidney, 5th ed. Philadelphia, W.B. Saunders, 1996, pp 2507–2575.
2. Gokal R, Alexander S, Ash S, et al: Peritoneal catheters and exit-site practices toward optimum peritoneal access: 1998 update. Perit Dial Int 18:11–33, 1998.
3. Golper T: Intermittent versus continuous antibiotics for PD-related peritonitis. Perit Dial Int 17:11–12, 1997.
4. Harwell CM, Newman LN, Cacho CP, et al: Abdominal catastrophe: Visceral injury as a cause of peritonitis in patients treated by peritoneal dialysis. Perit Dial Int 17:586–594, 1997.
5. Piraino B: Peritonitis as a complication of peritoneal dialysis. J Am Soc Nephrol 9:1956–1964, 1998.
6. Ramon RG, Carrasco AM: Hydrothorax in peritoneal dialysis. Perit Dial Int 18:5–10, 1998.
7. Vychytil A, Lorenz M, Schneider B, et al: New strategies to prevent *Staphylococcus aureus* infections in peritoneal dialysis patients. J Am Soc Nephrol 9:669–676, 1998.

49. RENAL TRANSPLANTATION: EPIDEMIOLOGY AND OUTCOMES

Donald E. Hricik, M.D.

1. How are patients selected for kidney transplantation?

All patients with end-stage renal disease are considered candidates for kidney transplantation unless they have a systemic malignancy, chronic infection, severe cardiovascular disease, or a neuropsychiatric disorder (including drug addiction) that precludes compliance with an immunosuppressive drug regimen. Renal transplantation can be performed before a patient requires dialysis. However, a patient cannot be listed for a cadaveric kidney transplant until creatinine clearance has fallen below 20 ml/minute. Ultimately, the patient is responsible for choosing between dialysis and transplantation as options for renal replacement therapy.

2. Is age a consideration?

Extremes of age are considered *relative* contraindications to renal transplantation. In neonates and children younger than 2 years, technical difficulties related to the small size of the recipient often preclude successful transplantation. Advanced age is no longer considered an absolute contraindication. In fact, high rates of success have been reported in patients between 60 and 70 years of age. For patients older than 70 years, transplantation should be considered only if the patient exhibits superb extrarenal health.

3. How many kidney transplants are being performed these days?

In recent years, between 10,000 and 12,000 kidney transplants have been performed annually in the United States. The growth rate has been minimal during the past 10 years, primarily because of the relatively fixed number of available donors. Although there has been steady growth in the number of kidney transplants performed using living donors during the same time period, heart-beating, brain-dead cadavers still serve as donors for more than 70% of the transplants performed in the United States. Growth in the number of transplants performed has not kept pace with the 6–8% annual increase in the number of patients with end-stage renal disease. As a consequence, the number of patients waiting for cadaveric renal allografts and the waiting times for these organs have increased dramatically.

4. Can anything be done to increase the donor pool?

The pool of living donors recently has been expanded by increased use of living, *unrelated* donors (e.g., spouses and friends). To increase the pool of cadaver donors, some centers have advocated acceptance of donors previously considered "marginal." Examples include the use of non–heart-beating cadavers and transplantation of two kidneys from donors who previously would have been excluded from single kidney donation on the basis of advanced age or renal impairment. Because family refusal to allow organ donation from otherwise suitable cadavers remains a common problem, public education continues to play an important role in maintaining or increasing rates of cadaveric organ donation.

5. How successful is kidney transplantation?

Short-term success (defined by 1-year allograft survival rates) has steadily increased during the past decade (see Figure). For the cohort of U.S. patients transplanted in 1994, 1-year allograft survival was 85.6% for recipients of cadaver donor allografts and 92.4% for recipients of living donor allografts.

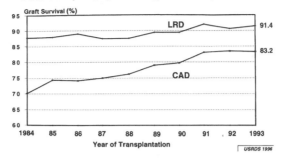

**One-Year Adjusted Medicare _Graft Survival_,
First Transplant, by Donor Type and Year, 1984-1993**

One-year allograft survival, first transplants adjusted for age, sex, race, by donor type, and year, 1985–1994. (From U.S. Renal Data Systems: 1997 Annual Report: VII: Renal transplantation: Access and outcomes. Am J Kidney Dis 30(suppl 1):S118–S127, 1997, with permission.)

6. How does kidney transplantation compare to dialysis in terms of patient survival?

Annual mortality rates for patients on dialysis in recent years have ranged from 21% and 25%. In contrast, mortality rates are now less than 8% per year for cadaveric transplant recipients and less than 4% per year for living-related transplant recipients. Any comparison of outcomes in patients treated with transplantation or dialysis must take into consideration that healthier patients generally are selected for transplantation. The fact that mortality rates of successfully transplanted patients are lower than those of patients maintained on dialysis while awaiting a kidney transplant suggests, however, that transplantation is associated with a clear-cut survival advantage.

7. What constitutes a good match between donor and recipient?

A person's "tissue type" is determined by cell surface antigens encoded for by the family of human leukocyte (HLA) genes located on the short arm of the sixth chromosome. The HLA-A and HLA-B loci encode for class I antigens expressed on the surface of most nucleated cells. The HLA-DR (D-related) locus encodes for class II antigens expressed on selected antigen-presenting cells and activated lymphocytes. With a complement of two chromosomes, each individual expresses 6 HLA antigens. Because disparities in the HLA antigen composition of the recipient and host may trigger the immunologic events leading to allograft rejection, these 6 antigens are referred to as major transplantation antigens. The "match" between two individuals can range from 0 to 6. Six is good!

Matching based on tissue typing should not be confused with crossmatching, a laboratory test that determines whether a potential transplant recipient has preformed antibodies against the HLA antigens of the potential donor. A potential kidney transplant recipient may have a relatively good match but still exhibit a positive crossmatch against the donor that precludes transplantation. Keep in mind that, generally speaking, potential kidney transplant recipients and donors must exhibit blood group ABO compatibility in order to allow successful transplantation.

8. What is the effect of HLA-matching on the outcome of kidney transplantation?

Data from large registries indicate that, the better the HLA-match, the better the long-term survival of the allograft. The benefits of matching are particularly noteworthy in recipients of kidneys from donors who match for 6 HLA antigens (or who exhibit no HLA antigen mismatches). The benefits of lesser degrees of matching have become less obvious with the use of newer and more potent immunosuppressive drugs. For any number of HLA matches, the long-term survival of allografts tends to be better in recipients of living unrelated transplants compared to recipients of cadaveric allografts, suggesting that elimination of "cold" ischemia required for the preservation of cadaveric organs may outweigh the influence of matching on long-term outcome (see Figure).

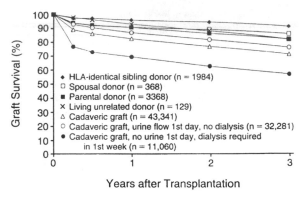

Years after Transplantation

Survival of first kidney grafts. (From Terasaki PI, Cecka JM, Gjerston DW, Takemoto S: High survival rates of kidney transplants from spousal and living unrelated donors. N Engl J Med 333:333–336, 1995, with permission.)

9. How are cadaveric renal allografts allocated to patients on the waiting list?

In the United States, organ allocation policies are dictated by the United Network for Organ Sharing (UNOS), a government-appointed agency that maintains a computerized list of all potential kidney transplant recipients and a post-transplant database that provides a source of information about outcomes after transplantation. Currently, the allocation of cadaveric kidneys is dictated by a point system that assigns organs harvested within regional organ procurement areas. The point system is most heavily weighted by the degree of HLA-matching between the potential recipient and donor and, to a far lesser extent, by other factors such as time on the waiting list. Current UNOS policy dictates that kidneys from 6-antigen–matched donors are exported within the continental U.S. to the recipient irrespective of the recipient's waiting time. This policy accounts for the occasional patient who receives a cadaveric kidney transplant after a relatively short period of waiting.

10. How long do kidney transplants last?

The average life span of a cadaveric renal allograft is currently about 8 years.

11. What factors influence the longevity of renal allografts?

Aside from HLA matching, factors that have been associated with decreased long-term allograft survival include the number of acute rejection episodes experienced by the recipient, delayed allograft function (defined by the need for at least one dialysis treatment after transplantation because of initially poor allograft function), black race, and extremes of donor age (< 5 or > 65 years of age).

12. What are the major causes of long-term renal allograft failure?

• Chronic rejection (see Chapter 51, Renal Transplantation: Classification and Consequences of Rejection)
• Death with a functioning allograft

13. What are the most common causes of death after kidney transplantation?

• Cardiovascular disease (i.e., myocardial infarction, stroke, complications of peripheral vascular disease)
• Infection

14. What about kidney transplants from animals?

Xenotransplantation (the transplantation of organs from one species to another) may become a reality before pigs fly. Until recently, the major barrier to transplantation between species was the presence of preformed antibodies directed against glycosylated cell surface proteins of the animal donor, which lead to immune destruction of the transplanted organ within minutes of revascularization. It is now known that this form of hyperacute rejection is mediated by complement. Genetic engineering has allowed for the procreation of animals that either express non-immunogenic glycosylated cell surface proteins or that overexpress molecules capable of preventing complement activation. Although this major hurdle has been overcome, the more traditional forms of rejection mediated by activated T cells tend to be severe after xenotransplantation and may not be prevented by currently available immunosuppressive drugs. In addition, there are serious concerns about the possibility that xenotransplants will result in the transmission of new infectious diseases to humans. Finally, it is not clear whether proteins (e.g., enzymes, hormones) synthesized by organs transplanted from different species will be capable of sustaining their physiologic functions in humans over long periods of time.

BIBLIOGRAPHY

1. Platt JL: Approaching the clinical application of xenotransplantation. Am J Med Sci 313:315–321, 1997.
2. Schulak JA, Mayes JT, Johnston KH, Hricik DE: Kidney transplantation in patients aged sixty years and older. Surgery 108:726–733, 1990.
3. Terasaki PI, Cecka JM, Gjerston DW, Takemoto S: High survival rates of kidney transplants from spousal and living unrelated donors. N Engl J Med 333:333–336, 1995.
4. Troppmann C, Gillingham KT, Benedetti E, et al: Delayed graft function, acute rejection, and outcome after cadaveric renal transplantation. Transplantation 59:962–968, 1995.
5. U.S. Renal Data Systems: 1997 Annual Report: VII: Renal transplantation: Access and outcomes. Am J Kidney Dis 30(suppl 1):S118–S127, 1997.

50. RENAL TRANSPLANTATION: DONOR AND RECIPIENT EVALUATION

Thomas C. Knauss, M.D.

1. What are the current sources of donor kidneys in the United States?
1. **Living related donors**
2. **Living unrelated donors:** Most often spouses or significant others
3. **Cadaveric donors:** The majority of these donors are brain-dead individuals who are taken to the operating room with artificial life support systems intact. Some transplant programs also use "non–heart-beating donors." These are usually individuals who do not meet criteria for brain death but are felt to have profound irreversible neurologic damage leading a family to request discontinuation of life support. The subject is taken to the operating room, and life support is discontinued. The organs are harvested after the development of asystole.

2. Does a signed donor card ensure that a brain-dead individual is legally approved to be an organ donor?
No. Currently, in the United States, organ donor cards express the wishes of the individual, but family members are always contacted to obtain approval for donating organs.

3. What are some of the exclusion criteria for cadaveric organ donation?
Absolute contraindications
• Systemic infection
• Malignancy
• Chronic kidney disease
• Long-standing diabetes mellitus
• Positive serologic test for human immunodeficiency virus (HIV)
Relative contraindications
• Extremes of age (< 5 years; > 65 years)
• History of risk factors for infectious diseases (e.g., intravenous drug abuse, sexual promiscuity, recent imprisonment)
• Long-standing hypertension
• Acute renal failure at the time of harvest

4. Which infectious agents can be transferred from donor to recipient through a kidney transplant?
• Bacteria (e.g., in bacterial pyelonephritis)
• Viruses that reside in renal tissue or passenger leukocytes (e.g., cytomegalovirus, Epstein-Barr virus, hepatitis B, hepatitis C, HIV, human herpesvirus 8)
• Fungi
• Mycobacteria

5. What is a crossmatch?
A crossmatch is performed by incubating donor lymphocytes (obtained from peripheral blood or from the spleen or lymph nodes) with recipient serum. The test determines whether the recipient serum contains preformed antibodies against the human leukocyte (HLA) antigens of the donor. Preformed antibodies can mediate hyperacute rejection (see Chapter 51, Renal Transplantation: Classification and Consequences of Rejection), and their presence is considered a contraindication to transplantation. A final crossmatch between donor and recipient is performed routinely just prior to transplantation irrespective of whether the donor is dead or alive.

6. Do kidney transplant donors and recipients need to have identical blood types?

Mismatching Rh types are not important in organ transplantation. However, the donor and recipient generally must be **ABO compatible**. This is true under one or more of the following conditions:

- The donor and recipient are ABO identical
- The donor has blood type O (universal donor)
- The recipient has blood type AB (universal recipient)

7. Are some HLA antigens more important than others in matching a donor and recipient for a kidney transplant?

The major histocompatibility complex (MHC) antigens measured routinely in most HLA laboratories include the class I antigens (A, B, and C) and class II antigens (D, including the subsets DP, DQ, and DR). Practically, the antigens used clinically for matching prior to a kidney transplant are A, B, and DR. Of the individual antigens, matching for DR antigens appears to result in the most favorable long-term outcome for the allograft.

8. What are the general principles involved in evaluating a prospective living kidney donor?

In general, the evaluation of a potential living donor is geared to determine (1) whether there is a medical condition that will put the donor at increased risk for complications for general anesthesia and surgery and (2) whether the removal of one kidney will increase the donor's risk for developing renal insufficiency.

9. What tests can be used to assess kidney function in potential kidney donors?

Serum creatinine concentration
Creatinine clearance
Radionuclide glomerular filtration rate

10. What is the minimal level of renal function required for a living kidney donor?

Most transplant centers require a minimum glomerular filtration rate of 70 ml/min in order for a subject to serve as a living kidney donor.

11. What other screening tests are performed routinely to rule out underlying renal disease in a prospective kidney donor?

- Urinalysis
- Urine culture
- Measurement of urine protein (either a 24-hour collection or measurement of a protein to creatinine ratio in a spot urine collection)

12. What medical conditions exclude living kidney donation?

- Renal parenchymal disease
- Conditions that may predispose to renal disease:
  History of multiple kidney stones
  History of frequent urinary tract infections
  Hypertension
- Conditions that increase the risks of anesthesia and surgery (i.e., significant cardiac, pulmonary, or hepatic disease)
- Recent malignancy

13. What tests are performed as part of the living donor evaluation?

- Complete blood count
- Blood chemistries
- Urinalysis

- Urine culture
- Chest x-ray
- Electrocardiogram
- Serologic studies for past exposures to infections (cytomegalovirus, hepatitis B and C, Epstein-Barr virus, syphilis, HIV)
- Renal imaging studies

Depending on the age of the potential donor and his or her medical history, other studies (e.g., in-depth cardiac evaluation, pulmonary functions tests) may be indicated.

14. Why are renal imaging studies performed in evaluating living renal donors?
- To ensure that the donor has two kidneys!
- To rule out neoplasia of the urinary tract
- To rule out structural abnormalities of the urinary tract
- To assess the vascular supply of the donor kidney

15. Which imaging studies are done to obtain this information?
Traditionally, an intravenous pyelogram has been done followed by a renal angiogram (usually a digital subtraction angiogram). However, some transplant programs use a single study such as spiral computed tomography (CT) with three-dimensional reconstruction.

16. Does donation of a kidney pose a long-term renal risk for the donor?
Obviously, the living kidney donor is forever at risk for developing end-stage renal disease if the remaining kidney is damaged by unforeseen parenchymal disease or trauma. Compensatory hypertrophy and glomerular hyperfiltration occur in the remaining kidney following unilateral nephrectomy, raising the theoretical concern that the procedure may increase the long-term risk of proteinuria, hypertension, and even renal failure. Although studies from some centers have suggested a slight risk of proteinuria and hypertension, meta-analyses of data from donors followed for more than 20 years generally have shown no statistically significant increase in the incidence of these complications.

17. At what level of renal dysfunction is it appropriate to evaluate a patient for kidney transplantation?
Discussions regarding transplantation as a renal replacement modality should be initiated early in the course of a renal disease if it is clearly progressing to end stage. If a medically acceptable living donor has been identified, elective renal transplantation ideally is performed just before dialysis is needed. If a living-donor transplant is not an option, patients can be evaluated for transplantation at any time but cannot officially be put on the list for transplantation ("listed") until the glomerular filtration rate falls below 20 ml/min.

18. What are some contraindications to renal transplantation?
The only **absolute** contraindication is the presence of severe vascular disease that precludes the arterial and venous anastomoses required for a technically successful transplant. There are many **relative** contraindications (for which individualized circumstances must be taken into consideration), including:
- Recent or current malignancy
- Coronary artery disease
- Active bacterial, fungal, or viral disease
- HIV positivity
- Social conditions that prevent compliance with medical follow-up

19. What medical evaluation is performed to determine if a patient is a suitable candidate for transplantation?
The "pretransplant" evaluation varies from one transplant center to another but generally includes a complete history, physical examination, and a number of tests designed to assess overall

health and to screen for occult malignancy and infection. At a minimum, this usually includes a complete blood count, blood chemistries, chest x-ray, electrocardiogram, urine culture, Pap smear, mammogram, examination of stool for occult blood, and serologic studies for cytomegalovirus, hepatitis B and C, HIV, and syphilis. The integrity of the aortoiliac circulation usually is assessed noninvasively (e.g., by duplex scanning). In many centers, a more complete cardiac evaluation (including echocardiography, stress testing, carotid studies, or myocardial perfusion scans) is performed in selected patients, including patients older than 50 years, those with diabetes mellitus, and those with symptoms suggestive of cardiovascular disease.

20. What is the role of the social worker in evaluating a patient for renal transplantation?

Transplantation involves a complex mix of psychosocial issues that are best evaluated by a social worker. Ability to pay for surgery, hospitalization, and immunosuppressant medications must be assessed in advance; surgical success of the transplant does not ensure overall success if the procedure leaves a patient and his or her family destitute. The psychological make-up of the potential recipient also should be assessed. The best indicator of noncompliance after a transplant is noncompliance before the transplant. Finally, family support may be critical to success, especially in the case of elderly or debilitated patients.

BIBLIOGRAPHY

1. Alexandre GPJ, Latinne D, Carlier M, et al: ABO-incompatibility and organ transplantation. Transplant Rev 5:230–241, 1991.
2. Bay WH, Hebert LA: The living donor in kidney transplantation. Ann Intern Med 106:719–727, 1987.
3. Hakim RM, Goldszer RC, Brenner BM: Hypertension and proteinuria: Long-term sequelae of uninephrectomy in humans. Kidney Int 25:930–936, 1984.
4. Jones J, Payne WD, Matas AJ: The living donor—risks, benefits, and related concerns. Transplant Rev 7:115–128, 1993.
5. Kasiske BL, Gaston RS, Bia MJ, et al: The evaluation of renal transplant candidates: Clinical guidelines. J Am Soc Nephrol 6:1–34, 1995.
6. Kasiske BL, Ravenscraft M, Ramos EL, et al: The evaluation of living renal transplant donors: Clinical practice guidelines. J Am Soc Nephrol 7:2288–2313, 1996.

51. RENAL TRANSPLANTATION: CLASSIFICATION AND CONSEQUENCES OF REJECTION

Donald E. Hricik, M.D.

1. What are the major forms of renal allograft rejection?
1. Hyperacute
2. Acute
3. Chronic

Older classification schemes differentiated histologic variants of rejection such as interstitial, cellular, or vascular. These latter terms have become increasingly obsolete as standardized criteria have evolved to classify allograft rejection histologically (see question 3).

2. What is hyperacute rejection?
Hyperacute rejection is mediated by a transplant recipient's preformed antibodies that recognize human leukocyte (HLA) antigens in the donor organ. Preformed anti-HLA antibodies generally occur as a consequence of previous blood transfusions, pregnancy, or a prior organ transplant. Occasionally, patients with autoimmune diseases may generate antibodies that cross-react with HLA antigens. In hyperacute rejection, fibrinoid necrosis typically occurs within minutes to hours leading to almost immediate destruction of the allograft. Modern crossmatching techniques are very sensitive to detecting anti-HLA antibodies and now are performed routinely prior to all kidney transplants, thus accounting for the current rarity of hyperacute rejection. A delayed form of hyperacute rejection may occur several days after transplantation. If recognized expeditiously, plasmapheresis may be beneficial in reversing the rejection process by eliminating the offending antibodies.

3. What is acute renal allograft rejection?
Acute rejection is mediated by activated T cells that proliferate and attack the allograft after recognizing antigens in the graft (1) directly (direct pathway) or (2) after being processed by recipient antigen-presenting cells that present donor antigens to CD4+ T cells within the grooves of surface class II HLA molecules (indirect pathway). (The cellular and intracellular events leading to T-cell activation are described in Chapter 52, Renal Transplantation: Immunosuppression.) Although subclinical cases undoubtedly occur, acute rejection in kidney transplant recipients is usually recognized clinically by the development of otherwise unexplained acute renal failure manifested by an acute rise in serum creatinine concentration and, in severe cases, by oliguria. Episodes of acute rejection can occur at any time after transplantation; however, most cases occur within the first 6 months following transplantation.

4. How common is acute rejection?
At least one episode of acute rejection occurred in 40–70% of cadaveric kidney transplant recipients maintained on cyclosporine, azathioprine, and steroids. Since 1994, the use of newer immunosuppressant drugs and drug combinations has been accompanied by acute rejection rates of 25% or less.

5. How is acute rejection treated?
Traditionally, first-line therapy of acute rejection has consisted of high doses of corticosteroids (i.e., "pulse" steroids) administered either intravenously or orally for 3–5 days. Doses range between 250 mg and 1000 mg daily of methylprednisolone or its equivalent. Steroid-resistant

rejection is usually treated with antilymphocyte antibodies including OKT3 (a monoclonal antibody directed against the CD3 complex on the surface of activated T cells) or various polyclonal antibody preparations (directed against multiple cell-surface structures on lymphocytes). Some centers prefer to choose between steroids and antilymphocyte antibodies for first-line therapy of acute rejection based on the severity of the rejection episode as determined by biopsy of the allograft. Some of the newer "maintenance" immunosuppressants, such as mycophenolate mofetil and tacrolimus, have proven to be effective in the treatment of acute rejection when used in high doses. Novel or unproven therapies for acute rejection include radiation of the allograft and photopheresis.

6. How successful is treatment for acute rejection?

More than 90% of acute rejection episodes occurring in the first 6 months after transplantation can be reversed. Treatment is less successful in patients with late acute rejection episodes (occurring more than 1 year after transplantation).

7. What is chronic renal allograft rejection?

Chronic rejection is clinically manifest by a slow and gradual decline in renal allograft function, usually beginning more than 6 months after transplantation, and typically accompanied by moderate to heavy proteinuria. Histologically, chronic rejection is characterized by glomerulosclerosis, interstitial fibrosis, and obliteration of arteriolar lumina. The vasculopathy is mediated initially by lymphocytic invasion of the intima followed by infiltration of macrophages and proliferation of smooth muscle cells that ultimately lead to intimal fibrosis reminiscent of atherosclerosis (see Figure). Because the pathophysiology of chronic rejection is poorly understood, treatment is unsatisfactory. Chronic rejection is currently the most common cause of long-term renal allograft failure.

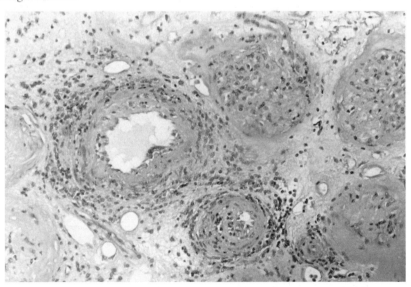

Light micrograph demonstrating the histologic changes of chronic renal allograft rejection including varying degrees of glomerulosclerosis and vascular intimal fibroplasia.

8. What is known about the pathophysiology of chronic rejection?

Both immune and nonimmune factors play a role. Because chronic rejection is most common in patients who have experienced multiple episodes of acute rejection, it has been suggested that chronic rejection results from "smoldering" or inadequately treated acute rejection. Nonimmune factors speculated to play a role in chronic rejection include:

• Systemic hypertension
• Hyperlipidemia
• Viral infections, especially cytomegalovirus
• Drug toxicity (e.g., cyclosporine, tacrolimus)
• Ischemic injury

9. Is there any treatment for chronic rejection?

Because chronic rejection is characterized histologically by sclerosis and fibrosis, recently there has been interest in the possibility that the disorder is mediated by the upregulation of fibrogenic growth factors. A number of drugs including angiotensin-converting enzyme (ACE) inhibitors, angiotensin receptor antagonists, and HMG coenzyme A (CoA)-reductase inhibitors are capable of inhibiting these growth factors and may prove to be effective in retarding the rate of progressive renal impairment in patients with chronic rejection.

10. Where is Banff? What are the Banff criteria?

A group of nephrologists and nephropathologists, apparently fond of the Canadian Rockies, has periodically convened in the lovely town of Banff, Alberta, to develop standardized histologic criteria for the diagnoses of acute and chronic renal allograft rejection. Each meeting has resulted in classification schemes that are increasingly complex. The simplified criteria for acute renal allograft rejection follow:

Banff Grade	Histology
I	Interstitial edema and tubulitis (i.e., lymphocytic invasion of tubular basement membranes)
II	More severe tubulitis with or without mild vasculitis characterized by intimal lymphocytic infiltrates
III	Severe vasculitis with fibrinoid necrosis

BIBLIOGRAPHY

1. Basadonna GP, Matas AJ, Gillingham KJ, et al: Early versus late acute renal allograft rejection: Impact on chronic rejection. Transplantation 55:993–998, 1993.
2. Hariharan S, Alexander JW, Schroeder TJ, First MR: Impact of first acute rejection episode and severity of rejection on cadaveric renal allograft survival. Clin Transplant 10:538–543, 1996.
3. Hricik DE, Almawi WY, Strom TB: Trends in the use of glucocorticoids in renal transplantation. Transplantation 57:979–989, 1994.
4. Leggat JE, Ojo AD, Leichtman AB, et al: Long-term allograft survival: Prognostic implication of the timing of acute rejection episodes. Transplantation 63:1268–1272, 1997.
5. Solez K, Axelson RA, Benediktsson H, et al: International standardization of criteria for the histologic diagnosis of renal allograft rejection: The Banff working classification of kidney transplant pathology. Kidney Int 44:411–422, 1993.
6. Tilney NL, Whitley DW, Diamond JR, et al: Chronic rejection: An undefined conundrum. Transplantation 52:389–398, 1991.

52. RENAL TRANSPLANTATION: IMMUNOSUPPRESSION

Donald E. Hricik, M.D.

1. What are the general principles underlying current immunosuppressive treatment strategies for kidney transplant recipients?

1. The benefits of a successful transplant outweigh the risks of chronic immunosuppression.

2. Immunosuppressive therapy is required indefinitely to maintain allograft function. Although a small fraction of transplant recipients develop immunologic tolerance to their allografts, no satisfactory tests confirm this state of tolerance. Complete withdrawal of immunosuppression, whether patient- or physician-directed, is associated with a prohibitive risk of potentially irreversible allograft rejection.

3. Multidrug regimens generally are employed to prevent rejection by inhibiting T-cell immunity through multiple mechanisms.

4. Large doses of immunosuppressant drugs are used in the early post-transplant period. In patients who remain free of rejection, doses are generally reduced with time. Complete elimination of one or more drugs from multidrug regimens is possible in many stable patients.

2. What are the risks associated with chronic immunosuppressive drug therapy?

Each of the currently prescribed immunosuppressive agents is associated with unique side effects (see question 10). The common risks of major concern are **infection** (especially opportunistic infections) and **malignancy** (especially lymphoproliferative disease).

3. What is Induction immunosuppressive therapy?

Induction therapy refers to the immunosuppressive drug therapy provided during the early post-transplant period (i.e., the first 1–3 weeks following transplant surgery). However, more commonly the term describes the use of anti–T-cell antibodies during this early post-transplant period.

4. What antibodies are used for induction therapy?

Polyclonal antibodies (that bind to multiple cell surface molecules)
• ATGAM
• Thymoglobulin
• Other noncommercial preparations derived from injection of human thymocytes or immunoblasts into horses, rabbits, or other animals

Monoclonal antibodies (that bind to specific cell surface molecules)
• OKT3
• Anti-CD25 (anti–interleukin-2 [IL-2] receptor) antibodies
  Basiliximab (Simulect)
  Daclizumab (Zenepax)

5. What is the rationale for induction therapy?

Theoretically, the use of induction antibodies prevents the development of acute rejection in the early postoperative period. Some, but not all, studies suggest that the use of these agents results in a lower incidence of subsequent rejection episodes and better long-term allograft survival. However, the benefits and risks of induction therapy have been a subject of debate. Some studies indicate that induction antibodies simply delay the time to onset of first rejection episodes. Any benefit of these expensive agents must be weighed against their potential to increase the risks of injection and malignancy. Many centers now limit use of these antibodies to transplant recipients deemed to be at high risk for rejection (i.e., African-American patients, second transplant recipients, patients who are highly sensitized as evidenced by high titers of human leukocyte [HLA] antibodies, and those with delayed allograft function following transplant surgery).

6. What is the immunologic basis for maintenance immunosuppression?

The T lymphocyte plays a central role in the acute rejection of allografts. Proliferation of T cells is initiated by recognition of antigens that are presented to the T-cell receptor–CD3 complex either directly as major histocompatibility complex (MHC) molecules on donor cells or indirectly as antigens that are processed and presented within the grooves of MHC molecules of the recipient's antigen presenting cells. Full activation of the T cell requires other costimulatory ligands between surface receptors on the lymphocyte and on antigen presenting cells. These cell surface ligands result in a cascade of intracellular events that ultimately stimulate nuclear transcription of IL-2 and other cytokines that promote the proliferation of antigen-specific clones of cytotoxic T cells that can directly injure the allograft. CD4-positive T cells are involved in the afferent antigen-recognition loop of this immune reaction, while CD8-positive T cells are cytotoxic cells that mediate the efferent cytodestructive loop of the reaction. The afferent and efferent loops of the reaction are shown schematically in the Figure, which also depicts the site of action of commonly used immunosuppressive drugs.

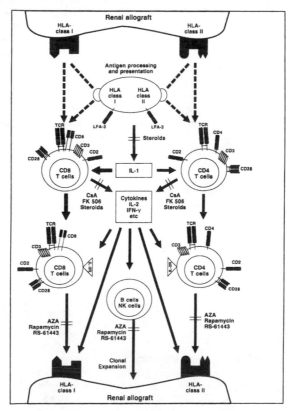

Abbreviations and drug names: HLA class I = HLA A, B, and C antigens; HLA class II = HLA DR and DQ antigens; TCR = T-cell receptor; AZA = azathioprine; IL-1 = interleukin 1; IL-2 = interleukin-2; IFN-γ = interferon-γ; NK cells = natural killer cells; RS-61443 = mycophenolate mofetil; FK506 = tacrolimus; CsA = cyclosporine; Rapamycin = sirolimus. (Adapted from Strom TB, Suthanthiran M: Mechanisms of graft rejection. In Sayegh MH, Turka LA (eds): ASTP Lectures in Transplantation. Philadelphia, CoMed Communications, 1996, with permission.)

7. What are the major classes of maintenance immunosuppressive drugs?

Classes of Maintenance Immunosuppressive Drugs

Immunophilin-binding agents	Antimetabolites
Calcineurin inhibitors	Purine inhibitors: nonselective
Cyclosporine	Azathioprine
Tacrolimus (FK506)	Purine inhibitors: lymphocyte selective
Calcineurin-independent agents	Mycophenolate mofetil (RS-61443)
Sirolimus (rapamycin)*	Mizoribine*
Glucocorticoids	Pyrimidine inhibitors
	Brequinar*
	Poorly understood mechanisms
	Deoxyspergualin*
	Leflunomide*

* Experimental or not yet approved by the Food and Drug Administration (FDA)

8. What is an immunophilin and how do immunophilin-binding agents work?

The term *immunophilin* refers to a group of cytosolic proteins that bind certain immunosuppressive agents (i.e., cyclosporine, tacrolimus, and sirolimus). The mechanism of the immunophilin-drug combination leading to inhibition of T-cell function is depicted in the Figure. On stimulation with antigens, the T-cell receptor–CD3 complex and the associated CD4 or CD8 proteins activate cytosolic tyrosine kinases. Tyrosine phosphorylation and activation of phospholipase C leads to hydrolysis of phosphatidylinositol 4,5-biphosphate and generation of inositol 1,4,5-triphosphate (IP_3) and diacylglycerol. IP_3 mobilizes intracellular calcium. Calcium activates the calmodulin-dependent phosphatase, calcineurin. Diacylglycerol stimulates protein kinase C activity. Calcineurin and protein kinase C either directly or indirectly modulate regulatory molecules, such as nuclear factor of activated T cells (NF-AT) and NF-κβ, that control the production of messenger RNA for IL-2, a cytokine that plays a key role in promoting growth and proliferation.

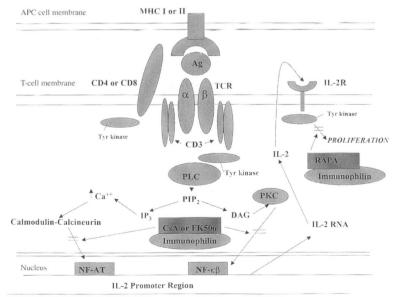

Abbreviations and drug names: Tyr kinase = tyrosine kinase; PLC = phospholipase C; TCR = T-cell receptor; PIP2 = phosphatidylinositol 4,5-biphosphate; IP3 = inositol 1,4,5-triphosphate; DAG = diacylglycerol; PKC = protein kinase C; IL-2 = interleukin-2; IL-2R = interleukin-2 receptor; NF-AT = nuclear factor of activated T cells; NF-κβ = nuclear factor-κβ; CsA - cyclosporine; FK506 = tacrolimus; RAPA = sirolimus.

Cyclosporine binds to an immunophilin called cyclophilin. Tacrolimus binds to a distinct immunophilin called FK-binding protein. The immunophilin-drug combination inhibit the actions of calcineurin and protein kinase C, thereby preventing the transcription of messenger RNA for IL-2 and other cytokines. Rapamycin also binds to FK-binding protein. However, this immunophilin-drug combination does not interfere with IL-2 production but somehow blocks signal transduction that is mediated by stimulation of the IL-2 receptor and that ultimately yields cell proliferation.

9. What are some commonly used combinations of maintenance immunosuppressive drugs?

The recent introduction of new immunosuppressive drugs has increased the number of possible drug combinations available to prevent rejection. Currently, most centers use a combination of glucocorticoids and either cyclosporine or tacrolimus for initial maintenance immunosuppression. Many centers add either mycophenolate mofetil or azathioprine to this combination for so-called triple therapy. Although sirolimus remains experimental, if approved by the FDA, it will be used primarily as a replacement for mycophenolate mofetil or azathioprine. Because sirolimus binds to the same immunophilin as tacrolimus, the two drugs are theoretically antagonists so that sirolimus will more likely be used in conjunction with cyclosporine. Because of the long-term side effects and expense of maintenance immunosuppression, a number of clinical trials are currently testing the safety and benefits of withdrawing single drugs from multidrug regimens in stable patients.

10. What are the common side effects of immunosuppressive drugs?

Side Effects of Glucocorticoids

Weight gain with cushingoid features	Cataracts
Hypertension	Dermatologic effects (acne, striae, easy bruisability, impaired wound healing)
Hyperlipidemia	Impaired growth
Osteopenia	Glucose intolerance

Side Effects of Immunophilin-binding Agents

SIDE EFFECT	CYCLOSPORINE	TACROLIMUS	SIROLIMUS
Nephrotoxicity	++	++	−
Neurotoxicity (tremor, seizures)	+	++	−
Hirsutism	++	−	−
Gingival hyperplasia	+	−	−
Hypertension	++	+	−
Hyperlipidemia	++	+/−	+++
Glucose intolerance	+	+++	−
Bone marrow suppression	−	−	++

Side Effects of Antimetabolites

SIDE EFFECT	AZATHIOPRINE	MYCOPHENOLATE MOFETIL
Bone marrow suppression	+++	++
Gastrointestinal (diarrhea, nausea)	+	++

Side Effects of Induction Antibodies

SIDE EFFECT	OKT3	POLYCLONALS	ANTI-CD25 AGENTS
Fever	+++	+	−
Headache	++	+	−
Myalgias	++	+	−
Gastrointestinal (diarrhea, nausea)	++	−	−
Respiratory distress	+	+/−	−

11. What does the future hold for new immunosuppressive strategies?

Specific immunologic tolerance, that is, tolerance to an allograft without the need for immunosuppressive drugs and without loss of immunity to other exogenous antigens, would allow organ transplantation without the need for toxic immunosuppressants. To date, it has not been possible to achieve true tolerance in humans. In some animal species, specific tolerance has been achieved using some combination of bone marrow ablation, donor-specific bone marrow transplantation, and anti–T-cell antibodies following transplantation of an allograft. It remains unclear whether similar strategies will be successful in humans. Other novel approaches to achieving states of immunologic hyporesponsiveness are currently being explored and include the administration of peptides derived from MHC molecules, use of antibodies that block costimulatory ligands between T cells and antigen-presenting T cells, and administration of antisense oligonucleotides.

BIBLIOGRAPHY

1. Germain RN: MHC-dependent antigen processing and peptide presentation: Providing ligands for T lymphocyte activation. Cell 76:287–299, 1994.
2. Miceli MC, Parnes JR: The role of CD4 and CD8 in T-cell activation. Semin Immunol 3:133–141, 1991.
3. Norman DJ: Antilymphocyte antibodies in the treatment of allograft rejection: Targets, mechanisms of action, monitoring, and efficacy. Semin Nephrol 12:315–324, 1992.
4. Strom TB, Suthanthiran M: Mechanisms of graft rejection. In Sayegh MH, Turka LA (eds): ASTP Lectures in Transplantation. Philadelphia, CoMed Communications, 1996.
5. Suthanthiran M, Morris RE, Strom TB: Immunosuppressants: Cellular and molecular mechanisms of action. Am J Kidney Dis 28:159–172, 1996.
6. Weiss A, Litman DR: Signal transduction by lymphocyte antigen receptors. Cell 76:263–264, 1994.

53. COMPLICATIONS OF RENAL TRANSPLANTATION

Thomas C.Knauss, M.D.

1. What percentage of kidney transplant recipients suffer from some type of infection (other than routine viral upper respiratory infections) in the first year?

Seventy-five percent of patients experience nontrivial infections during the first post-transplant year. Bacterial infections (e.g., wound infections, bladder infections) predominate in the early postoperative period. Opportunistic infections occur with increasing frequency thereafter.

2. What is the most common opportunistic infection in the first 6 months post-transplant?

Infection with cytomegalovirus (CMV) is the most common opportunistic infection occurring during the first 6 months following kidney transplantation.

3. Which transplant patients are at greatest risk for clinical CMV infection?

Individuals who are seronegative for CMV prior to the transplant and who then receive an organ from a CMV-positive donor are at highest risk. These patients have no protective antibody and become infected when CMV is transmitted from the donor organ at a time of maximal immunosuppression in the early transplant period. Of course, the lowest risk group would be CMV-negative recipients receiving transplants from CMV-negative donors. Intermediate risk is present when the donor and recipient are both CMV-positive.

4. What are some of the clinical presentations of CMV infection?

The most common features are fever, neutropenia, hepatitis, esophagitis, and gastritis. However, CMV may also cause retinitis, pneumonitis, colitis, and nephritis.

5. What other viral infections occur in transplant patients?

Infections caused by herpes simplex and herpes zoster were once common; however, the frequency of these diseases has decreased dramatically with the routine use of prophylactic antiviral drugs such acyclovir and ganciclovir.

6. What are the most common malignancies in transplant recipients?

The incidence of neoplasia is higher in transplant recipients than in the general population. Cancer of the skin (including the lip) accounts for over one third of all tumors. Unlike the nonimmunosuppressed individual, squamous cell skin cancer is more common than basal cell cancer. Lymphoma, cancer of the cervix, and Kaposi's sarcoma are examples of other malignancies that occur with greater frequency in transplant recipients than in the general population or in the dialysis population.

7. What is post-transplant lymphoproliferative disease (PTLD)?

PTLD is a neoplastic disorder that occurs as a complication of immunosuppressive therapy in solid-organ transplant recipients. Many cases result from proliferation of lymphocytes in response to reactivation of Epstein-Barr virus (EBV). The disorder sometimes presents as a mononucleosis-like syndrome with generalized lymphadenopathy. In such cases, lymph node pathology typically reveals a polyclonal proliferation of B lymphocytes that often regresses with reduction or temporary cessation of immunosuppression. More commonly, PTLD presents as frank lymphoma that demonstrates an unusual proclivity for involvement of extranodal sites such as the gastrointestinal tract or brain. In these cases, pathologic examination typically reveals a monoclonal B-cell lymphoma. Treatment usually includes chemotherapy and simultaneous reduction of overall immunosuppression.

8. What percentage of kidney transplant patients develop PTLD?

The overall incidence of PTLD is between 1.5% and 2.0%; however, there appears to be wide geographic variation in the reported incidence. At least half of the reported cases of PTLD are EBV-related. The incidence of lymphoma is higher in patients who have received antibody therapy (monoclonal or polyclonal) for either induction therapy or treatment of rejection. Other risk factors include age (higher risk in children), transplantation between an EBV-positive donor and an EBV-negative recipient, and very high cumulative doses of immunosuppressive drugs.

9. What percentage of kidney transplant patients develop de novo glucose intolerance?

Based on abnormal glucose tolerance curves, up to 40% of previously nondiabetic patients exhibit glucose intolerance. Between 8% and 20% of patients develop frank diabetes mellitus requiring therapy with insulin or oral hypoglycemic agents. The incidence is higher in African Americans and Hispanics than in whites. Other risk factors include significant weight gain after transplant, advanced age, and the use of corticosteroids or tacrolimus (FK-506) for immunosuppression.

10. What percentage of renal transplant recipients are hypertensive?

Approximately 70% of patients receiving corticosteroids with either cyclosporine or tacrolimus are hypertensive. The incidence approaches this level even in patients with excellent renal function. Aside from the effects of immunosuppressants, other causes include genetic predisposition, the effects of parenchymal renal disease resulting from acute and chronic rejection in the allograft or persistent disease in retained native kidneys, and, in some cases, renal artery stenosis.

11. What is the frequency of stenosis of the transplant renal artery?

The reported incidence varies between 1% and 12% with a mean of about 5%. Transplant renal artery stenosis may result from anastomotic strictures, from kinks in the allografted renal artery, or possibly from immune attack on the renal artery with subsequent scarring. In general, end-to-end arterial anastomoses (often performed in living-donor transplantation) are associated with a higher risk of subsequent stenosis than end-to-side anastomoses or anastomoses employing a Carrel aortic patch, which is applicable only in cadaveric kidney transplantation. Other risk factors include the use of pediatric or elderly cadaveric donors.

12. How common is hyperlipidemia after transplantation?

As many as 70% of kidney transplant recipients exhibit some combination of hypercholesterolemia or hypertriglyceridemia. Although dietary and genetic factors play a role, immunosuppressant drugs (especially steroids and cyclosporine) play a preeminent role in the pathogenesis of hyperlipidemia.

13. What bone diseases are common in transplant recipients?

Aseptic necrosis of bone is a well-known complication of high-dose corticosteroid use. Typically, it occurs in the hips and shoulders. This often occurs in the context of preexisting renal osteodystrophy, which further weakens bone. In individuals with severe neuropathy due to uremia or diabetes, bone calcium loss may be accelerated, leading to osteomalacia. Osteopenia, largely attributable to chronic steroid therapy, occurs in many renal transplant recipients within 6 months of the transplant surgery. Risk factors other than cumulative doses of corticosteroids include female gender and postmenopausal status.

14. What is the most common reason for failure of a kidney transplant?

Chronic rejection (see Chapter 51, Renal Transplantation: Classification and Consequences of Rejection) is now the leading cause of renal allograft failure beyond the first post-transplant year. Among kidney transplants that function for at least 1 year, half will fail by the ninth post-transplant year. This percentage is unchanged from that seen 15 years ago, well before the availability of cyclosporine or "newer" antirejection drugs. Clinically, patients become hypertensive and moderately proteinuric and exhibit a gradual decline in renal function.

15. What are the most common causes of death in patients with functioning renal allografts?

Atherosclerotic vascular occlusive disease, sepsis, malignancy, and hepatic failure. Mortality from coronary artery disease is at least five times higher than that seen in the general population.

BIBLIOGRAPHY

1. Braun WE: Long-term complications of renal transplantation. Kidney Int 37:1363–1378, 1990.
2. Curtis JJ: Hypertension following kidney transplantation. Am J Kidney Dis 23:471–475, 1994.
3. Fishman JA, Rubin RH: Infection in organ-transplant recipients. N Engl J Med 338:1741–1751, 1998.
4. Hill MN, Grossman RA, Feldman HI, et al: Changes in causes of death after renal transplantation: 1966 to 1987. Am J Kidney Dis 27:512–518, 1991.
5. Ho M: EBV infection and posttransplant lymphoproliferative disorders. Transplant Sci 2:88–92, 1992.
6. Jindal RM: Posttransplant diabetes mellitus—a review. Transplantation 58:1289–1298, 1997.
7. Julian BA, Quarles D, Niemann KM: Musculoskeletal complications after renal transplantation: Pathogenesis and treatment. Am J Kidney Dis 19:99–120, 1992.

VIII. Hypertension

54. ESSENTIAL HYPERTENSION

Mahboob Rahman, M.D., M.S.

1. How is hypertension defined and classified?

In adults aged 18 years or older, blood pressure less than 120/80 mmHg is defined as optimal blood pressure, and readings greater than 140/90 mmHg are defined as hypertensive. Normal, high normal, and stages 1–3 of hypertension are defined below:

Classification of Blood Pressure in Adults

CATEGORY	SYSTOLIC (mmHg)		DIASTOLIC (mmHg)
Optimal	< 120	*and*	< 80
Normal	< 130	*and*	< 85
High normal	130–139	*or*	85–89
Hypertension			
Stage 1	140–159	*or*	90–99
Stage 2	160–179	*or*	100–109
Stage 3	≥ 180	*or*	≥ 110

Data from National Institutes of Health: Sixth Report of the Joint National Committee on Prevention, Detection, Evaluation, and Treatment of High Blood Pressure. Bethesda, MD, NIH, 1997, NIH publication 98-4080.

2. What is the prevalence of hypertension in the United States? How well is blood pressure controlled in the general population?

An estimated 50 million Americans have high blood pressure. Hypertension is the leading cause of office visits to primary care physicians. Available evidence suggests that cardiovascular disease and all cause mortality increase progressively with higher blood pressure and that treatment of hypertension results in improved morbidity and mortality. However, even with widespread educational efforts, it is estimated that only 27% of patients with hypertension have blood pressure controlled to less than 140/90 mmHg.

3. What are the pathophysiologic mechanisms underlying essential hypertension?

Essential hypertension is a disorder of multifactorial etiologies resulting from a complex interaction of genetic factors, altered functional and structural mechanisms, and environmental factors. Most studies support the concept that inheritance of hypertension is polygenic, and a number of candidate genes are currently being investigated.

From a physiologic standpoint, all proposed mechanisms of essential hypertension have a final common pathway of increased peripheral vascular resistance. Increased sympathetic nervous system activity, alterations in the renin angiotensin system, imbalances in the production of vasoactive metabolites such as nitric oxide and endothelins, and alterations in intracellular cation metabolism are candidate mechanisms and the focus of active investigation. A number of environmental factors such as dietary salt intake, stress, and obesity have also been implicated in the development of hypertension.

4. What steps ensure that blood pressure is measured accurately?

Patients should be seated in a chair with their backs supported, feet on the ground, and arms bared and supported at heart level. They should refrain from smoking or ingesting caffeine during the 30 minutes preceding the measurement and be rested for at least 5 minutes before the procedure. The appropriate-sized cuff should be used. Unless the width of the cuff is more than 40% of the circumference of the mid-upper arm, the blood pressure reading will be increased artifactually. Two or more readings separated by 2 minutes should be averaged.

5. What is ambulatory blood pressure monitoring? When should it be used?

Ambulatory blood pressure monitoring is a technique where several blood pressure readings are obtained over a 24-hour period while the patient goes about his usual daily activities. Some patients have "white coat" hypertension; they have high blood pressure readings at the physician's office and significantly lower blood pressure measurements at home. Ambulatory blood pressure monitoring is helpful in deciding if antihypertensive therapy is indicated in these patients. Other circumstances where ambulatory blood pressure monitoring can be useful are in the evaluation of resistant hypertension, occurrence of hypotensive episodes, episodic hypertension, and autonomic dysfunction.

6. What are the goals of the initial evaluation of a hypertensive patient?

The evaluation should be designed to identify known secondary causes of high blood pressure, to assess the presence of target organ damage, and to identify other cardiovascular risk factors or concomitant disorders that may affect the prognosis or choice of drug therapy.

7. What are the key aspects of history and physical examination of the hypertensive patient?

The history should include assessment of coexistent conditions (e.g., cardiac disease, cerebrovascular disease, peripheral vascular disease), family history of cardiovascular disease, symptoms suggestive of secondary hypertension, use of over-the-counter medications, and dietary, psychosocial and environmental factors that influence blood pressure. Physical exam should include fundoscopic examination for hypertensive retinopathy, detection of bruits, assessment of the strength and symmetry of peripheral pulses, and palpation for thyromegaly.

8. What lab tests should be ordered in the initial evaluation of a hypertensive patient?

Laboratory tests help in determining the presence of target organ damage and other risk factors for cardiovascular disease. These include urinalysis, complete blood cell count (CBC), blood chemistry panel, total and high-density lipoprotein (HDL) cholesterol, and a 12-lead electrocardiogram (ECG). Other tests such as echocardiography and urinary microalbuminuria in patients with diabetes may be helpful in choosing antihypertensive therapy and determining goal blood pressure levels in selected patients.

9. What signs and symptoms suggest that a work-up for secondary hypertension is needed?

A work-up for secondary hypertension is indicated in the following circumstances:
- Patients whose blood pressure responds poorly to adequate drug therapy (three antihypertensive drugs at maximal dosage, including a diuretic)
- Patients who were well-controlled in the past and now have difficult-to-control hypertension
- Sudden onset of hypertension
- Onset of hypertension at a younger or older than usual age
- Signs and symptoms of known secondary causes of hypertension (see Chapter 58, Other Causes of Secondary Hypertension, and Chapter 59, Hypertensive Emergencies)

10. How is cardiovascular risk assessed in patients with hypertension? How does cardiovascular risk influence management of hypertension?

The presence of target organ damage and other concomitant risk factors influences the overall cardiovascular risk of hypertensive patients and, therefore, is used to stratify the risk in each individual and guide management of hypertension. Refer to the table below for the stratification scheme proposed in the Sixth Joint National Committee on Hypertension.

Risk Stratification and Treatment of Hypertension

BLOOD PRESSURE STAGES	RISK GROUP A (NO RISK FACTORS, NO TOD/CCD)	RISK GROUP B (AT LEAST 1 RISK FACTOR, NOT DIABETES: NO TOD/CCD)	RISK GROUP C (TOD/CCD AND/OR DIABETES WITH OR WITHOUT OTHER RISK FACTORS
High normal	Lifestyle modification	Lifestyle modification	Drug therapy
Stage 1	Lifestyle modification	Lifestyle modification	Drug therapy
Stages 2 and 3	Drug therapy	Drug therapy	Drug therapy

TOD = target organ damage; CCD = clinical cardiovascular disease
Data from National Institutes of Health: Sixth Report of the Joint National Committee on Prevention, Detection, Evaluation, and Treatment of High Blood Pressure. Bethesda, MD, NIH, 1997, NIH publication 98-4080.

The major risk factors to consider are smoking, dyslipidemia, diabetes, age older than 60 years, sex (men and postmenopausal females), and family history of cardiovascular disease. The presence of heart disease (left ventricular hypertrophy, angina or myocardial infarction, coronary revascularization, and heart failure), stroke or transient ischemic attack, nephropathy, peripheral arterial disease, and retinopathy is evidence of target organ damage, and prompt institution of drug therapy is indicated.

11. What lifestyle modifications are recommended for patients with essential hypertension?

Lifestyle modification is an important part of management of patients with hypertension. All patients should be counseled to maintain desirable body weight, limit alcohol intake to less than 1 oz/day, and increase aerobic physical activity. In addition, sodium intake should be restricted to less than 100 mmol/day, and adequate dietary intake of potassium, calcium, and magnesium should be maintained. Smoking cessation and reduced dietary intake of saturated fat should be encouraged in all patients to improve overall cardiovascular health.

12. What are the general principles of antihypertensive drug therapy?

In patients with stage 1 or 2 hypertension, drug therapy should be initiated with a low dose of a single agent, preferably once a day. The dose should be titrated upward as needed for blood pressure control. If the blood pressure remains greater than 140/90 after 1–2 months despite monotherapy, a second agent from a different class (particularly a diuretic if not already being used) should be added. If blood pressure is not controlled with adequate doses of three antihypertensive medications, a work-up for resistant hypertension should be started in consultation with a hypertension specialist. Once-daily dosing is generally preferred due to better adherence, smooth and persistent control of hypertension, and lower cost.

13. What are the main classes of antihypertensive drugs?

Diuretics	Angiotensin receptor antagonists
Beta blockers	Calcium channel antagonists
Alpha blockers	Centrally acting agents
Angiotensin-converting enzyme (ACE) inhibitors	Direct vasodilators

14. In patients with uncomplicated essential hypertension, which drugs are recommended for initial use?

Diuretics and beta blockers are the preferred drugs for initial therapy in patients with uncomplicated essential hypertension. These drugs are effective in lowering blood pressure, are generally well tolerated, and have been shown in several prospective trials to lower morbidity and mortality. Diuretics are particularly effective in African-American and elderly patients. They may cause some metabolic side effects including short-term increases in glucose and cholesterol levels, hypokalemia, and hyperuricemia. Therefore, these biochemical parameters should be monitored on a periodic basis in patients on diuretic therapy. There are several different types of beta blockers depending on their cardioselectivity, lipid solubility, and intrinsic sympathomimetic activity. This class of drugs is a good choice in patients with coexisting coronary artery disease because of its antianginal properties. Beta blockers are contraindicated in patients with bronchospasm or advanced heart block and may mask insulin-induced hypoglycemia in diabetic patients.

15. How do ACE inhibitors act? When should they be used and what are their side effects?

The renin angiotensin system is an important homeostatic mechanism involved in maintaining blood pressure and salt and water balance. ACE inhibitors act by inhibiting the enzyme that converts angiotensin I to angiotensin II, which is a potent vasoconstrictor that also promotes renal retention of sodium. Captopril, lisinopril, enalapril, ramipril, and quinapril are some of the commonly used ACE inhibitors.

Due to their unique effects on lowering intraglomerular pressure, ACE inhibitors are particularly useful in diabetics and those with mild to moderate chronic renal insufficiency. In addition, this class of drugs has been shown to reduce morbidity and mortality in patients with congestive heart failure. The side effect profile is attributed to reduced degradation of bradykinin and similar vasodilator metabolites. Angioedema and agranulocytosis are rare but serious side effects of ACE inhibitor therapy. A dry cough is the most common side effect, occurring in 10–15% of patients.

16. What is the mechanism of action of the angiotensin II receptor blockers? How do they differ from ACE inhibitors?

Recently, a new class of drugs has been introduced that acts by blocking the angiotensin II receptors (losartan, candesartan, valsartan, irbesartan). These products do not interfere with the production of angiotensin II but bind to the angiotensin I receptor preventing the actions of angiotensin II in the target tissues. In theory, these drugs should have all the beneficial effects of ACE inhibition; in addition, because they do not interfere with bradykinin metabolism, the incidence of cough is much lower than ACE inhibitors. Long-term studies with angiotensin II receptor antagonists are currently under way.

17. What are the commonly used calcium channel blockers and what are their common side effects?

The dihydropyridine calcium channel blockers, including amlodipine, nifedipine, and felodipine, act primarily as vasodilators and are effective antihypertensive agents. The short-acting formulations of nifedipine may be associated with excessive and rapid lowering of blood pressure and are not recommended for routine use. The long-acting formulations are well-tolerated and are among the most frequently prescribed antihypertensive medications in the United States currently. Ankle edema, flushing, and headache are the common side effects of these agents. The nondihydropyridine calcium channel blockers are diltiazem and verapamil. In addition to their antihypertensive efficacy, they also can depress cardiac contractility and inhibit atrioventricular node conduction. These are generally well tolerated but should be used with caution in patients with impaired systolic function or bradyarrhythmias.

18. What are some reasons for resistance to antihypertensive therapy?

Patients may not respond adequately to antihypertensive therapy for several reasons. Non-adherence to therapy is always a consideration in a chronic and asymptomatic condition such as hypertension. Educating patients about the disease and using simple, once-a-day, and affordable drug regimens can help to improve patient compliance. Volume overload and excessive salt intake, particularly in patients with impaired renal function, are common causes of poor blood pressure control and require appropriate diuretic therapy. Use of inadequate doses of antihypertensive drugs, ingestion of other medications such as nonsteroidal anti-inflammatory drugs (NSAIDs) and sympathomimetic agents, and associated conditions such as obesity, sleep apnea, and excessive ethanol intake can also contribute to poor blood pressure control.

19. What are the features of hypertension in African Americans?

The prevalence of hypertension in African Americans is among the highest in the world. Compared with whites, hypertension develops earlier in life, and average blood pressures and risk of target organ damage are much higher in African Americans. Diuretics are the agents of choice in hypertensive African Americans and should be used unless there are compelling indications for alternative drugs. ACE inhibitors may be less potent in this population but, at higher doses and in combination with diuretics, are still effective antihypertensive agents.

20. What are the clinical features of hypertension in elderly patients?

Hypertension is very common in patients older than 60 years with prevalence of 60–70%. These patients frequently have predominantly systolic hypertension, and systolic blood pressure has been shown to be a better predictor of cardiovascular events than diastolic blood pressure. Blood pressure can sometimes be falsely high due to arterial stiffness and should be evaluated using Osler's maneuver. In addition, older patients are more likely to have an orthostatic fall in blood pressure; therefore, blood pressure should always be measured in the standing and supine positions.

Diuretics have been shown to lower morbidity and mortality from hypertension in older patients and are, therefore, recommended as initial therapy. Calcium channel blockers can also be used as alternative therapy. The goal of treatment is the same as in younger persons (less than 140/90 mmHg), though an interim goal of systolic blood pressure less than 160 mmHg may be necessary in patients with marked systolic hypertension.

21. What are the treatment considerations in hypertensive patients who have coexistent cardiovascular disease?

Patients with coronary heart disease are at high risk for cardiovascular morbidity and mortality and will benefit from good control of blood pressure. Excessively rapid lowering of blood pressure, particularly associated with reflex tachycardia, should be avoided in these patients. In patients who have had a myocardial infarction (MI), beta blockers without sympathomimetic activity are the drugs of choice. If there is evidence of left ventricular systolic dysfunction following an MI, then ACE inhibitors are especially beneficial.

Left ventricular hypertrophy (LVH) is an independent risk factor for cardiovascular events. Most antihypertensive agents (except direct vasodilators such as hydralazine and minoxidil) are capable of reducing left ventricular mass and wall thickness. In some studies, ACE inhibitors, perhaps due to their actions on the local renin angiotensin systems, have been shown to be more effective in inducing regression of LVH. Whether regression of LVH reduces morbidity and mortality independent of blood pressure reduction has not been shown.

Hypertension is a leading factor in the development of congestive heart failure. ACE inhibitors, when used alone or in conjunction with diuretics or digoxin, are effective in lowering morbidity and mortality in patients with congestive heart failure. When ACE inhibitors are not tolerated, a combination of hydralazine and isosorbide dinitrate can be used. Angiotensin receptor antagonists have recently been shown to be beneficial in the treatment of congestive heart failure.

BIBLIOGRAPHY

1. Brown NJ, Vaughan DE: Angiotensin-converting enzyme inhibitors. Circulation 97:1411–1420, 1998.
2. Cutler JA, Follman D, Allender PS: Randomized trials of sodium reduction: An overview. Am J Clin Nutr 65(suppl):643S–651S, 1997.
3. Freis ED: Current status of diuretics, beta-blockers, alpha-blockers, and alpha-beta-blockers in the treatment of hypertension. Med Clin North Am 81:1305–1317, 1997.

4. Kaplan NM: Resistant hypertension: What to do after trying "the usual." Geriatrics 50:24–38, 1995.
5. Lever A, Ramsay LE: Treatment of hypertension in the elderly. J Hypertens 13:571–579, 1995.
6. National Institutes of Health: Sixth Report of the Joint National Committee on Prevention, Detection, Evaluation, and Treatment of High Blood Pressure. Bethesda, MD, NIH, 1997, NIH publication 98-4080.
7. Perloff D, Grim C, Flack J, et al: Human blood pressure determination by sphygmomanometry. Circulation 88:2460–2467, 1993.
8. Rahman M, Douglas JG, Wright JT Jr: Pathophysiology and treatment implications of hypertension in the African American population. Endocrinol Metab Clin North Am 26:125–144, 1997.

55. RENAL PARENCHYMAL HYPERTENSION

Michael C. Smith, M.D.

1. How common is renal parenchymal hypertension?
Hypertension due to chronic renal parenchymal disease is the most common form of secondary hypertension. Five percent to 6% of all patients with high blood pressure have underlying renal disease.

2. Does hypertension occur in patients with acute renal disease? What are its causes?
Hypertension can complicate acute poststreptococcal glomerulonephritis, acute tubular necrosis, and minimal change disease. Twenty percent to 30% of adults with minimal change disease are hypertensive at initial presentation, while 40% of patients with acute tubular necrosis and 80% of those with acute poststreptococcal glomerulonephritis exhibit hypertension at some time during their clinical course. Evidence to date suggests that the majority of hypertensive patients with acute renal disease demonstrate volume-dependent hypertension that improves with resolution of the underlying disease or with salt removal during dialysis. In some, however, vasoconstrictor mechanisms (i.e., angiotensin II, activation of the sympathetic nervous system) contribute to the increase in blood pressure.

3. What is the prevalence of hypertension in chronic renal parenchymal disease?
Estimates of hypertension in various chronic renal diseases range from 35% to 80% (see Table).

Renal Disease	*Percent of Patients with Hypertension*
Chronic glomerular disease	
Focal glomerulosclerosis	75–80
Membranoproliferative glomerulonephritis	65–70
Diabetic nephropathy	65–70
Membranous nephropathy	40–50
Mesangioproliferative glomerulonephritis	35–40
IgA nephropathy	30–35
Polycystic kidney disease	60
Chronic interstitial nephritis	35

Hypertension is less prevalent early in the course of most renal diseases but is present in 80–90% of patients with end-stage renal disease.

4. What factors are causally related to the development of hypertension in patients with chronic renal disease?
Renal parenchymal hypertension results from the integrated interaction of multiple factors that affect cardiac output, peripheral resistance, or both. Although alterations in the production of natriuretic peptides, prostaglandins, and endothelin have been implicated in the genesis of experimental renal hypertension, their relevance to renal hypertension in humans is unclear. On the other hand, a positive salt balance, increased activity of the renin-angiotensin-aldosterone system, and stimulation of the sympathetic nervous system are important contributors to human renal parenchymal hypertension.

5. What evidence supports a central role for salt balance in renal hypertension?

Patients with renal parenchymal hypertension demonstrate increased total exchangeable sodium and an increase in plasma and extracellular fluid volume that correlates with blood pressure. In addition, dietary salt loading increases blood pressure in these patients while salt restriction or salt removal with diuretics decreases blood pressure in the majority. Finally, in patients with end-stage renal disease, salt subtraction and reduction to dry weight with dialysis normalizes blood pressure in most patients without need for pharmacologic therapy.

6. What evidence supports a role for the renin-angiotensin-aldosterone system in renal parenchymal hypertension?

Plasma renin activity and angiotensin II are increased and correlate with blood pressure in hypertensive patients with mild to moderate renal dysfunction. In addition, interruption of the renin-angiotensin axis with angiotensin-converting enzyme (ACE) inhibitors or angiotensin receptor blockers decreases blood pressure in proportion to baseline plasma renin activity. Finally 10–20% of patients with end-stage renal disease demonstrate hypertension that is resistant to salt removal but normalizes with ACE inhibition. Hence, the renin-angiotensin-aldosterone system is causally related to hypertension in many, but not all, hypertensive patients with renal disease.

7. What evidence supports an etiologic role for the sympathetic nervous system in renal parenchymal hypertension?

Early in the course of renal disease, plasma concentrations of norepinephrine are elevated and correlate with arterial pressure. In patients with end-stage renal disease, selective postganglionic sympathetic blockade normalizes blood pressure in hypertensive dialysis patients. Furthermore, accumulating data suggest that postganglionic sympathetic nerve activity is increased in hemodialysis patients who retain their native kidneys. It is hypothesized that afferent sympathetic nerves from diseased kidneys signal the anterior hypothalamus with a consequent increase in peripheral sympathetic activity thus increasing blood pressure. This evidence strongly suggests that increased sympathetic nerve activity contributes to renal parenchymal hypertension.

8. What effect does hypertension have on renal function in patients with renal parenchymal disease?

Over the past several decades, the concept that hypertension accelerates the loss of renal function has become well accepted. Glomerular filtration rate declines more rapidly in hypertensive patients with renal parenchymal disease compared with their normotensive counterparts. Poor blood pressure control contributes to the progressive decline in glomerular filtration rate in both diabetic and nondiabetic kidney disease.

9. How does systemic hypertension accelerate the decline in renal function?

Accumulating data suggest that multiple interrelated mechanisms including impaired autoregulation of renal blood flow, glomerular capillary hypertension, and glomerular hypertrophy are causally related to the progressive loss of kidney function in hypertensive patients with renal disease. The normal kidney maintains a relatively constant glomerular filtration rate and renal blood flow over a wide range of systemic blood pressures by modulating afferent arteriolar tone. Kidney disease impairs autoregulation of renal blood flow so that even slightly elevated systemic blood pressures are transmitted to the glomerulus, increase intraglomerular pressure with consequent hydraulically mediated injury, and result in increased proteinuria, glomerulosclerosis, and loss of renal function. In addition, the mitogenic effects of angiotensin II, endothelin, and other fibrogenic cytokines increase mesangial cell proliferation and cause glomerular scarring that further worsens renal function.

10. Does control of blood pressure retard the rate of decline in glomerular filtration rate?

Reduction of systemic blood pressure limits glomerular damage and slows the rate of loss of kidney function in animal models of renal disease. Further, numerous prospective clinical trials have shown that excellent blood pressure control slows the progression of human renal parenchymal disease. Current recommendations suggest that reduction of blood pressure to a level of 130/80–85 mmHg should be a minimum goal in patients with chronic renal disease. Hypertensive patients with urine protein excretion greater than 1 gm/day, and especially those with greater than 3 gm/day, have a slower progression of renal disease with even lower blood pressure (i.e., 125/75 mmHg).

11. What is the approach to treatment of hypertension in patients with advanced chronic renal failure?

Abnormal salt metabolism is a central etiologic factor in the development of renal parenchymal hypertension. Sodium excretion is limited not only because of the decrease in glomerular filtration rate but also because of the direct salt-retaining effects of the activated renal-angiotensin-aldosterone axis and the sympathetic nervous system. Consequently, dietary salt restriction (80–90 mmol/day) and diuretic therapy are essential for adequate control of blood pressure. Diuretics should be titrated upward until the patient is free of edema. Because thiazide diuretics are ineffective in patients with creatinine clearances less than 25–30 ml/minute, loop diuretics, usually administered twice or three times/day, are often required to achieve adequate salt subtraction. The majority of patients, however, require additional drug therapy for control of blood pressure. Of the available classes of antihypertensive agents, ACE inhibitors, angiotensin receptor blockers, calcium channel antagonists, and centrally acting sympatholytics (e.g., clonidine) are preferable. Irrespective of the drugs selected, dosage should be adjusted to decrease blood pressure to a goal of 130/80–85 mmHg.

12. Are certain classes of antihypertensive agents uniquely renoprotective?

A large body of experimental and clinical data suggests that both ACE inhibitors and calcium channel blockers slow the progression of renal disease to a greater extent than other classes of antihypertensive drugs. Most, but not all, studies in patients with diabetic nephropathy show that ACE inhibitors retard the progression of renal disease compared with non–calcium channel blocker–based conventional antihypertensive therapy. Similar data are emerging in nondiabetic kidney disease; most studies show a greater renoprotective effect with ACE inhibitors. However, two long-term prospective studies comparing ACE inhibitors and calcium channel blockers in patients with nondiabetic kidney disease showed that both drug classes slowed the decline in renal function to a similar extent. Hence, the available data support the notion that both of these drug classes slow the progression of kidney disease compared with alternative antihypertensive regimens. It remains to be determined whether this beneficial effect is due to unique renoprotective properties or greater antihypertensive efficacy.

13. What is the approach to the treatment of hypertension in patients with end-stage renal disease?

Eighty percent to 90% of hypertensive dialysis patients become normotensive if sufficient salt and water are removed by dialysis to achieve a true dry weight. The remaining patients require nondiuretic antihypertensive therapy. Because the pathogenesis of hypertension in dialysis patients is similar to that in patients with advanced chronic renal failure, selection of pharmacologic agents should be comparable. In this regard, ACE inhibitors, centrally acting sympatholytics, and calcium channel antagonists are logical and effective selections.

BIBLIOGRAPHY

1. Epstein M: Calcium antagonists and renal disease. Kidney Int 54:1771–1784, 1998.
2. Giatras I, Lau J, Levey A: Effect of angiotensin-converting enzyme inhibitors on the progression of non-diabetic renal disease: A meta-analysis of randomized trials. Ann Intern Med 127:337–345, 1997.
3. Ihle BU, Whitworth JA, Shahinfar S, et al: Angiotensin-converting enzyme inhibition in nondiabetic renal insufficiency: A controlled double-blind trial. Am J Kidney Dis 27:489–495, 1996.

4. Klahr S, Levey AS, Beck GJ, et al: The effects of dietary protein restriction and blood pressure control on the progression of chronic renal disease. N Engl J Med 330:877–894, 1994.
5. Maki DD, Ma JZ, Louis TA, Kasiske BL: Long-term effects of antihypertensive agents on proteinuria and renal function. Arch Intern Med 155:1073–1080, 1995.
6. Maschio G, Alberti D, Janin G, et al: Effect of the angiotensin-converting inhibitor benazepril on the progression of chronic renal insufficiency. N Engl J Med 334:939–945, 1996.
7. Peterson JC, Adler S, Burkhart JM, et al: Blood pressure control, proteinuria, and the progression of renal disease. The modification of diet in renal disease study. Ann Intern Med 123:754–762, 1995.
8. Rahman M, Smith MC: Chronic renal insufficiency. Arch Intern Med 158:1743–1752, 1998.
9. Smith MC, Dunn MJ: Hypertension associated with renal parenchymal disease. In Schrier RW, Gottschalk CW (eds): Diseases of the Kidney, 6th ed. Vol. 2. Boston, Little, Brown, 1997, pp 1333–1365.
10. Weir MR, Dworkin LD: Antihypertensive drugs, dietary salt, and renal protection: How low should you go and with which therapy? Am J Kidney Dis 32:1–22, 1998.
11. Zucchelli P, Zuccala A, Borghi M, et al: Long-term comparison between captopril and nifedipine in the progression of renal insufficiency. Kidney Int 42:452–458, 1992.

56. RENOVASCULAR HYPERTENSION

Donald E. Hricik, M.D.

1. What is renovascular hypertension?

The term *renovascular hypertension* refers to high blood pressure caused by occlusive disease of one or both main renal arteries or their branches. A diagnosis of renovascular hypertension can be made with certainty only by showing that high blood pressure is improved or cured after correction of the occlusion. However, decisions to proceed with interventions to correct occlusive renal arterial disease are based on a tentative diagnosis that requires anatomic or functional tests.

2. What is the pathophysiology of renovascular hypertension?

Renovascular hypertension results from activation of the renin-angiotensin-aldosterone axis mediated by ischemia. Decreased perfusion to the affected kidney results in the release of renin, which, in turn, accelerates the conversion of angiotensinogen to angiotensin I. Angiotensin-converting enzyme (ACE) converts angiotensin I to angiotensin II, a peptide with potent vasoconstrictor properties. Angiotensin II also stimulates the adrenal gland to release aldosterone, leading to renal sodium retention.

The pathophysiology of renovascular hypertension varies depending on whether renal occlusive disease occurs in one kidney in a patient with two kidneys and a normal contralateral kidney ("two-kidney, one-clip model") or in a solitary kidney in a patient with no contralateral kidney ("one-kidney, one-clip model"). In the two-kidney model, the ischemic kidney secretes renin and retains salt and water, but the normal contralateral kidney exhibits a pressure natriuresis that actually leads to negative sodium balance, further exacerbating the release of renin. The clinical analogy is unilateral renal artery stenosis in a patient with two kidneys. In the one-kidney model, absence of a contralateral kidney prevents sodium loss. Extracellular volume expansion ensues, plasma renin activity is suppressed, and hypertension persists largely because of volume overload. Clinical analogies include renal artery stenosis in a patient with a solitary kidney and bilateral renal artery stenoses in a patient with two kidneys.

3. What are the causes of renovascular hypertension?

Common Causes of Renovascular Hypertension (~ 95% of all cases)
- Atherosclerosis
- Fibromuscular dysplasia

Rare Causes of Renovascular Hypertension (~ 5% of cases)
- Neurofibromatosis
- Extrinsic compression
- Congenital anomalies
- Radiation fibrosis
- Arterial thromboembolism
- Vasculitis

4. How common is renovascular hypertension?

The reported prevalence of renovascular hypertension varies widely depending on the population being studied and the type of tests performed to make the diagnosis. Autopsy studies suggest that as many as 40% of adults have at least mild narrowing of the renal arteries, but many cases may be clinically insignificant. Among severely hypertensive patients referred to tertiary care centers, the prevalence of renovascular hypertension may exceed 20% in patients studied with angiography. Most authorities agree, however, that renovascular disease probably accounts for high blood pressure in no more than 5% of the general population of patients with hypertension.

5. What is fibromuscular dysplasia?

Fibromuscular dysplasia is a nonarteriosclerotic occlusive vascular disease of unknown etiology. The disorder occurs most commonly in young or middle-aged adult women and is uncommon in African Americans. The dysplastic process primarily involves the renal arteries, but other vascular beds (e.g., cerebral vessels) can be involved. Four pathologic variants have been described. **Medial fibroplasia** is the most common (accounting for 70% of all cases) and is recognized angiographically by the classic "string of beads" appearance (see Figure). The less common variants are **intimal**, **perimedial**, and **adventitial fibrous dysplasia**.

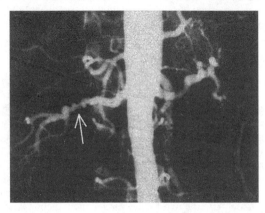

Renal angiogram demonstrating medial fibrous dysplasia in a main renal artery.

6. What clinical characteristics are typical of patients with renovascular hypertension?

In most cases, renovascular hypertension cannot be differentiated clinically from essential hypertension. However, the following clinical features should increase suspicion and prompt diagnostic evaluation for possible renovascular disease:
- Progression in the severity of chronic hypertension
- Recent onset of hypertension
- Malignant hypertension
- Moderate hypertension in a patient with diffuse vascular disease (especially if the patient is a smoker)
- Early (age < 25 years) or late (age > 60 years) onset
- Renal failure during treatment with an ACE inhibitor or angiotensin receptor blocker
- Abdominal or flank bruit
- Recurrent episodes of "flash" pulmonary edema

7. What tests are used to make a diagnosis of renovascular hypertension?

Angiography remains the gold standard for determining whether a patient has occlusive disease of the renal arteries. Digital subtraction angiography is preferred in some centers in an effort to minimize the amount of administered contrast dye. However, digital studies may not provide adequate images of the peripheral branches of the arterial tree. Angiographic techniques can detect anatomic abnormalities, but they do not provide information about the functional significance of a renal artery stenosis. Most clinicians would agree, however, that luminal narrowing of 70% or greater is usually clinically significant. Other noninvasive tests that have been used to screen for renovascular disease include:

Duplex ultrasonography
Magnetic resonance angiography
ACE-inhibitor–stimulated renography
ACE-inhibitor–stimulated peripheral renin activity

8. How do angiotensin inhibitors cause renal failure in patients with renovascular disease?

ACE inhibitor–induced renal failure was first described in patients with bilateral renal artery stenosis or renal artery stenosis involving a solitary kidney. Under circumstances in which the entire renal mass is hypoperfused as a consequence of arterial occlusion, intrarenal hemodynamics are altered such that autoregulation of glomerular filtration rate becomes critically dependent on the effects of angiotensin II on the efferent (postglomerular) capillaries. When angiotensin II is inhibited by an ACE inhibitor (or by an angiotensin receptor blocker), postglomerular resistance decreases. In theory, renal blood flow is maintained or increased, but glomerular filtration rate may fall dramatically. The hemodynamic pattern is best described as a dissociation in the autoregulation of renal blood flow and glomerular filtration rate.

The same phenomenon forms the basis for ACE inhibitor renography. In this diagnostic test, glomerular filtration rate is estimated by the clearance of a radioisotope under baseline conditions and again after administration of an ACE inhibitor. A decrease in the glomerular filtration rate suggests the presence of a functionally significant occlusion.

9. What are the objectives of therapy in patients with renovascular disease?

1. Control systemic blood pressure
2. Preserve renal function

10. What treatments are available for patients with renovascular hypertension?

1. Medical therapy (i.e., antihypertensive drugs)
2. Percutaneous transluminal angioplasty (with or without stenting)
3. Surgery

11. What are the management principles underlying the choice of therapy for patients with renovascular hypertension?

The choice of therapy depends on the severity of the systemic hypertension, the pathologic process (i.e., atherosclerosis vs. fibromuscular dysplasia), the presence or absence of renal impairment, location of the lesion (see question 14), and the presence of comorbid conditions (e.g., coronary or cerebrovascular disease) that may affect life expectancy. Medical therapy may adequately control blood pressure but will not likely decrease the risk of progressive renal impairment resulting from renal ischemia. In fact, medical therapy may contribute to progressive ischemic injury by reducing systemic pressure and further reducing perfusion to the affected kidney. For patients who are candidates for invasive therapy, percutaneous transluminal angioplasty is preferred because it can be performed without general anesthesia or prolonged hospitalization. The main limitations of angioplasty are technical failures, vascular accidents (e.g., dissection or rupture), and recurrence of stenoses. Angioplasty has emerged as the treatment of choice for patients with fibromuscular dysplasia.

12. What are the indications for medical therapy in patients with renovascular hypertension?

Medical therapy is reasonable in patients:
• With bilateral or segmental lesions deemed to be nondilatable and inoperable
• With high operative risks (e.g., elderly patients with concomitant coronary or cerebrovascular disease)
• Who refuse invasive therapy

13. How does the location of an atherosclerotic renal artery stenosis influence therapy?

Angioplasty is technically difficult to perform in atherosclerotic lesions in the proximal portion of the renal artery, especially if the lesion involves the renal ostium. Furthermore, such lesions tend to recur with great frequency. Bypass surgery is preferred in such cases if the patient is an operative candidate. Angioplasty is more successful in the management of atherosclerotic lesions involving the distal two thirds of the main renal artery.

14. What are the indications for surgery in patients with renovascular hypertension?
- Ostial or near-ostial atherosclerotic lesions (usually treated with a bypass graft)
- Occlusive lesions in distal branches of the renal arterial tree (may require bench surgery or nephrectomy)
- Progressive fibrous dysplastic lesions not responsive to angioplasty (usually occurring in patients with the adventitial or intimal variants)
- Progressive hypertension or renal failure despite transient improvements with angioplasty

BIBLIOGRAPHY

1. Davidson RA, Wilcox CS: Newer tests for the diagnosis of renovascular disease. JAMA 268:3353–3358, 1992.
2. Hricik DE, Dunn MJ: Angiotensin-converting enzyme inhibitor–induced renal failure: Causes, consequences, and diagnostic uses. J Am Soc Nephrol 1:845–858, 1990.
3. Mann SJ, Pickering TG: Detection of renovascular hypertension: State of the art, 1992. Ann Intern Med 117:845–853, 1992.
4. Martinez-Maldonado M: Pathophysiology of renovascular hypertension. Hypertension 17:707–719, 1991.
5. Plouin PF, Darne B, Chantellier G, et al: Restenosis after a first percutaneous transluminal angioplasty. Hypertension 21:89–96, 1993.
6. Rimmer JM, Gennari FJ: Atherosclerotic renovascular disease and progressive renal failure. Ann Intern Med 118:712–719, 1993.
7. Ying CY, Tift CP, Gavras H, Chobanian AV: Renal revascularization in the azotemic hypertensive patient resistant to therapy. N Engl J Med 311:1070–1075, 1984.

57. PHEOCHROMOCYTOMA

Ashwin Dixit, M.D.

1. What is a pheochromocytoma?

Pheochromocytoma is a catecholamine-producing tumor derived from chromaffin cells (staining with chromium salts) of the sympathetic nervous system. Over 90% of these tumors are located in the adrenal gland. The remainder are derived from chromaffin cells of neural crest origin and can be found in locations such as the carotid body and the abdominal sympathetic ganglia—including the organ of Zuckerlandl, which consists of ganglia at the bifurcation of the aorta. Most tumors are benign, but 10% are malignant with the potential to metastasize.

2. What are the clinical manifestations of pheochromocytoma?

The most common finding is **hypertension**, which occurs in more than 90% of patients and which is paroxysmal in character in 20–25% of cases. Paroxysmal episodes of hypertension are typically associated with other signs and symptoms of catecholamine excess: tremor, tachycardia, hyperhydrosis, headache, and pupillary dilatation. Orthostatic hypotension may occur as a result of decreased sympathetic reflexes reflecting downregulation of adrenergic receptors. Weight loss may result from chronic hypermetabolism.

3. What catecholamines are produced by pheochromocytomas?

Synthesis of catecholamines begins with the amino acid tyrosine derived either from the diet or from hydroxylation of phenylalanine. The metabolism of tyrosine within the sympathetic nervous system is shown in the Figure.

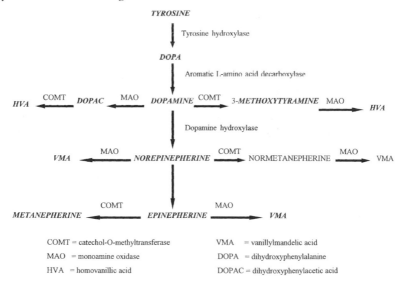

COMT = catechol-O-methyltransferase   VMA = vanillylmandelic acid
MAO = monoamine oxidase   DOPA = dihydroxyphenylalanine
HVA = homovanillic acid   DOPAC = dihydroxyphenylacetic acid

Norepinephrine is the catecholamine secreted predominantly by most pheochromocytomas. Tumors that predominantly secrete epinephrine or dopamine are less common and more often are malignant or extra-adrenal in location.

4. How common is pheochromocytoma?

Pheochromocytomas are rare tumors. They are responsible for hypertension in less than 0.1% of all patients with high blood pressure.

5. What conditions are associated with pheochromocytoma?
1. von Recklinghausen's disease (neurofibromatosis)
2. von Hippel-Lindau disease
3. Multiple endocrine neoplasia (MEN) syndromes
   • MEN type 2: pheochromocytoma (often bilateral), parathyroid adenoma, medullary carcinoma of the thyroid
   • MEN type 3: pheochromocytoma (often bilateral), medullary carcinoma of the thyroid, mucosal neuromas, abdominal gangliomas, marfanoid body habitus

6. What is the ten percent rule?
Each of the following accounts for 10% of all pheochromocytomas:
• Bilateral (in adrenal glands)
• Extra-adrenal
• Malignant
• Familial (associated with MEN syndromes)
• Pediatric

7. Which patients should be evaluated?
Consider evaluation in patients with:
• Sustained or paroxysmal hypertension associated with the triad of headache, palpitations, and diaphoresis
• Hypertension and a family history of pheochromocytoma
• Features of MEN type 2 or 3
• Refractory hypertension—especially if associated with weight loss
• Hypertensive crises during surgical procedures
• An incidentally discovered adrenal mass

8. Elaborate on the biochemical screening for pheochromocytoma.
Measurement of catecholamines and their metabolites in the plasma and urine are recommended for screening. Small tumors (< 50 gm) may exhibit rapid turnover rates and release mainly unmetabolized catecholamines. Larger tumors often exhibit slower turnover rates associated with higher concentration of catecholamine metabolites in plasma and urine. Resting plasma catecholamine concentrations greater than 2000 pg/ml suggest a pheochromocytoma while values less than 500 pg/ml are normal. Intermediate values (500–2000 pg/ml) are equivocal and mandate additional testing if clinical suspicion is high. Urine screening consists of measuring metanephrines, vanillylmandelic acid, and free catecholamines in a 24-hour urine collection.

9. What are potential sources of error in chemical screening tests?
Plasma catecholamine levels may be elevated falsely with any kind of stress. In patients with paroxysmal hypertension, urinary concentrations of catecholamines and their metabolites may be normal if the 24-hour urine is collected when the patient is normotensive and asymptomatic.

Drugs that Effect Chemical Screening

METABOLITE	DRUG	EFFECT
Free catecholamines	Methyldopa	False increase
	L-dopa	False increase
Metanephrines	Monoamine oxidase (MAO) inhibitors	Increase
Vanillylmandelic acid	MAO inhibitors	Decrease
	Clofibrate	False decrease
	Nalidixic acid	False increase

10. What tests should be performed in equivocal cases?

A number of provocative pharmacologic tests can be performed:

Test	Rationale
Regitine (phentolamine) test	Phentolamine is an alpha blocker, and a reduction in blood pressure suggests catecholamine excess. Not very sensitive or specific.
Glucagon stimulation test	Glucagon stimulates catecholamine release. Associated with risk of precipitating a hypertensive crisis.
Clonidine suppression test	Clonidine decreases central sympathetic outflow but does not suppress autonomous production by a tumor. Failure to suppress plasma norepinephrine by more than 50% after administration of clonidine suggests a pheochromocytoma.

11. What studies are used to localize a pheochromocytoma?

Computed tomography (CT) scan or magnetic resonance imaging (MRI) of the abdomen are the imaging studies of choice. I-metaiodobenzylguanidine (MIBG) scintigraphy employs an isotope with an affinity for chromaffin tissue and can be used to detect extra-adrenal tumors or to confirm that an adrenal mass is a pheochromocytoma. When imaging studies are equivocal, selective venous sampling of the vena cava at various levels can help to locate the tumor.

12. What is the treatment of choice?

Surgical resection is the treatment of choice and is curative in 90% of cases. Medical therapy is used mainly for perioperative management.

13. Describe the perioperative management.

Blood pressure should be well controlled for 1–4 weeks prior to surgery in order to minimize perioperative hemodynamic instability. Alpha blockers are the agents of choice and phenoxybenzamine, a long-acting noncompetitive alpha blocker, is preferred. The newer competitive alpha blockers (e.g., prazosin, terazosin) have a shorter duration of action and are used less commonly. If beta blockers are required to treat cardiac arrhythmias, they should only be administered after alpha blockade is achieved in order to prevent unopposed alpha receptor stimulation. Rapidly acting agents such as phentolamine or nitroprusside should be readily available in order to manage perioperative hypertensive crises.

14. What about treatment for malignant pheochromocytoma?

Malignant pheochromocytomas are slow growing and respond poorly to radio- or chemotherapy. Surgical debulking may be necessary to decrease catecholamine synthesis. Radioactive MIBG has been used with some success to ablate primary and metastatic sites. Alpha methyltyrosine, an inhibitor of tyrosine hydroxylase, can inhibit catecholamine synthesis and has been tried in inoperable cases.

BIBLIOGRAPHY

1. Bravo EL: Pheochromocytoma: New concepts and future trends. Kidney Int 40:544–556, 1991.
2. Kebebew E, Duh QY: Benign and malignant pheochromocytoma: Diagnosis, treatment, and follow-up. Surg Oncol Clin North Am 7:765–789, 1998.
3. Russell WJ, Metcalf IR, Tonkin AL, Frewin DB: The preoperative management of phaeochromocytoma. Anaesth Intensive Care 26:196–200, 1998.
4. Sheps SG, Jiang NS, Klee GG, vanHeerden JA: Recent developments in the diagnosis and treatment of pheochromocytoma. Mayo Clin Proc 65:88–95, 1990.
5. Young WF: Pheochromocytoma and primary aldosteronism: Diagnostic approaches. Endocrinol Metab Clin North Am 26:801–827, 1997.

58. OTHER CAUSES OF SECONDARY HYPERTENSION

Mahboob Rahman, M.D., M.S.

1. What are some of the relatively uncommon causes of secondary hypertension?

Primary aldosteronism
Cushing's syndrome
Coarctation of the aorta
Hypothyroidism
Acromegaly
Sleep apnea
Drugs
    cyclosporine
    erythropoietin
    estrogens
    cocaine
    anabolic steroids
    glucocorticoids
    monoamine oxidase (MAO) inhibitors
    bromocriptine

2. What are the clinical features of primary aldosteronism?

Primary aldosteronism is a rare cause of secondary hypertension. It is usually seen in patients between the ages of 30 and 50 years and in women more frequently than in men. The typical clinical features of this syndrome are hypertension associated with hypokalemia, excessive urinary potassium excretion, and metabolic alkalosis. This clinical picture may be due to an aldosterone-producing adenoma or, less commonly, due to bilateral adrenal hyperplasia or adrenal carcinoma.

3. What laboratory tests are helpful in diagnosis of primary aldosteronism?

Unexplained hypokalemia is usually the first marker suggesting the possibility of underlying primary aldosteronism. The excretion of greater than 30 mEq/day of potassium in the presence of hypokalemia confirms urinary potassium wasting and supports a diagnosis of primary aldosteronism.

The plasma aldosterone (PA) and plasma renin activity (PRA) are important biochemical markers in the diagnosis of primary aldosteronism. The PA/PRA ratio is normally 10; patients with primary aldosteronism frequently have a ratio of greater than 20. Ideally, this test should be done in the absence of drug therapy such as diuretics, beta blockers, or angiotensin-converting enzyme (ACE) inhibitors, which can affect these measurements.

Once an abnormal PA/PRA ratio is seen, it is important to document whether the excessive aldosterone production is autonomous or responsive to normal homeostatic mechanisms. This can be accomplished either by saline infusion or by the captopril suppression test. If the elevated aldosterone levels are not suppressed by these maneuvers, it is likely that an aldosterone production is autonomous.

4. What radiologic tests are helpful in the diagnosis of this condition?

Both computed tomography (CT) and magnetic resonance imaging (MRI) are effective in visualizing aldosterone-producing adenomas greater than 1 cm in diameter. Adrenal scintigraphy and adrenal venous sampling are useful in special circumstances.

5. What are the therapeutic options in patients with primary aldosteronism?

The treatment depends on the type of adrenal pathology. Surgical removal is the treatment of choice for patients with adrenal adenomas or carcinomas, and medical therapy with spironolactone is recommended for those with bilateral adrenal hyperplasia. Spironolactone is an aldosterone antagonist and is used in doses ranging between 50 and 200 mg/day. Impotence and gynecomastia are common side effects of long-term therapy with aldosterone.

6. What is glucocorticoid remediable aldosteronism?

Glucocorticoid remediable aldosteronism is a genetic disorder in which there is excess secretion of aldosterone due to ectopic production in the zona fasciculata of the adrenal gland resulting in all the clinical manifestations described above. This secretion is regulated by adrenocorticotrophic hormone (ACTH); therefore, suppression of ACTH by administration of exogenous steroids results in complete resolution of the symptoms. The diagnosis can be confirmed by genetic analysis.

7. What clinical signs and symptoms suggest a diagnosis of Cushing's syndrome?

Cushing's syndrome is another relatively rare cause of secondary hypertension. The typical clinical features include truncal obesity, facial plethora ("cushingoid facies"), hirsutism, striae, easy bruising, neuropsychiatric disturbances, osteopenia, and glucose intolerance. Hypertension is present in 80% of patients with Cushing's syndrome.

8. What are the common screening tests used in the diagnosis of Cushing's syndrome?

An overnight dexamethasone suppression test is a good screening test in patients with suspected Cushing's syndrome. After a bedtime dose of 1 mg of dexamethasone is given, the plasma cortisol is measured at 8:00 the next morning. A level of less than 5 µg/dl indicates normal suppression. If the screening test is abnormal, further testing is needed to establish the cause of the syndrome, i.e., adrenal hyperplasia, ectopic ACTH production, or pituitary disease.

9. What are the treatment options in Cushing's syndrome?

Hypertension can be difficult to treat in patients with Cushing's syndrome. A diuretic, in combination with spironolactone, is usually the first choice with additional antihypertensive therapy as needed. After definitive therapy of the underlying cause of Cushing's syndrome, the hypertension usually resolves. The definitive therapy depends on the underlying disease. Surgical removal is the treatment of choice for benign adrenal tumors. For adrenal cancers and ectopic ACTH production, adjuvant chemotherapy may be required. Transsphenoidal removal is the treatment of choice for pituitary tumors.

10. What signs suggest coarctation of the aorta?

Hypertension in the arms with weak femoral pulses in a young person is suggestive of coarctation of the aorta. The chest x-ray will typically show the "3 sign" from the dilatation of the aorta above and below the constriction and notching of the ribs by enlarged collateral vessels. The diagnosis is usually made by echocardiography and by color-flow Doppler imaging.

11. Why should thyroid function tests be considered in hypertensive patients?

Hypothyroidism is associated with elevated diastolic pressure due to increased peripheral vascular resistance. Blood pressure can improve when patients are treated with thyroid hormone replacement therapy.

12. What are the symptoms of sleep apnea? What is its association with hypertension?

Patients with obstructive sleep apnea present with excessive snoring, daytime somnolence, and nocturia. The diagnosis is confirmed by an overnight sleep study. It is important to keep this diagnosis in mind, particularly in obese hypertensive patients. The pathogenesis of hypertension in sleep apnea is not clear; however, correction of the defect by surgery or by continuous positive airway pressure (CPAP) is associated with improvement in blood pressure.

13. What are some of the neurologic disorders associated with hypertension?
Patients with intracranial brain tumors, quadriplegia, or severe head injury may have hypertension due to excessive sympathetic nervous system activity.

14. What is the relationship among oral contraceptives, estrogen replacement therapy, and hypertension?
Hypertension is reported to be two to three times more common in women taking oral contraceptives, especially in obese and older women, than in those not taking oral contraceptives. Blood pressure should be monitored every 6 months in patients taking oral contraceptives. If hypertension develops, oral contraceptives should be stopped, and blood pressure will normalize in most cases in a few months. Hypertension is not a contraindication for postmenopausal hormone replacement therapy. However, a few women may experience rise in blood pressure attributable to hormone replacement therapy. Therefore, all women treated with hormone replacement therapy should have their blood pressure monitored periodically.

15. Does cocaine use cause hypertension?
There is no evidence that ongoing cocaine use causes chronic hypertension. However, it can cause an acute rise in blood pressure and can be associated with ischemia from coronary and cerebral vasoconstriction or acute renal failure from rhabdomyolysis.

BIBLIOGRAPHY

1. Bravo EL: Primary aldosteronism. Issues in diagnosis and management. Endocrinol Metab Clin North Am 23:271–283, 1994.
2. Dluhy RG, Lifton RP: Glucocorticoid remediable aldosteronism (GRA): Diagnosis, variability of phenotype, and regulation of potassium homeostasis. Steroids 60:48–51, 1995.
3. Danese RD, Aron DC: Cushing's syndrome and hypertension. Endocrinol Metab Clin North Am 23:299–324, 1994.
4. Kaplan NM: Other forms of secondary hypertension. In Kaplan NM (ed): Clinical Hypertension. Baltimore, Williams & Wilkins, 1988, pp 395–406.

59. HYPERTENSIVE EMERGENCIES

Mahboob Rahman, M.D., M.S.

1. What constitutes a hypertensive emergency?

A hypertensive emergency is a clinical situation characterized by marked elevation of blood pressure associated with progressive target organ damage that requires immediate reduction of blood pressure. These include:

- Hypertensive encephalopathy
- Hypertension associated with acute left ventricular failure
- Subarachnoid or intracerebral bleed
- Aortic dissection
- Acute myocardial infarction or unstable angina
- Adrenergic crises
- Malignant hypertension
- Eclampsia

It is important to emphasize that evidence of new or progressive target organ damage and not the absolute levels of blood pressure determine the urgency of treatment. For example, relatively modest acute increases in blood pressure may lead to target organ damage in previously normotensive patients (as in eclampsia) and in those with accompanying medical conditions (aortic dissection or myocardial infarction). Elevated blood pressure alone, in the absence of symptoms or new or progressive target organ damage, rarely requires emergency therapy.

2. What is malignant hypertension?

Malignant hypertension is a syndrome of severe elevation of arterial pressure (usually, but not always, the diastolic pressure exceeds 140 mmHg) associated with vascular damage manifested by retinal hemorrhages, exudates, and papilledema. *Accelerated hypertension* is the term used for a similar syndrome without papilledema.

3. What are the clinical circumstances associated with malignant hypertension?

Patients presenting with malignant hypertension may have a history of severe and inadequately treated essential hypertension and frequently are smokers. It is important to evaluate these patients for secondary hypertension because renovascular and renal parenchymal disease can be present in many patients presenting with malignant hypertension.

4. What is the pathophysiology leading to development of malignant hypertension?

A rapid and progressive rise in blood pressure causes endothelial damage in the blood vessels, leading to platelet and fibrin deposition and fibrinoid necrosis. In addition, due to tissue ischemia, there is increased production of angiotensin II, which is a potent vasoconstrictor. Due to the higher blood pressure, a pressure natriuresis promotes volume depletion and further activation of the renin angiotensin axis. These events form a positive feedback loop and result in progressive elevation of blood pressure and the vascular sequelae seen in malignant hypertension.

5. What are the typical pathologic lesions seen in malignant hypertension?

The vascular lesions consist predominantly of myointimal proliferation and fibrinoid necrosis. Vascular smooth muscle hypertrophy and collagen deposition contribute to medial thickening, which, accompanied by cellular intimal proliferation, results in the onion skin appearance of the small vessels.

6. What are the clinical features of malignant hypertension?

The blood pressure is usually, but not always, markedly elevated (diastolic > 140 mmHg). The presence of hemorrhages, exudates, and papilledema on funduscopic exam is typical in patients with malignant hypertension. Neurologic symptoms may include headache, confusion, somnolence, visual loss, seizures, or coma. Renal involvement is common, and patients may have oliguria or azotemia. Generalized weakness, nausea, vomiting, and malaise may be present. Microangiopathic hemolytic anemia with red cell fragmentation can be seen in association with fibrinoid necrosis. The urine may contain protein and red cells.

7. What are the principles of antihypertensive therapy in patients with hypertensive emergencies?

Patients with hypertensive emergencies should be admitted to intensive care settings. An intra-arterial line should be placed to monitor the response to therapy. Parenteral antihypertensive therapy should be initiated as early as possible. It is important to avoid abrupt falls and excessive lowering of blood pressure to minimize precipitating cardiac or cerebral ischemia. Patients with chronic hypertension and elderly patients have impaired ability to autoregulate blood flow and are at greater risk for hypoperfusion. The initial goal of therapy in hypertensive emergencies is to reduce mean arterial pressure by no more than 25% (within minutes to 2 hours) then toward 160/100 mmHg within 2–6 hours. Once blood pressure is controlled, oral antihypertensive drugs should be introduced and intravenous therapy weaned.

8. What drugs are available for treatment of hypertensive emergencies?

Sodium nitroprusside is the drug of choice in many hypertensive emergencies due to its rapid onset and efficacy in lowering blood pressure. In addition, the antihypertensive effect disappears within minutes of the drug being stopped, making it easier to titrate therapy. It is an arterial and venous dilator, reducing cardiac preload and afterload and myocardial oxygen consumption. Nitroprusside is metabolized to thiocyanate and excreted in the urine. Prolonged administration of nitroprusside can result in thiocyanate toxicity, which manifests as blurred vision, confusion, tinnitus, and hyperreflexia. Therefore, use of nitroprusside should be limited to a rate of less than 3 μg per minute for less than 72 hours.

Labetalol is a combined alpha and beta blocker and reduces peripheral resistance without increasing cardiac output. It can be used as repeated IV boluses or as a continuous infusion and is contraindicated in bradycardia, heart block, bronchospasm, or congestive heart failure. IV nitroglycerin, due to its properties of afterload reduction and improved myocardial perfusion, is the treatment of choice in patients with myocardial ischemia. Esmolol is a short-acting beta blocker that is particularly useful in the treatment of hypertension associated with aortic dissection to reduce the shear stress in the vessel wall. Details of these and other agents are listed in the Table.

Parenteral Therapy for Hypertensive Emergencies

DRUG	ONSET OF ACTION	DOSE	COMMENTS
Sodium nitroprusside	Immediate	0.25–10 μg/kg/min as IV infusion	Effective in most hypertensive emergencies; caution with high intracranial pressure or azotemia
Nitroglycerin	2–5 minutes	5–100 μg/min IV	Particularly useful in hypertension associated with coronary ischemia
Nicardipine	5–10 minutes	5–15 mg/hr IV	Avoid in acute heart failure and coronary ischemia
Enalaprilat	15–30 minutes	1.25–5 mg q 6 hr IV	Useful in acute left ventricular failure; avoid in acute myocardial infarction

Table continued on next page

Parenteral Therapy for Hypertensive Emergencies (Cont.)

DRUG	ONSET OF ACTION	DOSE	COMMENTS
Labetalol	5–10 minutes	20–80 mg IV bolus every 10 minutes; 0.5–2.0 mg/min IV infusion	Avoid in acute heart failure
Esmolol	10–20 minutes	250-500 µg/kg/min for 1 min, then 50–100 µg/kg/min for 4 min, may repeat sequence	Particularly useful in aortic dissection and perioperative hypertension

9. What is the long-term prognosis and outcome of patients with malignant hypertension?

Patients with untreated malignant hypertension have a high mortality rate with a 1-year survival rate as low as 10–20% reported in a series in 1958. However, with improved antihypertensive therapy, survival has improved considerably in the last few years. The presence of renal failure at the time of initial presentation is associated with a poorer prognosis. After the initiation of vigorous antihypertensive therapy, renal function may deteriorate transiently but usually improves with good blood pressure control. In fact, several studies show that some patients recover enough renal function to allow withdrawal of dialysis.

10. What are the clinical features of hypertensive encephalopathy?

Patients with hypertensive encephalopathy can present with headache, somnolence, seizures, or focal neurologic abnormalities. Funduscopic exam usually shows stage 3 or 4 hypertensive retinopathy, and there is frequently evidence of prior target organ damage in the kidneys or the heart. Definitive diagnosis of hypertensive encephalopathy requires exclusion of other neurologic processes, usually by computed tomography (CT) scan and other diagnostic work-up.

11. How do patients with aortic dissection present? How is hypertension treated in the presence of aortic dissection?

A history of severe hypertension and inherited disorders of connective tissue such as Marfan syndrome or Ehlers-Danlos syndrome increase the risk for developing an aortic dissection. Patients usually present with severe chest or upper back pain, which may radiate into the arms or upper abdomen and is associated with difference in blood pressure between the two arms. In addition, a murmur of aortic regurgitation, a pericardial rub, or evidence of a pleural effusion may be present. The diagnosis is confirmed by CT scan or transesophageal echocardiography.

The goal of treatment of hypertension in the setting of an aortic dissection is to reduce the shear force of the pressure upstroke. The combination of intravenous beta blockade and sodium nitroprusside is the treatment of choice, and blood pressure should be maintained as low as possible. Definitive treatment depends on the location of the dissection. Lesions before the aortic arch (type A) require immediate surgery, whereas those distal to the arch (type B) can have a trial of medical therapy.

12. What are the clinical features of hypertension associated with acute left ventricular failure and pulmonary edema? How is this condition treated?

Patients present with severe shortness of breath associated with a cough producing a frothy pink-tinged sputum. The blood pressure is markedly elevated, neck veins are distended, and crackles or wheezes are present in both lung fields. An S_3 or S_4 gallop may be heard. The chest x-ray shows bilateral cephalization, hilar congestion, and pulmonary edema. Treatment should be initiated immediately with oxygen, intubation, or, if necessary, intravenous furosemide. IV nitroglycerin is very effective because it lowers preload and afterload, improves coronary perfusion, and, therefore, is the treatment of choice in this setting. IV morphine is also helpful as an adjunctive measure.

13. What is an adrenergic crisis? How is it treated?

Adrenergic crises are clinical situations characterized by abrupt increases in alpha-adrenergic tone and plasma catecholamine levels. These can occur due to withdrawal of clonidine, cocaine and amphetamine overdose, and monoamine oxidase–tyramine syndrome. Alpha blockers such as phentolamine, phenoxybenzamine, and combined alpha and beta blockers such as labetalol are effective antihypertensive agents in this scenario. Sodium nitroprusside can be used if necessary.

BIBLIOGRAPHY

1. Gifford RW: Management of hypertensive crises. JAMA 266:829–835, 1991.
2. Kitiyakara C, Guzman NJ: Malignant hypertension and hypertensive emergencies. J Am Soc Nephrol 9:133–142, 1998.
3. National Institutes of Health: Sixth Report of the Joint National Committee on Prevention, Detection, Evaluation, and Treatment of High Blood Pressure, Bethesda, MD, NIH, 1997, NIH publication 98-4080.
4. Phillips RA, Krakoff LR: Hypertensive Emergencies. True and False. New York, American Society of Hypertension, 1997.

60. CHILDHOOD HYPERTENSION

Ira D. Davis, M.D.

1. What is the definition of hypertension in children?

Hypertension is based on the normal distribution of systolic and diastolic blood pressure in the general population for children of comparable age, weight, and height. High normal blood pressure is defined as pressures between the 90th and 95th percentile; significant hypertension is defined as pressures greater than the 95th–99th percentile; severe hypertension is defined as pressures greater than the 99th percentile (see Tables).

90th and 95th Percentiles of Blood Pressure (BP) for Girls

AGE (YEARS)	BP PERCENTILE	SYSTOLIC BP (mmHg) BY PERCENTILE OF HEIGHT			DIASTOLIC BP (mmHg) BY PERCENTILE OF HEIGHT		
		25%	75%	95%	25%	75%	95%
2	90th	100	103	105	58	59	61
	95th	104	107	109	62	63	65
4	90th	103	106	108	64	65	67
	95th	107	109	111	68	69	71
8	90th	110	112	114	71	72	74
	95th	113	116	118	75	76	78
10	90th	114	116	118	73	75	76
	95th	117	120	122	77	79	80
14	90th	121	124	126	78	79	81
	95th	125	128	130	82	83	85

90th and 95th Percentiles of Blood Pressure (BP) for Boys

AGE (YEARS)	BP PERCENTILE	SYSTOLIC BP (mmHg) BY PERCENTILE OF HEIGHT			DIASTOLIC BP (mmHg) BY PERCENTILE OF HEIGHT		
		25%	75%	95%	25%	75%	95%
2	90th	100	104	106	56	58	59
	95th	104	108	110	60	62	63
4	90th	105	109	111	63	65	66
	95th	109	113	115	67	69	71
8	90th	110	114	116	72	74	75
	95th	114	118	120	76	78	80
10	90th	113	117	119	74	76	78
	95th	117	121	123	79	80	82
14	90th	123	126	128	77	79	80
	95th	127	130	132	81	83	85

Adapted from National High Blood Pressure Education Program Working Group on Hypertension Control in Children and Adolescents: Update on the 1987 task force report on high blood pressure in children and adolescents: A working group report from the National Blood Pressure Education Program. Pediatrics 98:649–658, 1996.

2. When should the blood pressure be checked in the pediatric patient?

The American Academy of Pediatrics recommends that annual blood pressure screening should begin at 3 years of age.

3. Does essential hypertension occur in children?

Essential hypertension accounts for only 10–20% of the cases of hypertension in children younger than 10 years. On the other hand, essential hypertension accounts for about 35% of cases of hypertension in the adolescent population. The majority of hypertension in the pediatric population is due to secondary or identifiable causes.

4. What is the primary cause of hypertension in newborn infants?

The most frequent cause of hypertension in this population is renovascular disease associated with renal arterial thromboemboli or renal artery stenosis. Other causes include coarctation of the aorta, congenital renal malformations such as obstructive uropathy or polycystic kidney disease, and bronchopulmonary dysplasia.

5. What are the most common causes of hypertension in infants through preschool age children?

Hypertension secondary to renal parenchymal disease, renal artery stenosis, or coarctation of the aorta occurs most frequently in this age group.

6. What are the most common causes of hypertension in children aged 6–10 years?

Hypertension secondary to either renal parenchymal disease or renal artery stenosis occurs most frequently in this age group.

7. What are the most common causes of secondary hypertension in the adolescent population?

The primary cause of secondary hypertension in adolescence is renal parenchymal disease. Etiologies include acute or chronic forms of glomerulonephritis and renal scarring associated with a remote history of pyelonephritis.

8. Which clinical characteristics are commonly associated with essential hypertension?

Typical characteristics include mild blood pressure elevations to the 95th percentile with significant variability in measurements, a strong family history, and obesity.

9. What important features of the patient history need to be assessed when evaluating a child with hypertension?

A careful family history including the age of onset of hypertension and the presence of complications such as myocardial infarction, kidney failure, heart failure, stroke, and peripheral vascular disease in first- and second-degree relatives is essential. The patient's growth pattern and neonatal history should also be assessed. Patients should also be questioned regarding the intake of foods and medications (including over-the-counter and illicit drugs including caffeine, nicotine, sodium, sympathomimetics, steroids, cocaine, and amphetamines) that cause elevations in blood pressure. The patient should also be questioned regarding the presence of symptoms suggestive of hypertension, renal disease, or other acute or chronic illnesses.

10. What are the symptoms of hypertension in children?

Children with essential hypertension or mildly elevated blood pressure due to secondary causes are usually asymptomatic. Severe hypertension may be associated with headaches, epistaxis, dizziness, blurred vision, nausea, changes in mental status, or seizures. Neonates with hypertension may present with poor feeding, irritability, lethargy, respiratory distress, seizures, or apnea.

11. What are the important features of the physical exam when evaluating a child with hypertension?

These include:
- Growth assessment
- Four extremity blood pressure measurements for evidence of coarctation of the aorta
- Funduscopic exam and a careful neurologic exam
- Neck exam for evidence of thyromegaly
- Cardiopulmonary exam for evidence of congestive heart failure or murmurs
- Abdominal exam for masses or bruits
- Skin exam looking for manifestations of rheumatologic diseases (such as systemic lupus erythematosus) or neurocutaneous syndromes (such as neurofibromatosis or tuberous sclerosis)
- Genitalia

12. What is the initial approach to the laboratory evaluation of hypertension in children?

All patients with hypertension require a urinalysis, serum chemistries, blood urea nitrogen (BUN), and creatinine determination. Patients with suspected essential hypertension should have a fasting lipid profile checked. Those with suspected secondary hypertension due to urologic abnormalities or pyelonephritis should have a urine culture. Children with severe hypertension and all children younger than 13 years should undergo a renal ultrasound. Patients with tachycardia or thyromegaly should have thyroid function studies. Echocardiography should be performed in patients with blood pressure above the 95th percentile and when pharmacotherapy is being considered.

13. What are the nonpharmacologic approaches to the treatment of hypertension in children?

Weight reduction, aerobic exercise, and dietary modifications (low salt and low fat) are standard approaches for the treatment of essential hypertension in the adolescent with high normal blood pressure or significant hypertension

14. When are the pharmacologic approaches necessary in treating childhood hypertension?

The indications for pharmacologic therapy include:
- Presence of significant hypertension unresponsive to nonpharmacologic approaches
- Presence of symptoms
- Presence of end-organ injury evidenced by increased left ventricular mass or left ventricular dysfunction on echocardiogram
- Presence of severe hypertension

The goal of treatment is to reduce the blood pressure below the 95th percentile.

BIBLIOGRAPHY

1. Coody DK, Yetman RJ, Portman RJ: Hypertension in children. J Pediatr Health Care 9:3–11, 1995.
2. National High Blood Pressure Education Program Working Group on Hypertension Control in Children and Adolescents: Update on the 1987 task force report on high blood pressure in children and adolescents: A working group report from the National High Blood Pressure Education Program. Pediatrics 98:649–658, 1996.
3. Sadowski RH, Falkner B: Hypertension in pediatric patients. Am J Kidney Dis 27:305–358, 1996.
4. Sinaiko AR: Hypertension in children. New Engl J Med 335:1968–1973, 1996.
5. Task Force on Blood Pressure Control in Children: Report of the second task force on blood pressure control in children—1987. Pediatrics 79:1–25, 1987.

IX. Acid-Base and Electrolyte Disorders

61. METABOLIC ACIDOSIS

Jay B. Wish, M.D.

1. What is pH and why is it important?

pH is the negative logarithm of the hydrogen ion concentration of a solution, expressed in equivalents per liter. The concentration in free hydrogen ion in body fluids is approximately 40×10^{-9} equivalents per liter or 40 nanoequivalents per liter. This corresponds to a pH of approximately 7.40. When the extracellular fluid pH deviates significantly from normal, cellular enzymatic and electrochemical processes break down, which can be rapidly fatal. The body defends pH by recruiting a number of extracellular and intracellular buffers, including bicarbonate, proteins, and bone. The most important buffer system is the bicarbonate–carbonic acid buffer pair in the extracellular fluid.

2. What are the major sources and disposition of metabolic acids?

The body produces both organic and mineral acids as a product of normal metabolic processes. The oxidation of carbohydrates, amino acids, and fatty acids results in the formation of approximately 15,000 mmoles of carbon dioxide per day, which are rapidly excreted by the lungs. Body cells also metabolize certain nutrients to generate approximately 1 mEq/kg body weight or 60–70 mEq of mineral acid per day. These mineral acids consist of sulfates, which are derived from sulphur-containing amino acids in the diet, and phosphates, which are abundant in most foodstuffs. Because the concentration of free hydrogen ion in the body is approximately 40×10^{-9} equivalents per liter, it is obvious that even a slight accumulation of the $60–70 \times 10^{-3}$ equivalents of hydrogen ion produced daily would be rapidly fatal. Therefore, endogenously produced mineral acids must be immediately buffered so that free hydrogen ion does not accumulate in body fluids. The kidney's role in acid-base balance is to excrete the mineral ion associated with the endogenously produced mineral acids and to regenerate the 60–70 mEq of bicarbonate consumed daily in buffering the endogenous acid load.

3. Distinguish the roles of the proximal and distal renal tubules in maintaining acid-base balance.

The proximal tubule reabsorbs the majority of filtered bicarbonate (approximately 85%), thereby conserving the extracellular bicarbonate buffer pool. The proximal tubule also defends extracellular bicarbonate concentration by rejecting filtered bicarbonate in excess of the normal extracellular fluid bicarbonate concentration of 25–28 mEq/L, so that bicarbonate cannot accumulate to abnormally high levels in the plasma. Under normal circumstances, by the time the glomerular filtrate has reached the end of the distal tubule, most if not all of the filtered bicarbonate has been reabsorbed. In the cortical collecting duct, hydrogen ion is secreted against a gradient into the tubular lumen, acidifying the urine to a pH of around 5.0. This process of urinary acidification does not increase the amount of free hydrogen ions enough to maintain hydrogen ion balance (at a pH of 5, there are only 10×10^{-6} equivalents of hydrogen ion per liter compared to the $60–70 \times 10^{-3}$ equivalents of hydrogen ion that must be excreted to maintain acid balance). Rather, the purpose of acidifying the urine is to promote the proteination of buffers that are present in the glomerular filtrate, such as phosphate, uric acid, and creatinine. These "titratable acids" constitute approximately one third of net acid excretion under normal circumstances.

Urinary ammonium, which is produced by both proximal and distal tubular cells, comprises the remaining two thirds of net acid excretion. By metabolizing one molecule of glutamine, renal tubular cells produce two molecules of ammonium and one molecule of alpha-ketoglutarate. As the alpha-ketoglutarate (a divalent anion) is further metabolized to CO_2 and water through the Krebs cycle or to glucose through gluconeogenesis, it takes on two hydrogen ions from intracellular carbonic acid, leaving two bicarbonate molecules behind. These two bicarbonates are then returned to the extracellular fluid, regenerating the bicarbonate that was consumed in the initial process of buffering the mineral acids. As every milliequivalent of ammonium excreted represents a milliequivalent of bicarbonate regenerated by the kidney to replenish the bicarbonate buffer pool, every milliequivalent of titratable acid excreted also represents a milliequivalent of bicarbonate regenerated by the kidneys. Net acid excretion equals the total of ammonium and titratable acid excreted minus any bicarbonate present in the urine. In order to maintain acid-base homeostasis, daily net acid excretion must equal daily mineral acid production.

4. What is metabolic acidosis?

Metabolic acidosis is an acid-base disturbance characterized by a primary decrease in plasma bicarbonate concentration leading to a reduced arterial pH.

5. What is the difference between acidosis and acidemia?

An acidosis (which can be metabolic or respiratory) is a process that, if unopposed, will lead to a decrease in arterial pH. Acidemia refers only to an arterial pH that is less than normal, irrespective of the processes that may lead to this change. A simple metabolic or respiratory acidosis will invariably produce an acidemia. However, there are circumstances in which more than one acid-base disorder may be present. If an acidosis coexists with an alkalosis, the resulting arterial pH may be normal, below normal (acidemia), or above normal (alkalemia), depending on the relative magnitude of the acidosis and alkalosis.

6. What are the three major processes that can result in a metabolic acidosis?

1. Acid production in excess of the kidneys' ability to excrete the acid and regenerate bicarbonate

2. Decreased ability of a diseased kidney to excrete acid and regenerate bicarbonate

3. Loss of bicarbonate from the extracellular fluid through either the kidneys or the gastrointestinal tract

7. What is the anion gap and how does it help to distinguish the causes of metabolic acidosis?

The anion gap is computed by the difference between the sum of the serum chloride and bicarbonate concentrations and the serum sodium concentration (see Figure).

$$\text{Anion gap} = Na^+ - (Cl^- + HCO_3^-)$$

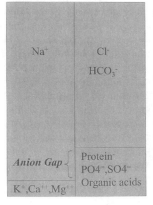

Cations   Anions

Na⁺   Cl⁻

HCO₃⁻

Anion Gap { Protein⁻
PO4⁻, SO4⁻
K⁺,Ca⁺⁺,Mg⁺⁺   Organic acids

Constituents of normal extracellular fluid used in calculating the anion gap. Note that the gap actually reflects the difference between "unmeasured" anions and cations although it is calculated based on commonly measured electrolytes (i.e., Na^+, Cl^-, and HCO_3^-).

A normal anion gap is 10–14 mEq/L. An elevated anion gap generally indicates the presence of a metabolic acidosis, but an anion gap less than 20 mEq/L can be observed in other acid-base disorders. A metabolic acidosis with an elevated anion gap generally results from the overproduction of endogenously produced organic acids, such as lactic acid and keto acids, or the generation of acid metabolites from the ingestion of certain toxins, such as salicylates, methanol, and ethylene glycol. Advanced renal failure can also lead to a metabolic acidosis with an elevated anion gap because of the decreased ability of the kidneys to keep up with the normal production of endogenously produced acids. A metabolic acidosis with a normal anion gap is generally due to bicarbonate loss from the extracellular fluid (through the kidneys or gastrointestinal tract) or the administration of a chloride-containing acid.

8. What is the urinary anion gap and how is it used in the differential diagnosis of metabolic acidosis?

The urinary anion gap is the difference between the urine chloride concentration and the sum of the urine sodium and potassium concentrations. In the setting of a metabolic acidosis with a normal serum anion gap, a negative urine anion gap correlates with urine ammonium excretion and implies a normal urinary acidification response to extrarenal bicarbonate loss or hydrochloric acid administration. A positive urinary anion gap in this setting suggests impaired urinary acidification as in type I (distal) renal tubular acidosis.

9. What is the osmolal gap and what is its role in the differential diagnosis of metabolic acidosis?

The osmolal gap is the difference between the measured serum osmolality and the calculated serum osmolality, which is determined by the formula:

$$\text{Serum osmolality} = 2 \times [\text{Na+(mEq/L)}] + \frac{[\text{glucose (mg/dl)}]}{180} + \frac{[\text{blood urea nitrogen (mg/dl)}]}{18}$$

The osmolality as determined by the laboratory should not exceed the calculated osmolarity by greater than 10 mOsm/kg. An elevated osmolal gap in the setting of a metabolic acidosis with an increased anion gap suggests intoxication with a low–molecular-weight substance such as methanol or ethylene glycol.

10. What are the four major factors that affect renal tubular bicarbonate reabsorption?

Renal tubular bicarbonate reabsorption (T_m bicarbonate) is increased in the setting of decreased extracellular fluid volume, hypokalemia, increased Pa_{CO_2}, and increased mineralocorticoid activity. Conversely, renal tubular bicarbonate reabsorption is suppressed by expanded extracellular fluid volume, hyperkalemia, decreased Pa_{CO_2}, and decreased mineralocorticoid activity.

11. Compare and contrast type I (distal) renal tubular acidosis (RTA) and type II (proximal) RTA.

By definition, type I and type II RTA are metabolic acidoses that are a result of a renal tubular disorder; therefore, glomerular filtration rate must be normal. In type I RTA, a defect in urinary acidification and renal ammoniagenesis results in a failure of net acid excretion to keep pace with mineral acid production. Consequently, there is an accumulation of acids within body fluids, a downward titration of extracellular bicarbonate, and recruitment of nonbicarbonate buffers such as bone. Buffering of hydrogen ions by bone buffers results in the release of calcium, which is filtered through the kidneys and easily precipitated in the tubules because of the failure of urinary acidification to keep it in solution. As a result, patients with type I RTA often develop chronic progressive renal failure as a result of nephrocalcinosis. Finally, in type I RTA, there is an augmentation of renal potassium secretion in exchange for sodium in the distal nephron. This leads to profound hypokalemia. Muscle weakness due to hypokalemia is a common presenting symptom in type I RTA. Once the diagnosis is made, type I RTA is not difficult to treat. Because many of these patients present with both profound hypokalemia and metabolic acidosis, it is important to replace the potassium first, because alkalinization of the plasma will lead to a shift of potassium into cells, which may aggravate the hypokalemia to a life-threatening degree. Once serum potassium levels are stabilized, alkali can be administered to restore plasma pH and serum bicarbonate levels to normal. Once the serum bicarbonate has been normalized, the maintenance bicarbonate dose is merely that required to buffer the daily excess of mineral acid production over net urinary acid excretion. Even if a patient with type I RTA had zero net acid excretion, which would be most unusual, his or her daily bicarbonate requirement would only be required to neutralize the 1 mEq/kg body weight (60–70 mEq) of mineral acid produced daily.

In type II RTA, a major defect is in the proximal tubular reabsorption of filtered bicarbonate. As a result, bicarbonate is lost in the urine, the extracellular bicarbonate buffer pool is reduced, and plasma bicarbonate concentration decreases. However, as the filtered load of bicarbonate decreases to a point that matches the degree of reduction in proximal bicarbonate absorption, a new steady state of bicarbonate filtration and reabsorption is achieved, bicarbonate disappears from the urine, and plasma bicarbonate remains stable at a reduced level. Unlike patients with type I RTA, patients with type II RTA are not in a continuous state of net acid accumulation, and long-term metabolic consequences from type II RTA are minimal. However, correcting the reduced plasma bicarbonate level in patients with type I RTA is very difficult, because the administration of exogenous bicarbonate will again cause the filtered load of bicarbonate to exceed the proximal tubular capacity to reabsorb bicarbonate. Administered bicarbonate is promptly excreted in the urine along with potassium, which may induce hypokalemia.

12. What are the indications for bicarbonate therapy in patients with acute metabolic acidosis?

Bicarbonate therapy should be reserved for patients with severe metabolic acidosis, characterized by hemodynamic instability, blood pH less than 7.15, or serum bicarbonate less than 12 mEq/L. Bicarbonate therapy is most beneficial in patients with metabolic acidosis that is due to bicarbonate loss from the body (such as severe diarrhea). It is generally not indicated if accumulated bicarbonate precursors (such as lactic acid or keto acids) can be metabolized to generate bicarbonate once the underlying metabolic abnormality is corrected. The goal of bicarbonate therapy is not to normalize serum bicarbonate but to improve hemodynamic and central nervous system function and severe acidemia. Bicarbonate dose should be calculated to increase the serum bicarbonate to 15 mEq/L or blood pH to 7.15, but no higher. In more severe metabolic acidosis, as nonbicarbonate buffers are recruited, the volume of distribution for administered bicarbonate increases. If the serum bicarbonate is greater than 10 mEq/L, the volume of distribution in liters for administered bicarbonate is 0.5 times the body weight in kilograms. If the serum bicarbonate is 5–10 mEq/L, then the volume of distribution of administered bicarbonate is 0.75 times the body weight in kilograms. If the serum bicarbonate is less than 5 mEq/L, then the volume of distribution of administered bicarbonate is 1.0 times the body weight in kilograms. Bicarbonate dose should be equal to the body weight × the volume distribution × (15 − the initial bicarbonate concentration). Fifty percent of the calculated bicarbonate dose should be administered immediately by intravenous bolus, with the remainder administered over 6–12 hours by intravenous infusion. Ongoing generation of acid may require frequent monitoring of the response to bicarbonate administration and adjustment of the dosage accordingly.

13. What are the causes of lactic acidosis and their implications regarding management and prognosis?

Type A lactic acidosis is associated with decreased delivery of oxygen to the tissues, as a result of either hypoxemia or hypotension. Patients with ongoing sepsis may have shunting of blood flow away from capillaries, leading to tissue hypoxia in the absence of overt hypotension, and also fall into the type A lactic acidosis group. Type B lactic acidosis is due to abnormalities of cellular metabolism, frequently associated with an uncoupling of oxidative phosphorylation, as may be seen in the setting of disseminated malignancy or certain toxins, including cyanide, phenformin, metformin, and salicylates. Prognosis of lactic acidosis depends on reversal of the underlying illness. If the underlying illness cannot be identified or corrected, as is more often the case in type B lactic acidosis, then the prognosis for survival tends to be very poor.

14. Should bicarbonate be administered to patients with lactic acidosis?

The role of bicarbonate therapy in patients with lactic acidosis is controversial. No study has demonstrated a relationship between the amount of bicarbonate administered to patients with lactic acidosis and the eventual outcome. Some experimental studies have demonstrated that bicarbonate administration results in the paradoxic acidification of the cerebrospinal fluid (because the CO_2 generated from some of the administered bicarbonate diffuses into the cerebrospinal fluid faster than the bicarbonate itself), results in the generation of more carbon dioxide and a higher $PaCO_2$, and actually increases lactic acid production by the cells—all resulting in a potential exacerbation rather than amelioration of the acidosis. However, because the goal of alkali administration in the setting of metabolic acidosis is stabilization of the cardiovascular system, raising the pH to greater than 7.15 may improve cardiac performance and enhance tissue oxygen delivery, thus decreasing lactate production.

15. What is the expected respiratory compensation in metabolic acidosis?

The $PaCO_2$ should fall by 1–1.3 mmHg for every 1 mEq/L fall in plasma bicarbonate.

16. What is the pathophysiology and treatment of the metabolic acidosis in patients with chronic renal failure?

A major defect in acid-base homeostasis in patients with chronic renal failure is decreased renal ammoniagenesis resulting from the decrease in functioning nephron mass. As a result of decreased net acid excretion, the rate of renal bicarbonate regeneration falls short of the rate of mineral acid production, and the patient goes into a state of positive acid balance, leading to titration of bicarbonate and nonbicarbonate buffers and a metabolic acidosis. Dietary protein restriction has been advocated to decrease the imbalance between acid production and excretion, which thereby ameliorates the acidosis of chronic renal failure. As is the case in patients with type I RTA, a shortfall between real bicarbonate regeneration and acid production can be made up with exogenous alkali administration.

17. What is type IV RTA?

A subset of patients with chronic renal failure who have hyperkalemia and metabolic acidosis out of proportion to their degree of renal function impairment carry a diagnosis of type IV RTA. This condition appears to be more common in patients whose renal disease is due to diabetic nephropathy, chronic interstitial nephritis, obstructive uropathy, sickle cell nephropathy, and chronic transplant rejection. Many of these patients will prove to have a subnormal plasma renin and aldosterone response to diuretic-induced volume depletion and upright posture, a condition known as *hyporeninemic hypoaldosteronism*. Because the hyperkalemia in this condition tends to be more problematic than the metabolic acidosis, therapy is primarily directed at augmenting renal potassium excretion with loop diuretics and exogenous mineralocorticoid. These therapies tend to have a modest effect on correcting the metabolic acidosis.

BIBLIOGRAPHY

1. Arieff A: Indications for use of bicarbonate in patients with metabolic acidosis. Br J Anaesth 67:165–177, 1991.
2. Battle DC, Hizon M, Cohen E, et al: The use of the urinary anion gap in the diagnosis of hyperchloremic metabolic acidosis. N Engl J Med 318:594–599, 1988.
3. Gabow PA: Disorders associated with an altered anion gap. Kidney Int 27:472–483, 1985.
4. Garella S, Dana C, Chazan J: Severity of metabolic acidosis is a determinant of bicarbonate requirements. N Engl J Med 289:121–126, 1973.
5. Halperin ML, Vasuvattakul S, Bayoumi A: A modified classification of metabolic acidosis: A pathophysiologic approach. Nephron 60:129–133, 1992.
6. Madias NE: Lactic acidosis. Kidney Int 29:752–774, 1986.
7. Narins RG, Emmett M: Simple and mixed acid-base disorders: A practical approach. Medicine 59:161–187, 1980.
8. Schelling JR, Howard RL, Winter SD, Linas SL: Increased osmolal gap in alcoholic ketoacidosis and lactic acidosis. Ann Intern Med 113:580–582, 1990.
9. Stacpoole PW: Lactic acidosis: The case against bicarbonate therapy. Ann Intern Med 105:276–279, 1986.

62. METABOLIC ALKALOSIS

Jay B. Wish, M.D.

1. What is metabolic alkalosis?
Metabolic alkalosis is an acid-base disturbance characterized by an increased blood pH primarily due to an increase in plasma bicarbonate concentration.

2. What factors influence renal handling of bicarbonate?
Under normal circumstances, absorption of filtered bicarbonate plateaus at the normal serum bicarbonate concentration of 25–28 mEq/L. At higher levels of serum bicarbonate, the incremental bicarbonate present in the glomerular filtrate is rejected by the renal tubules and appears in the urine. This phenomenon is known as the tubular transport maximum (Tm) for bicarbonate. Four factors may increase the Tm for bicarbonate, allowing for tubular reabsorption of increased amounts of filtered bicarbonate and the maintenance of elevated serum bicarbonate concentrations:
1. Extracellular volume depletion
2. Hypokalemia
3. Hypercapnia
4. Increased mineralocorticoid activity

3. Distinguish between the generation and maintenance of metabolic alkalosis.
The generation of metabolic alkalosis refers to the condition that results in the initial elevation in serum bicarbonate concentration. In most circumstances, this is due to a net loss of hydrogen ions from the body, resulting in the accumulation of unneutralized bicarbonate molecules. However, the mere accumulation of bicarbonate in the extracellular fluid is not sufficient to sustain a metabolic alkalosis, because a normal Tm for bicarbonate would cause the additional bicarbonate to be excreted rapidly in the urine. In order for a metabolic alkalosis to be maintained, one or more of the factors described in question 2 must be present to raise the Tm of bicarbonate above normal, maintaining a higher-than-normal serum bicarbonate concentration. The factor or factors that raise the Tm for bicarbonate and perpetuate the elevated serum bicarbonate concentration maintain the metabolic alkalosis.

4. What conditions may lead to the generation of a metabolic alkalosis?
The etiologies of metabolic alkalosis fall into three major categories:
1. Extracellular volume depletion accompanied by the loss of chloride-rich fluid from the body
2. A primary increase in mineralocorticoid or mineralocorticoid-like activity
3. Administration of alkali in a patient with renal insufficiency.

Extracellular volume depletion, in association with the loss of a chloride-rich fluid from the body, occurs in vomiting (where hydrochloric acid is lost), the use of diuretics (which inhibit chloride reabsorption in the loop of Henle and early distal nephron), and villous adenoma of the colon (which secretes a chloride-rich diarrheal fluid). The kidney reacts to the loss of such fluid by attempting to conserve sodium to maintain extracellular fluid volume. The kidney always chooses to maintain sodium and extracellular fluid balance over preservation of acid-base balance. With less chloride available for reabsorption with sodium, the renal tubule will reabsorb more of the filtered sodium with bicarbonate, the serum bicarbonate will rise, and a metobolic alkalosis will be maintained. It is important to note that the metabolic alkalosis will be maintained through this mechanism long after the initial loss of chloride-rich fluid has ceased, as long as exogenous chloride is not provided to replace the deficit.

The second major mechanism by which metabolic alkalosis can be generated is through a primary acceleration of the mineralocorticoid-dependent sodium-hydrogen exchange in the distal nephron. The increase in hydrogen ion excretion by distal tubular cells is accompanied by the production of additional bicarbonate, which accumulates in the extracellular fluid. At the same time, sodium-potassium exchange in the distal nephron also is accelerated, leading to potassium losses in the urine and hypokalemia. The metabolic alkalosis is maintained both by hypokalemia and by the effect of the mineralocorticoid on the renal tubule. The primary increase in sodium reabsorption by the distal nephron usually leads to expansion of extracellular intravascular fluid volume and hypertension.

Metabolic alkalosis due to excessive alkali administration in the setting of renal insufficiency is much less common than the etiologies described above. It may occur in patients with renal insufficiency who are given alkali-rich intravenous fluid such as Ringer's lactate or intravenous hyperalimentation. It also may occur in a condition known as the *milk-alkali syndrome*, in which excessive consumption of milk and calcium-containing antacids for treatment of dyspepsia leads to renal insufficiency due to nephrocalcinosis and impaired alkali excretion.

5. What is "paradoxical aciduria"?

One might question why the body does not simply use the endogenously produced metabolic acids to neutralize a metabolic alkalosis. To do so would require the kidney to sacrifice the reabsortion of sodium in exchange for secreted hydrogen in the distal nephron. Because sodium conservation remains the overriding priority of the kidney, acid excretion continues and urine pH remains "paradoxically" low despite systemic alkalemia.

6. What is the major laboratory tool for the differential diagnosis of metabolic alkalosis?

Urinary chloride concentration can be very useful in distinguishing the causes of metabolic alkalosis associated with the loss of chloride-rich fluid from those causes associated with excessive mineralocorticoid-like activity. In the former group, the extracellular volume depletion causes increased sodium and chloride reabsorption in the proximal tubule, exhausting tubular chloride and leading to a low urinary chloride concentration (0–10 mEq/L). In contrast, patients with metabolic alkalosis due to excess mineralocorticoid activity have extracellular volume expansion, leading to suppression of sodium and chloride reabsorption of the proximal tubule. Some of the sodium that escapes proximal reabsorption is reabsorbed in the distal portions of the nephron under the influence of increased mineralocorticoid activity, but the chloride escaping proximal reabsorption is excreted in the urine, leading to a urinary chloride concentration that is generally greater than 20 mEq/L.

7. What is the treatment for metabolic acidosis?

Treatment for metabolic acidosis depends on the mechanism by which the alkalosis was generated and maintained. In patients with metabolic alkalosis associated with extracellular volume depletion and excessive loss of chloride-containing fluids, the obvious treatment would be the restoration of effective extracellular fluid volume through the administration of chloride-containing solutions. These patients may have a secondary increase in mineralocorticoid activity due to the volume depletion. Consequently, sodium-potassium exchange in the distal nephron is accelerated, leading to urinary potassium losses and hypokalemia. Treatment often includes administration of potassium chloride to correct the hypokalemia and sodium-containing solutions to correct the hypovolemia. In rare patients, for whom there is a contraindication to the administration of sodium chloride (e.g., cardiac failure) or potassium chloride (e.g., hyperkalemia due to advanced renal insufficiency), chloride can be administered to correct the metabolic alkalosis in the form of intravenous hydrochloric acid, ammonium chloride, or arginine hydrochloride.

The treatment for metabolic alkalosis secondary to an increase in mineralocorticoid or mineralocorticoid-like activity is to eliminate or antagonize the mineralocorticoid activity. The differential diagnosis includes primary hyperaldosteronism due to renal adenoma or adrenal hyperplasia, Cushing's disease and Cushing's syndrome, and exogenous administration of agents with mineralocorticoid activity such as corticosteroids and natural licorice. These forms of metabolic alkalosis are often called chloride-resistant, because administration of chloride will not correct the alkalosis. Treatment of choice is to remove the source of mineralocorticoid-like activity. If it is due to a surgically resectable adenoma, then efforts should be made to excise the adenoma. In the case of adrenal hyperplasia, spironolactone, a direct antagonist of the action of aldosterone, is the treatment of choice. These patients are often profoundly hypokalemic because of the increased urinary potassium excretion. Large doses of oral potassium supplements may be required to correct the hypokalemia.

The treatment of metabolic acidosis due to excessive alkali administration in the setting of renal insufficiency is obviously to decrease the alkali administration. In most of these situations, the kidney will eventually excrete the excessive bicarbonate, returning plasma bicarbonate pH to normal.

BIBLIOGRAPHY

1. Harrington JT: Metabolic alkalosis. Kidney Int 26:88–97, 1984.
2. Knutsen OH: New method for administration of hydrochloric acid in metabolic alkalosis. Lancet 1:53–55, 1983.
3. Koch SM, Taylor RW: Chloride ion in intensive care medicine. Crit Care Med 20:227–240, 1992.
4. Rimmer JM, Gennari FJ: Metabolic alkalosis. J Intensive Care Med 78:482–485, 1985.
5. Vaziri ND, Byrne C, Barton CH, et al: Prevention of metabolic alkalosis induced by gastric fluid loss using H_2 receptor antagonists. Gen Pharmacol 16:141–144, 1985.

63. RESPIRATORY ACIDOSIS

Ashwin Dixit, M.D.

1. What is respiratory acidosis?

Respiratory acidosis is an acid-base disturbance characterized by a primary elevation in $Paco_2$ leading to reduced arterial pH of blood.

2. How is CO_2 produced and eliminated by the body?

CO_2 is produced by endogenous metabolism and is mainly eliminated by the lungs.

3. How is the arterial $Paco_2$ regulated?

The arterial $Paco_2$ (normally 40 ± 4 mmHg) and Pao_2 are closely linked and determined by alveolar ventilation. An increase in $Paco_2$ stimulates chemosensitive areas of the medulla by an increase in cerebral interstitial pH. Hypoxemia increases ventilation by stimulating chemoreceptors in carotid bodies.

4. What is the pathophysiology of respiratory acidosis?

Under steady-state conditions, the rate of elimination of $Paco_2$ matches the rate of $Paco_2$ production. Thus:

$$Paco_2 = 0.863 \times Vco_2/Va$$

where $Vco_2 = CO_2$ production, Va = alveolar ventilation, and 0.863 = a constant.

Hypercapnia can result either from increased CO_2 production or decreased alveolar ventilation. Increased CO_2 production is an uncommon cause of respiratory acidosis because the body can normally raise ventilatory rate to match almost any increase in CO_2 production. Thus, hypercapnia and respiratory acidosis are usually the results of decreased alveolar ventilation.

5. What is the pathophysiology of decreased alveolar ventilation?

Alveolar ventilation is expressed as:

Alveolar ventilation = Minute ventilation – Dead space ventilation

Decreased alveolar ventilation results from decreased minute ventilation in states of central nervous system depression, advanced neuromuscular disease, and respiratory muscle fatigue. Increased dead space ventilation mainly results from disorders associated with ventilation perfusion mismatching.

6. How does the body respond to an acute increase in $Paco_2$?

An acute increase in $Paco_2$ results in an immediate increase in plasma HCO_3^- based on the following equilibrium:

$$CO_2 + H_2O \rightleftharpoons H_2CO_3 \rightleftharpoons HCO_3^- + H^+$$

The H^+ combines with intracellular buffers. This chemical adaptation is complete in 5–10 minutes.

7. In acute respiratory acidosis, what is the change in serum HCO_3?

Plasma HCO_3^- increases by about 1 mEq/L for each 10-mm rise in $Paco_2$. The overall limit of adaptation is small. The maximum concentration of HCO_3^- reached during compensation for acute hypercapnia is about 30 mEq/L.

8. What is the adaptive response seen in chronic respiratory acidosis?

The adaptive response to chronic respiratory acidosis is an increase in plasma HCO_3^- generated mainly by the kidney.

9. **How do the kidneys generate bicarbonate in chronic respiratory acidosis?**
The kidneys generate bicarbonate by the following mechanisms:
- Increased net urinary acid excretion (as ammonium and titratable acids)
- Increased renal bicarbonate reabsorption

10. **In chronic respiratory acidosis, how does serum HCO_3^- change in response to an increase in Pa_{CO_2}?**
The serum HCO_3^- increases by about 3 mEq/L for every 10-mmHg rise in Pa_{CO_2}. This physiologic adaptation usually requires 3–5 days.

11. **What are the causes of acute respiratory acidosis?**
  1. Central nervous system disorders
       Head trauma
       Drugs (e.g., opiates, sedatives, anesthetics)
       Cerebrovascular accident
       Central sleep apnea
  2. Neuromuscular disorders
       High spinal cord injury
       Guillain-Barré syndrome
       Myasthenic crisis
       Drugs (e.g., aminoglycosides, succinylcholine)
       Hypokalemic or hyperkalemic paralysis
  3. Restriction to ventilation
       Flail chest
       Pneumothorax, hemothorax
  4. Upper airway dysfunction
       Aspiration of foreign body, food
       Laryngospasm
       Obstructive sleep apnea
  5. Alveolar causes
       Severe pneumonia
       Adult respiratory distress syndrome
  6. Impaired pulmonary perfusion
       Massive pulmonary embolism
       Cardiac arrest
  7. Iatrogenic
       Complications of mechanical ventilation

12. **What are the causes of chronic respiratory acidosis?**
  1. Central nervous system disorders
       Pickwickian syndrome (obesity-hypoventilation syndrome)
       Brain tumor
       Chronic use of sedatives, opiates
  2. Neuromuscular disorders
       Poliomyelitis
       Multiple sclerosis
       Myxedema
       Amyotrophic lateral sclerosis
  3. Restrictive to ventilation
       Kyphoscoliosis
       Extreme obesity
       Fibrothorax
       Hydrothorax

4. Upper airway obstruction
   Vocal cord paralysis
   Tracheal stenosis after prolonged intubation
5. Lower airway obstruction
   Chronic obstructive pulmonary disease (COPD)

13. What are the neurologic manifestations of respiratory acidosis?

The neurologic manifestations depend on the magnitude and rapidity with which respiratory acidosis develops and on the degree of accompanying hypoxemia. Patients may present with irritability, confusion, headaches, agitation, delirium, or hallucinations. Extreme elevations of $Paco_2$ are associated with myoclonic jerks, tremors, and even coma. Deep tendon reflexes are increased with lesser degrees of hypercapnia and are depressed in patients with severe hypercapnia. Pupillary constriction also may be observed.

14. What are cardiovascular manifestations of respiratory acidosis?

Mild to moderate respiratory acidosis is associated with an increase in cardiac output and blood pressure. Myocardial contractility may be impaired in patients with severe hypercapnia with a resulting decrease in cardiac output and blood pressure. Cardiac arrythmias, mainly supraventricular arrythmias, may be observed, but probably reflect not just the elevated $Paco_2$ but a combination of factors such as hypoxemia, electrolyte imbalance, sympathetic overactivity, and concomitant drug use.

15. What is the treatment for acute respiratory acidosis?

The mainstays of treatment of acute respiratory acidosis are to identify and treat the underlying cause with emphasis on maintaining airway patency and to use bronchodilators, corticosteroids, and antibiotics when clinically indicated. Alkali therapy is generally not used because it can be associated with the risk of volume overload and depression of ventilation mediated by an increase in pH. Alkali therapy may have a useful role in severe asthma in order to prevent barotrauma, which may result from attempts to improve pH by mechanical ventilation.

BIBLIOGRAPHY

1. Adrogue HJ, Madias NE: Management of life-threatening acid-base disorders. N Engl J Med 378:107–111, 1998.
2. Cohen JJ: Acid-Base. In Kassirer JP, Hricik DE, Cohen JJ (eds): Repair of Body Fluids: Principles and Practices. Philadelphia, W.B. Saunders, 1989, pp 130–168.
3. Madias NE, Wolf CJ, Cohen JJ: Regulation of acid-base equilibrium in chronic hypercapnia. Kidney Int 27:538–543, 1985.

64. RESPIRATORY ALKALOSIS

Ashwin Dixit, M.D.

1. What is respiratory alkalosis?

Respiratory alkalosis is an acid-base disturbance characterized by a primary decrease in $Paco_2$ leading to an elevated arterial pH.

2. What is the pathophysiologic basis for respiratory alkalosis?

Under steady state conditions, $Paco_2$, is directly proportional to the rate of CO_2 production and inversely related to alveolar ventilation, as follows:

$$Paco_2 = 0.863 \times Vco_2/Va$$

where 0.863 = constant, Vco_2 = CO_2 production, and Va = alveolar ventilation
Respiratory alkalosis can result from increased alveolar ventilation (most common), decreased CO_2 production, or both. Hyperventilation, in turn, can result from hypoxemia that stimulates peripheral chemoreceptors, direct stimulation of the respiratory center, and/or secondary signals arising from the lungs.

3. How does the body respond to acute respiratory alkalosis?

The adaptation to acute respiratory alkalosis occurs within 5–10 minutes by an immediate decrease in plasma HCO_3^-, based on the following equilibrium:

$$H^+ + HCO_3^- \rightleftharpoons H_2CO_3 \rightleftharpoons CO_2 + H_2O$$

When $Paco_2$ acutely decreases, hydrogen ions (H^+) are released from intracellular buffers and combine with extracellular HCO_3^- in a chemical response to generate more CO_2.

4. How much does the plasma HCO_3^- decrease in response to an acute decrease in $Paco_2$?

The plasma HCO_3^- decreases by approximately 2 mEq/L for every 10 mmHg decrease in $Paco_2$.

5. What other electrolyte abnormalities can be seen in acute respiratory alkalosis?

The small decrease in plasma bicarbonate is balanced by a small increase in plasma chloride, lactate, and other unmeasured ions.

6. What is the physiologic response to chronic respiratory alkalosis?

The response to chronic respiratory alkalosis is mediated mainly by a decrease in H^+ secretion by the kidney. The complete adaptation requires 2–3 days and is manifested by decreased ammonium secretion and loss of bicarbonate in the urine.

7. What is the magnitude of change in plasma HCO_3^- in chronic respiratory alkalosis?

The plasma HCO_3^- decreases by approximately 4–5 mEq/L for every 10 mmHg decrease in $Paco_2$.

8. What are the causes of respiratory alkalosis?
1. Hypoxemia
   High altitude
   Ventilation perfusion mismatch (e.g., pneumonia, pulmonary embolism)
   Cyanotic heart disease
2. Pulmonary disorders
   Pneumonia

Obstructive airway disease (e.g., asthma, chronic obstructive pulmonary disease [COPD])
Other parenchymal lung disease
3. Central nervous system stimulation
   Pain
   Anxiety
   Fever
   Structural brain lesions (e.g., stroke, tumors)
4. Drugs
   Salicylates
   Progesterone
5. Others
   Mechanical ventilation
   Gram-negative sepsis
   Pregnancy
   Liver failure

9. What are the clinical manifestations of respiratory alkalosis?

Acute respiratory alkalosis produces clinical manifestations more commonly than chronic respiratory alkalosis does. Hypocapnea-induced cerebral vasoconstriction has been implicated in the pathogenesis of the neurologic manifestations that include paresthesias, circumoral numbness, light-headedness, tetany, and seizures. A variety of supraventricular arrythmias may occur, particularly in critically ill patients.

10. What is the treatment for respiratory alkalosis?

Treatment is directed at management of the underlying cause. In anxiety-induced hyperventilation, reassurance, sedatives, or rebreathing into a closed system (e.g., paper bag) may help increase the $PaCO_2$. Patients on mechanical ventilation may require skeletal muscle paralysis if respiratory alkalosis is severe.

BIBLIOGRAPHY

1. Adrogue HJ, Madias NE: Management of life-threatening acid-base disorders. N Engl J Med 338:107–111, 1998.
2. Gennari FJ, Kassirer JP: Respiratory alkalosis. In Cohen JJ, Kassirer JP (eds): Acid-Base. Boston, Little, Brown, 1982, pp 349–376.
3. Krapf R, Beeler I, Hertner D, Hutler HN: Chronic respiratory alkalosis: The effect of sustained hyperventilation on renal regulation of acid-base equilibrium. N Engl J Med 324:1394–1401, 1991.

65. HYPONATREMIA AND HYPERNATREMIA

Linda Zarif, M.D.

1. What does hyponatremia indicate about a patient's salt and water balance?

With few exceptions (see question 2), a low serum sodium concentration reflects low osmolality of extracellular fluids. Hypo-osmolality, in turn, generally indicates either a relative or absolute excess of water in extracellular fluid. The osmolality of extracellular fluid can be estimated by the following formula:

$$\text{Osmolality (mOsm/kg)} = \{[Na^+] (mEq/L) + [K^+] (mEq/L)\} +$$
$$[\text{Urea (mg/dl)}/2.8] + [\text{Glucose (mg/dl)}/18]$$

The serum sodium concentration does not reflect the state of sodium balance. In fact, patients with hyponatremia may have sodium excess (volume overload) or a sodium deficit (volume depletion) or may appear to be relatively euvolemic.

2. What is pseudohyponatremia?

Sodium is confined to the aqueous phase of plasma. Its concentration in serum is decreased if plasma water content is lowered by other molecules such as lipids and proteins that are distributed in the nonaqueous phase of plasma. This phenomenon explains why normal plasma sodium concentration is approximately 154 mEq/L while normal serum sodium concentration is approximately 145 mEq/L (reflecting normal amounts of lipids and proteins in serum). Patients with severe hyperlipidemia or hyperproteinemia may exhibit pseudohyponatremia characterized by a low serum sodium and normal plasma sodium concentration. The plasma osmolality of patients with pseudohyponatremia is normal. Measurement of serum sodium by ion specific electrodes is much less influenced by hyperlipidemic or hyperproteinemic states.

3. What is spurious hyponatremia?

Spurious hyponatremia refers to a low serum sodium concentration with an *elevated* serum osmolality and occurs whenever high concentrations of low–molecular-weight solutes are present in extracellular fluid. This phenomenon is most commonly observed in patients with uncontrolled diabetes mellitus and hyperglycemia.

4. What is the correction factor for spurious hyponatremia in the face of hyperglycemia?

For each 100 mg/dl increase in serum glucose concentration above 100 mg/dl, serum sodium concentration should be corrected by 1.6 mEq/L. For example, in a patient presenting with a serum glucose of 1,000 mg/dl and a measured serum sodium concentration of 125 mEq/L, plasma sodium concentration can be assumed to be: 125 mEq/L + (9 × 1.6) mEq/L = ~140 mEq/L.

5. What is the syndrome of inappropriate antidiuretic hormone secretion (SIADH)?

Patients with SIADH exhibit either a sustained autonomous release of antidiuretic hormone (ADH) or an enhanced renal response to normal circulating levels of ADH that lead to hypotonic volume expansion. SIADH is a diagnosis of exclusion that can be considered only in hyponatremic patients in whom volume depletion, volume overload, renal failure, and hypothyroidism or hypoadrenalism have been excluded as causes of hypo-osmolality. SIADH was first described in patients with small cell lung cancer. Other causes include central nervous system disorders (e.g., stroke, tumors, brain abscess), pulmonary disorders (e.g., tuberculosis, pneumonia), and a variety of drugs (see Table).

Drugs Associated with Hyponatremia

AUGMENTED RENAL ACTION OF ADH	ENHANCED RELEASE OF ADH
Chlorpropamide	Carbamazapine
Tolbutamide	Vincristine
Nonsteroidal anti-inflammatory drugs	Vinblastine
	Cyclophosphamide
	Opiates
	Barbiturates
	? Thiazides

6. What are the clinical features of SIADH?

Patients with SIADH generally appear to be euvolemic on examination but, in fact, are hypotonically volume expanded. The blood urea nitrogen (BUN) and serum creatinine concentration tend to be low as a consequence of glomerular hyperfiltration resulting from the volume expansion. Urine sodium concentration tends to be relatively high (> 30 mEq/L) because of volume expansion but may be lower in patients consuming a low-salt diet. A low serum uric acid concentration often is noted and reflects enhanced uric acid clearance that is linked to reduced tubular reabsorption of sodium.

7. What is the differential diagnosis of hyponatremia?

Differential Diagnosis of Hyponatremia

TYPE OF HYPONATREMIA	POSSIBLE CAUSE
Euosmolar hyponatremia	Profound hyperlipidemia
	Profound hyperproteinemia
Hyperosmolar hyponatremia	Hyperglycemia
	Mannitol infusion
Hypo-osmolar hyponatremia	Hypovolemic
	Hemorrhage
	Gastrointestinal losses
	Diuretic therapy
	Adrenal insufficiency
	Third spacing
	Hypervolemic
	Congestive heart failure
	Cirrhosis
	Nephrotic syndrome
	End-stage renal failure
	Euvolemic
	Myxedema
	SIADH

8. How common is hyponatremia?

Among patients admitted to medical and surgical services, serum sodium concentrations less than 135 mEq/L occur in 15–22%. Concentrations less than 130 mEq/L occur in 1–4% of such patients.

9. What are the symptoms of hyponatremia?

Symptoms attributable to hyponatremia vary with the etiology, the absolute magnitude of the reduction in serum sodium concentration, and the rapidity with which the sodium concentration falls. The serious consequences of hypo-osmolality result from brain edema and include anorexia, nausea, vomiting, delirium, seizures, and coma. These symptoms usually are not observed until the serum sodium concentration has fallen below 120 mEq/L. When hyponatremia of this magnitude develops within 24 hours, mortality rate approaches 50%. By contrast, patients may be relatively asymptomatic when the sodium concentration is lowered to comparable levels over days or weeks.

10. What are the risk factors for hyponatremia-associated cerebral edema?
Risk factors for hyponatremia-associated cerebral edema include female gender, psychiatric disorders, and accompanying hypoxia. Cerebral edema appears to be particularly common in young women following surgery or anesthesia. Elderly women receiving thiazides also are at high risk.

11. What general principles should be considered when assessing a patient for treatment of hyponatremia?
 • The rapidity with which hyponatremia has developed
 • The magnitude of the reduction in serum sodium concentration
 • Presence or absence of symptoms
 • Volume status of the patient

12. How is hyponatremia treated?
 • For **hypovolemic hyponatremia**, correct volume depletion.
 • For **hypervolemic hyponatremia**, restrict water intake and correct the underlying disorder.
 • For **SIADH**, restrict water intake, replace urinary sodium losses, and treat the underlying cause. In chronic cases, demeclocycline or lithium may antagonize the effects of ADH on distal renal tubules and help to prevent severe hyponatremia.

13. How rapidly should hyponatremia be corrected?
Overly rapid correction of hyponatremia has been associated with pontine and extrapontine myelinolysis, resulting in a potentially fatal neurologic syndrome characterized by spastic quadriparesis, pseudobulbar palsies, and mental changes ranging from confusion to coma. A low serum sodium concentration should therefore not be corrected at a rate exceeding 2 mEq/L/hour. Most authorities recommend correction rates of 1.0–1.5 mEq/L/hour. In patients with acute symptomatic hyponatremia, these rates of correction should be employed until the serum sodium concentration exceeds 120 mEq/L. Thereafter, even slower rates of correction are appropriate.

14. What does hypernatremia indicate about a patient's salt and water balance?
Hypernatremia invariably signifies the presence of a hyperosmolar state. With the exception of patients receiving hypertonic fluids, most patients with hypernatremia are frankly volume-depleted (i.e., sodium-depleted) but have a deficit of water out of proportion to the deficit of sodium.

15. How does one calculate the water deficit in a patient with hypernatremia?
The water deficit is calculated from the observed serum sodium concentration and an estimate of total body water (TBW), assumed to be 60% of body weight. For example, the amount of free water needed to correct serum sodium concentration to 140 mEq/L can be calculated as follows:

$$\text{Water deficit} = (\text{Observed } [Na^+]/140 \times TBW) - TBW$$

Thus, in a 70-kg patient with a serum sodium of 170 mEq/L:

$$\text{Water deficit} = (170/140 \times 0.6 \times 70) - (0.6 \times 70) = 9L$$

16. What are the serious consequences of hypernatremia?
The major clinical manifestations of hypernatremia involve the central nervous system. Patients with acute hypernatremia may present with nausea, vomiting, seizures, coma, and virtually any type of neurologic syndrome. Fever, presumably related to impaired thermoregulation, also has been described.

17. What is diabetes insipidus?

Diabetes insipidus results from a deficiency in the production, secretion, or action of antidiuretic hormone (ADH). **Central** diabetes insipidus results from complete or partial defects in the hypothalamic secretion of ADH. **Nephrogenic** diabetes results from renal tubular resistance to the effects of circulating ADH. In either case, patients present with polyuria, polydipsia, and a tendency to develop hypernatremia when access to water is impeded. Central diabetes insipidus is idiopathic in nature in approximately 50% of cases. Other conditions associated with central and nephrogenic diabetes are shown in the table.

Some Causes of Diabetes Insipidus

TYPE OF DIABETES INSIPIDUS	CAUSE
Central diabetes insipidus	Idiopathic
	Head trauma
	Vascular lesions (aneurysms, thromboses)
	Brain tumors (primary or metastatic)
	Infections (encephalitis, meningitis)
	Sarcoidosis
	Guillain-Barré syndrome
Nephrogenic diabetes insipidus	Idiopathic
	Renal disease
	Acute tubular necrosis (recovery phase)
	Postobstructive diuresis
	Amyloidosis
	Multiple myeloma
	Sickle cell nephropathy
	Sjögren's syndrome
	Electrolyte disturbances
	Hypercalcemia
	Severe hypokalemia
	Pharmacologic agents
	Demeclocycline
	Lithium
	Amphotericin
	Methoxyflurane

18. How rapidly should hypernatremia be corrected?

Cerebral edema can occur when severe hypernatremia is corrected in less than 24 hours. Thus, fluids should be administered with the intention of correcting hypernatremia over a period of 48–72 hours. Isotonic saline can be administered initially to resuscitate a patient with severe volume depletion. Thereafter, further repair of the water deficit can be accomplished by administration of hypotonic fluids.

BIBLIOGRAPHY

1. Anderson RJ, Chung HM, Kluge R, et al: Hyponatremia: Prospective analysis of its epidemiology and the pathogenic role of vasopressin. Ann Intern Med 102:164–172, 1985.
2. Ayus JC, Arieff AI: Abnormalities of water metabolism in the elderly. Semin Nephrol 16:177–188, 1996.
3. Fried LF, Pavelsky PM: Hyponatremia and hypernatremia. Med Clin North Am 81:585–609, 1997.
4. Lauriat SM, Berl T: The hyponatremic patient: Practical focus on therapy. J Am Soc Nephrol 8:1599–1607, 1997.
5. Muloy AL, Carvana RJ: Hyponatremic emergencies. Med Clin North Am 79:155–168, 1995.
6. Pavelsky PM, Bhagrath R, Greenberg A: Hypernatremia in hospitalized patients. Ann Intern Med 124:197–203, 1996.

66. HYPOKALEMIA AND HYPERKALEMIA

Thomas C. Knauss, M.D.

1. Describe normal potassium homeostasis.
Total body potassium stores range between 3000 mmol and 4000 mmol. Approximately 98% of total body potassium is intracellular. Potassium absorption and excretion are regulated primarily by the gastrointestinal tract and the kidneys, respectively. Extracellular potassium concentration also depends critically on shifts of the cation between the intra- and extracellular pools. As a corollary, hypokalemia or hyperkalemia do not necessarily reflect total body potassium stores.

2. What factors can cause hypokalemia by shifting potassium into cells?
Increased insulin
Endogenous catecholamines
Beta-agonist drugs

3. What factors can cause hyperkalemia by shifting potassium out of cells?
Insulin deficiency (hyperglycemia)
Beta blockade
Metabolic acidosis
Hypertonicity
Muscle depolarizing agents such as succinylcholine
Exercise

4. What electrocardiographic changes occur in patients with hypokalemia?
Flattened T waves
Prominent U waves
ST segment depression

5. What electrocardiographic changes occur in patients with hyperkalemia?
• Initially, peaked, narrow T waves
• Subsequently, prolonged P waves, PR prolongation, QRS widening, and ST segment elevation or depression
• Eventually, cardiac standstill

6. What are some of the signs and symptoms of hypokalemia?
Paresthesias
Muscle weakness progressing to rhabdomyolysis
Paralytic ileus resulting in constipation

7. What are some of the signs and symptoms of hyperkalemia?
Paresthesias
Muscle weakness
Cardiac arrest

8. What is pseudohyperkalemia and what are some of its causes?
Pseudohyperkalemia is an elevated measured blood potassium level that does not reflect the true blood potassium value. It can be caused by release of potassium in the blood-drawing tube in patients with very high platelet counts. It also is seen when blood is drawn with prolonged tourniquet time or muscle clenching. If red blood cells hemolyze due to shaking of the blood-drawing tube, an artifactually elevated potassium level can result.

9. How can one determine if an elevated serum potassium level is an artifact due to thrombocytosis?

Blood can be drawn in a nonclotting tube using an anticoagulant such as heparin.

10. Does pseudohypokalemia also exist?

Yes. It can be seen in patients with leukemia and markedly elevated white blood cell counts. If blood drawn from such patients is not processed quickly, the white blood cells may reabsorb the potassium and artifactually lower the serum potassium concentration.

11. What two physiologic factors are needed to facilitate renal potassium secretion?

1. Adequate delivery of sodium to the distal nephron
2. Presence of aldosterone

12. What conditions would decrease distal delivery of volume and sodium?

1. Decreased glomerular filtration rate
2. Decreased distal tubular delivery of sodium

13. What conditions stimulate release of aldosterone?

Volume depletion or renal ischemia activate the renin-angiotensin system. Angiotensin II stimulates release of aldosterone from the zona fasciculata of the adrenal cortex. Hyperkalemia itself also directly stimulates aldosterone release from the adrenal gland.

14. How do diuretics cause renal potassium loss?

All diuretics cause sodium and volume loss leading to activation of the renin-angiotensin-aldosterone axis. They also increase distal delivery of volume and sodium to the distal portion of the nephron in which potassium is secreted.

15. What is the mechanism for hyperkalemia in patients with hyporeninemic hypoaldosteronism (type IV renal tubular acidosis)?

Decreased production of renin leads to decreased generation of angiotensin I and thus less angiotensin II. Less angiotensin II results in impaired stimulation of aldosterone synthesis and release and thus a defect in secretion of potassium. In addition, most of these patients have at least mild intrinsic renal scarring and end-organ resistance to aldosterone, further limiting potassium excretion.

16. What are some other causes of hypoaldosteronism?

Low aldosterone levels and hyperkalemia also can occur in the case of congenital adrenal aldosterone synthetic enzyme deficiencies, diffuse medical disease of the adrenals (Addison's disease), surgical removal of the adrenals, or acquired blockade of aldosterone synthesis.

17. What medication commonly used in hospitalized patients to prevent or treat clotting disorders partially blocks aldosterone synthesis?

Heparin. Even the low-dose heparin used for deep venous thrombosis prophylaxis can cause hyperkalemia, probably by impairing tubular responsiveness to aldosterone.

18. Which class of diuretics can result in hyperkalemia?

Potassium-sparing diuretics either competitively inhibit aldosterone (e.g., spironolactone) or block the sodium channel (e.g., amiloride or triamterene) and can result in hyperkalemia.

19. What is the treatment of choice for life-threatening hyperkalemia?

Intravenous calcium gluconate or calcium chloride will antagonize the cardiac effects of hyperkalemia. It works within 5 minutes with a duration of 30–60 minutes. This drug does not correct the hyperkalemia but stabilizes the cell membrane and provides time for more definitive therapy.

20. What other acute treatments can be used for management of severe hyperkalemia?

Administration of insulin causes potassium to shift into cells from the extracellular compartment. Glucose is given simultaneously to prevent hypoglycemia. These drugs can be given either by intravenous bolus or by constant infusion to achieve a more sustained effect. An alternative approach is to use beta-agonist drugs (inhaled or intravenous). This requires doses higher than those typically used for bronchodilator therapy and may cause cardiac irritability. If the patient is acidotic, infusion of sodium bicarbonate may have some beneficial effect. Potassium can be removed from the body with cation exchange resins (e.g, Kayexalate) given orally with a cathartic such as sorbitol. Ischemic lesions in the colon may complicate rectal use of this drug. If some renal function remains, loop diuretics and saline infusion may help. If renal function is minimal, dialysis may be required.

21. What is the value in measuring a urine potassium level?

Hypokalemia can develop with excessive losses in the urine or through extrarenal losses. In hypokalemic patients ingesting a "normal sodium" diet (> 100 mEq/day), the urine potassium should be less than 20 mEq/day with extrarenal potassium losses. In contrast, hypokalemic patients with active renal losses of potassium generally excrete more than 20 mEq of potassium daily.

22. What are common causes of extrarenal potassium loss?

The extra-renal conditions are categorized by those that cause:
- Acidosis (e.g., diarrhea, lower gastrointestinal fistulas)
- Alkalosis (diuretics, vomiting, nasogastric suction)
- Normal acid-base status (e.g., profuse sweating, cathartics)

BIBLIOGRAPHY

1. De Fronzo RA: Hyperkalemia and hyporeninemic hypoaldosteronism. Kidney Int 17:118–134, 1980.
2. Kassirer JP: Potassium. In Kassirer JP, Hricik DE, Cohen JJ (eds): Repairing Body Fluids: Principles and Practices. Philadelphia, W.B. Saunders, 1989, pp 46–72.
3. Rabelink TJ, Koomans HA, Hene RJ, Dourhout Mees EJ: Early and late adjustment to potassium loading in humans. Kidney Int 38:942–949, 1990.
4. Sterns RH, Cox M, Feig PU, Singer I: Internal potassium balance and the control of the plasma potassium concentration. Medicine 60:339–351, 1981.

67. HYPOCALCEMIA AND HYPERCALCEMIA

Lavinia A. Negrea, M.D.

1. What are the most common causes of hypocalcemia?
Chronic renal failure
Vitamin D deficiency
Hyperphosphatemia
Hypoalbuminemia (artifactual)
Hypomagnesemia
Hypoparathyroidism
Pseudohypoparathyroidism

2. What are the clinical manifestations of hypocalcemia?
Neuromuscular manifestations include tetany, muscle spasm, cramps, carpopedal spasm, irritability, and seizures. Cardiovascular manifestations include arrhythmias, hypotension, and congestive heart failure.

3. Describe the vitamin D–related causes of hypocalcemia.
- Vitamin D deficiency associated with inadequate exposure to ultraviolet light, poor dietary intake, or malabsorption
- Abnormalities of vitamin D metabolism: either reduced hydroxylation of vitamin D to 25-hydroxyvitamin D in chronic liver diseases or reduced hydroxylation of 25-hydroxyvitamin D to 1,25-dihydroxyvitamin D in renal failure
- Resistance to the actions of vitamin D (e.g., vitamin D–dependent rickets type I [deficiency of renal 1α-hydroxylase], and type II [molecular defects in the vitamin D receptor])

Anticonvulsant use is associated with decreased levels of 25-hydroxyvitamin D through an uncertain mechanism.

4. Explain how hypocalcemia can result from hyperphosphatemia.
Hyperphosphatemia can abruptly induce hypocalcemia through an increase in calcium × phosphorus product with subsequent spontaneous precipitation of calcium phosphate salts in soft tissues. This commonly occurs with excessive enteral or parenteral phosphate administration (during treatment of hypophosphatemia) or with massive release of intracellular phosphate in patients with tumor lysis syndrome or acute rhabdomyolysis.

5. What factors contribute to hypocalcemia in chronic renal failure?
The factors responsible for hypocalcemia in chronic renal failure are hyperphosphatemia, decreased levels of 1,25-dihydroxyvitamin D, and skeletal resistance to the calcemic action of parathyroid hormone (PTH).

6. How does hypoalbuminemia cause hypocalcemia?
Reduction in serum albumin will result in a reduction in the total serum calcium, while the ionized portion (the physiologically important one) remains normal. A reduction in albumin concentration of 1 gm/dl is associated with a fall in total serum calcium concentration of approximately 0.8 mg/dl.

7. How does hypomagnesemia cause hypocalcemia?
Hypomagnesemia is a common cause of functional hypoparathyroidism, resulting from impaired secretion of PTH and from resistance to the action of PTH on the end-organs.

8. What are some causes of hypoparathyroidism?

Idiopathic hypoparathyroidism may be due to absence of the parathyroid glands, branchial dysembryogenesis (DiGeorge syndrome) or a polyglandular autoimmune disorder. Acquired hypoparathyroidism can result from surgery, neck irradiation, or infiltrative disease (hemochromatosis, amyloidosis, thalassemia).

9. What is pseudohypoparathyroidism?

In contrast to hypoparathyroidism, in which the synthesis or secretion of hormone (PTH) is impaired, in pseudohypoparathyroidism target tissues are unresponsive to the actions of PTH. Chronic hypocalcemia in this disorder leads to hyperplastic parathyroid glands and increased levels of PTH.

10. Can hypocalcemia be associated with malignant disease?

Yes. Osteoblastic metastases, most commonly associated with cancer of the prostate or breast, can cause hypocalcemia as a consequence of accelerated bone formation. The osteoblastic lesions are usually evident on plain radiography, and the serum alkaline phosphatase is generally elevated.

11. What laboratory tests are helpful in the evaluation of hypocalcemia?

Once true hypocalcemia is confirmed, serum magnesium should be measured to exclude hypomagnesemia. If this is not present, measurement of intact PTH should help differentiate between hypoparathyroidism (low PTH) and conditions associated with elevated PTH levels, such as pseudohypoparathyroidism and vitamin D deficiency. Serum phosphorus is elevated in pseudohypoparathyroidism and decreased in vitamin D deficiency.

12. What is the treatment for acute symptomatic hypocalcemia?

Acute symptomatic hypocalcemia requires therapy with intravenous calcium. This can be given as 10–20 ml of calcium gluconate (90 mg Ca^{++} per 10-ml ampule), infused at no more than 2 ml/min. This should be repeated as needed to keep the patient free of symptoms.

13. What are the most common causes of hypercalcemia?

Hyperparathyroidism
Malignancy
Granulomatous diseases (e.g., sarcoidosis, tuberculosis)
Thyrotoxicosis
Immobilization
Vitamin D intoxication

14. What are the clinical manifestations of hypercalcemia?

Common clinical manifestations of hypercalcemia include lethargy, confusion, irritability, stupor, coma, anorexia, nausea, vomiting, constipation, polyuria, and hypertension.

15. Describe the mechanisms leading to hypercalcemia in primary hyperparathyroidism.

Primary hyperparathyroidism is the most common cause of hypercalcemia, accounting for over 50% of all cases. PTH causes hypercalcemia by stimulating osteoclastic bone resorption and by decreasing renal calcium excretion. PTH also increases 1,25-dihydroxyvitamin D synthesis, which leads to increased calcium absorption from the gut.

16. What is the association between hypercalcemia and malignancy?

Malignancy is the second most common cause of hypercalcemia. *Humoral hypercalcemia of malignancy* refers to hypercalcemia that results from secretion of PTH-related peptide (PTH-rP) by tumors including squamous cell carcinomas of the lung, head, or neck and renal cell carcinoma. PTH-rP mimics the actions of PTH by binding to the same receptor. Other tumors secrete either bone-resorbing cytokines (such as lymphotoxin, interleukin-1, and interleukin-6 in some patients with multiple myeloma) or 1,25-hydroxyvitamin D (certain lymphomas), with resultant hypercalcemia. In addition to these mechanisms, local osteolytic hypercalcemia is believed to result from resorption by cancer cells, either directly or by secreting osteoclast-activating factors such as prostaglandins.

17. What are the mechanisms responsible for hypercalcemia in granulomatous disorders?

Hypercalcemia in sarcoidosis, tuberculosis, and other granulomatous diseases results from increased production of 1,25-hydroxyvitamin D by the macrophage, a prominent constituent of the sarcoid granuloma.

18. How does thyrotoxicosis lead to hypercalcemia?

The thyroid hormones thyroxine and triiodothyronine stimulate osteoclastic bone resorption.

19. How does hypercalcemia occur during immobilization?

Immobilization regularly leads to accelerated bone resorption and hypercalcemia in individuals with high rates of bone turnover (e.g., adolescents, patients with Paget's disease). Hypercalcemia is preceded by hypercalciuria, which may lead to renal stones. Hypercalcemia promptly reverses with the resumption of normal weight bearing.

20. What medications have been associated with hypercalcemia?

The hypercalcemia of vitamin D intoxication usually develops in vitamin faddists and has gastrointestinal, renal, and skeletal components. Vitamin A intoxication, more commonly seen today with dermatologic or oncologic use of vitamin A analogues, causes hypercalcemia mediated by osteoclast-mediated bone resorption. Excessive oral ingestion of calcium-containing compounds can occasionally result in hypercalcemia. Thiazide diuretics can cause mild and usually transient hypercalcemia by increased renal calcium reabsorption.

21. What is the milk-alkali syndrome?

This syndrome consists of hypercalcemia, hyperphosphatemia, metabolic alkalosis, and renal failure. It was most commonly observed years ago in patients who were treated for peptic ulcer disease with large doses of calcium carbonate and milk. Renal failure was mediated by metastatic calcification of the kidney resulting from excessive calcium and phosphorus absorption. Renal failure accounted for impairment of bicarbonate excretion.

22. Which laboratory tests are helpful in the evaluation of hypercalcemia?

In patients with normal renal function, an elevated serum intact-PTH level will diagnose primary hyperparathyroidism in over 90% of cases. Serum phosphorus is usually decreased in PTH or PTH-rP–mediated hypercalcemias and elevated in 1,25-dihydroxyvitamin D–mediated hypercalcemias. Elevated serum levels of PTH-rP can be helpful in diagnosing hypercalcemia of malignancy. Elevated levels of 1,25-dihydroxyvitamin D are detected in patients with certain lymphomas and granulomatous diseases. Elevated serum levels of 25-hydroxyvitamin D suggest vitamin D intoxication.

23. What are the general therapeutic interventions in the management of hypercalcemia?

In symptomatic patients, general measures that facilitate urinary calcium excretion include administration of intravenous saline, followed by furosemide. The latter is calciuric and helps prevent pulmonary congestion. Patients with impaired renal function who are unable to excrete the sodium load may require hemodialysis against a low calcium bath.

24. What specific treatment should be employed in hypercalcemia associated with granulomatous disease?

Glucocorticoids are the mainstay of therapy. These agents inhibit the macrophage hydroxylation reaction and prompt a decrease in the circulating levels of 1,25-dihydroxyvitamin D.

25. What specific treatment should be employed in hypercalcemia of malignancy?

Hypercalcemia of malignancy almost always is associated with increased osteoclastic bone resorption. Osteoclast activity is best inhibited by drugs such as calcitonin (effect often transient) or biphosphonates (etidronate, pamidronate).

BIBLIOGRAPHY

1. Lebowitz MR, Moses AM: Hypocalcemia. Semin Nephrol 12:146–158, 1992.
2. Mallette LE: The hypercalcemias. Semin Nephrol 12:159–190, 1992.
3. Mundy GR, Reasner CA: Hypercalcemia. In Jacobson HR, Striker GE, Klahr S (eds): The Principles and Practice of Nephrology, 2nd ed. St. Louis, Mosby, 1995, pp 977–986.
4. Mundy GR, Reasner CA: Hypocalcemia. In Jacobson HR, Striker GE, Klahr S (eds): The Principles and Practice of Nephrology, 2nd ed. St. Louis, Mosby, 1995, pp 971–977.
5. Shane E: Hypercalcemia: Pathogenesis, clinical manifestations, differential diagnosis, and management. In Favus MJ (ed): Primer on the Metabolic Bone Diseases and Disorders of the Mineral Metabolism, 3rd ed. Philadelphia, Lippincott-Raven, 1996, pp 177–181.
6. Shane E: Hypocalcemia: Pathogenesis, differential diagnosis, and management. In Favus MJ (ed): Primer on the Metabolic Bone Diseases and Disorders of Mineral Metabolism, 3rd ed. Philadelphia, Lippincott-Raven, 1996, pp 217–219.

68. PHOSPHORUS

Chokchai Chareandee, M.D., and Donald E. Hricik, M.D.

1. What is the chemical relationship between phosphorus and phosphate?

Phosphorus circulates in serum as a constituent of both organic (i.e., phospholipids) and inorganic molecular species. The term *inorganic phosphate* refers to ionic species derived either from pyrophosphoric acid (a component of bone) or orthophosphoric acid (H_3PO_4). The equilibrium shown in the equation below is governed by pH. Within the pH range of blood, the concentrations of undissociated phosphoric acid and trivalent phosphate are extremely small.

$$H_3PO_4 \rightleftharpoons H^+ + H_2PO_4^- \rightleftharpoons H^+ + HPO_4^{2-} \rightleftharpoons H^+ + PO_4^{3-}$$

At the normal plasma pH of 7.4, the molar ratio of $H_2PO_4^-$ to HPO_4^{2-} is 1.4, and the average valence of the mixture is 1.8. Because variations in plasma pH alter the molar ratio and average valence, the milliequivalent is not a convenient term for expressing phosphate concentration. Instead, concentrations of inorganic phosphate are conventionally expressed in terms of elemental phosphorus. Each millimole of phosphate contains 31 mg of elemental phosphorus.

2. Describe normal phosphate homeostasis.

The average adult consumes 800–1200 mg of phosphate per day, largely in the form of meats, cereals, and dairy products. Approximately 80% of ingested phosphate is absorbed in the small bowel under the influence of vitamin D. About 40% of the dietary intake is excreted in the stool, suggesting that intestinal phosphate excretion contributes to phosphate balance. However, the kidney is primarily responsible for regulating serum phosphorus levels. Normally, 80–90% of the inorganic phosphate filtered through glomeruli is reabsorbed by the renal tubules. Tubular transport of phosphates is influenced by a number of hormones; parathyroid hormone and 1,25-dihydroxyvitamin D_3 decrease phosphate reabsorption, whereas growth hormone and thyroxine increase reabsorption.

Impairment of renal function per se is by far the most common underlying cause of phosphate retention. The distribution of phosphate within body compartments also is influenced by acid-base balance. Respiratory and metabolic alkalosis are accompanied by a fall in serum phosphorus that results from the intracellular migration of phosphate in exchange for organic acids destined to buffer the alkalosis. Considering the large number of factors that influence the internal distribution of phosphorus, it is clear that serum phosphorus levels, like serum levels of any predominantly intracellular ion, may not reflect total body stores.

3. What are the causes of phosphate depletion?

Three categories of disturbances may cause hypophosphatemia, phosphate depletion, or both:
1. Decreased intestinal absorption
    Prolonged, inadequate dietary intake
    Vitamin D deficiency
    Malabsorption
    Chronic administration of magnesium- or aluminum-containing antacids
2. Increased urinary losses
    Diuretic therapy
    Hyperparathyroidism
    Fanconi syndrome
    Vitamin D deficiency
    Diabetic ketoacidosis
    Volume expansion
        saline infusion
        aldosteronism

3. Transcellular redistribution
    Chronic alkalosis
    Increased insulin levels
        exogenous administration
        after glucose loads
        following refeeding after prolonged starvation
        hyperalimentation
In many cases, some combination of the above factors can be implicated in patients with hypophosphatemia. For example, in diabetic ketoacidosis, phosphate depletion can occur in part because of urinary losses related to osmotic diuresis and also because of transcellular shifts that occur after administration of insulin. In patients with severe burns, hypophosphatemia can result from excessive urinary losses during the diuresis that follows an initial period of fluid retention and from incorporation of phosphorus into new tissues during the healing phase.

4. What mechanisms account for hypophosphatemia in alcoholic patients?
Hypophosphatemia occurs in up to 50% of hospitalized patients with chronic alcoholism. A number of factors may play a role: poor dietary intake, diarrhea, vomiting, use of antacids, and the effects of refeeding. In addition, it has been speculated that alcoholic ketoacidosis may serve to decompose organic phosphates within cells and lead to urinary loss of phosphate analogous to that observed in diabetic ketoacidosis.

5. Grade the severity of hypophosphatemia.
In adults, normal serum concentration of phosphorus ranges from 2.5–4.5 mg/dl. **Moderate** hypophosphatemia (serum phosphorus concentration between 1.0 and 2.5 mg/dl) usually is not associated with signs or symptoms. By contrast, **severe** hypophosphatemia (concentration < 1.0 mg/dl) may be associated with serious clinical derangements. The most common causes of severe hypophosphatemia are:
 • Hyperalimentation
 • Nutritional recovery syndrome (refeeding)
 • Diabetic ketoacidosis
 • Alcoholism
 • Chronic respiratory alkalosis
 • Severe burns
 • Excessive use of phosphate-binding antacids

6. What are the serious consequences of hypophosphatemia?
Hematologic:
    Hemolysis
    Leukocyte dysfunction: impaired chemotaxis and phagocytosis
    Platelet dysfunction
Neuromuscular:
    Myalgias
    Weakness that may progress to paralysis
    Rhabdomyolysis
    Metabolic encephalopathy
Cardiac: decreased contractility or heart failure
Skeletal:
    Osteomalacia
    Bone pain
    Pathologic fractures

7. How is hypophosphatemia treated?
Potential side effects of intravenously administered phosphate include tetany (resulting from precipitation of calcium leading to hypocalcemia), metastatic soft tissue calcification, and hyper-

kalemia (if potassium is used). Thus, intravenous preparations should be given only to patients with severe, symptomatic hypophosphatemia. The apparent space of distribution for phosphorus varies widely among hypophosphatemic patients, and treatment is empiric. In normal individuals, intravenous administration of phosphorus in a dose of 7 mg/kg will raise the serum phosphorus concentration approximately 1 mg/dl. In hypophosphatemic patients, up to 23 mg/kg may be required to achieve the same increment. To be safe, the recommended initial dose of sodium phosphate or potassium phosphate is 2.5–5.0 mg/kg over 6 hours.

Oral phosphate salts are preferred for the treatment of moderate hypophosphatemia. Keep in mind that milk contains approximately 1 gm of phosphorus per liter. All of the commercially available oral phosphate salts can cause diarrhea. Regardless of the preparation used, the starting dose is 1–2 gm daily in three divided doses.

8. What are the causes of hyperphosphatemia?
Decreased renal excretion
   Acute or chronic renal failure
   Hypoparathyroidism, pseudohypoparathyroidism
   Acromegaly
Increased phosphate load
   Ingestion of phosphate salts
   Vitamin D intoxication
Transcellular redistribution
   Acidosis
   Insulin deficiency
   Increased catabolism
   Neoplasia, tumor lysis syndrome

9. What are the consequences of hyperphosphatemia?
Hypocalcemia and tetany
Metastatic soft tissue calcification
Secondary hyperparathyroidism

10. How is hyperphosphatemia treated?
Emergent management of severe hyperphosphatemia in patients without renal failure includes volume expansion and diuretic therapy. As in the emergency treatment of hyperkalemia, administration of glucose and insulin will cause a temporary fall in the serum phosphorus level. In patients with severe hyperphosphatemia and hypocalcemic tetany, intravenous administration of calcium and removal of phosphate by dialysis may be required. In patients with renal failure, treatment with phosphate-binding antacids usually is required to control hyperphosphatemia.

BIBLIOGRAPHY

1. Bushinsky DA: Disorders of phosphorus homeostasis. In Greenberg A (ed): Primer on Kidney Diseases, 2nd ed. San Diego, Academic Press, 1998, pp 111–113.
2. Hricik DE: Phosphate. In Kassirer JP, Hricik DE, Cohen JC (eds): Repairing Body Fluids: Principles and Practice. Philadelphia, W.B. Saunders, 1989, pp 100–117.
3. Hruska KA, Kovach KL: Phosphate balance and metabolism. In Jacobson HR, Striker GE, Klahr S (eds): The Principles and Practice of Nephrology, 2nd ed. St. Louis, Mosby, 1995, pp 986–992.
4. Knochel JP: Hypophosphatemia and rhabdomyolysis. Am J Med 92:445–447, 1992.
5. Knochel JP: The pathophysiology and clinic characteristics of severe hypophosphatemia. Arch Intern Med 137:203–220, 1977.
6. Lentz RD, Brown DM, Kjellstrand CM: Treatment of severe hypophosphatemia. Ann Intern Med 89:941–944, 1978.

69. MAGNESIUM

Chokchai Chareandee, M.D., and Donald E. Hricik, M.D.

1. Describe normal magnesium homeostasis.

Magnesium is predominantly an intracellular cation. Total body stores in the average adult are on the order of 2000 mEq (~ 60% in bone, ~ 40% in soft tissues). Less than 1% of total body magnesium is contained in extracellular fluid. Thus, the serum magnesium concentration may not be an accurate reflection of total body magnesium. Magnesium balance is influenced by gastrointestinal absorption and renal excretion. The cation is absorbed mainly in the proximal jejunum and ileum. Following glomerular filtration, approximately 15% of magnesium is absorbed by the proximal tubule, 70% by the cortical thick ascending limb of Henle, and 10% by the distal tubule. Less than 5% of the filtered load is excreted. Normally, serum magnesium concentration is maintained between 1.4 and 2.0 mEq/L.

2. How is magnesium deficiency diagnosed?

A serum magnesium concentration less than 1.4 mEq/L usually indicates some degree of total body magnesium depletion. In equivocal cases, magnesium depletion can be recognized by measuring the retention of magnesium after either an oral (50 mg elemental magnesium) or intravenous (2.4 mg/kg over 4 hours) load. Normal subjects excrete 80% of the magnesium in the urine within 24 hours. Magnesium-deficient patients excrete less than 40% of the load. This test is not valid and potentially dangerous in patients with renal impairment and is clearly not applicable to patients in whom magnesium depletion is a consequence of renal magnesium wasting.

3. What are the most common causes of hypomagnesemia?

Common Causes of Hypomagnesemia

DECREASED GASTROINTESTINAL ABSORPTION	INCREASED RENAL EXCRETION	INTERNAL REDISTRIBUTION
External losses	Acute ethanol consumption	Treatment of diabetic ketoacidosis
Vomiting or nasogastric suction	Osmotic diuresis	Refeeding after starvation
gastric suction	Saline diuresis	Intravenous glucose or amino acids
Biliary or intestinal	Primary hyperaldosteronism	Acute pancreatitis (through
fistula	Interstitial renal disease	saponification)
Diarrhea	Drugs: diuretics, aminoglycosides,	
Negative net absorption	amphotericin B, cisplatin, cyclo-	
Low oral intake	sporine, pentamidine, foscarnet	
Malabsorption	Renal tubular disorders: Bartter's	
Ileal bypass or	syndrome, Gitelman's syndrome	
resection	Primary renal magnesium wasting	

4. What are the major consequences of hypomagnesemia?
Electrolyte disturbances
  Hypocalcemia (tetany)
  Hypokalemia (weakness)
Cardiovascular effects
  Electrocardiogram (ECG) abnormalities (flattened T waves, prolonged PR and QT intervals, broadened QRS complexes)
  Enhanced digitalis toxicity

Neurologic

Apathy	Ataxia
Agitation	Asterixis
Nystagmus	Myoclonus
Vertigo	

5. How does magnesium depletion cause hypocalcemia and hypokalemia?

The pathogenesis of the hypocalcemia is complex. An acute fall in serum magnesium stimulates the synthesis of parathyroid hormone; however, prolonged magnesium depletion inhibits parathyroid hormone release. Experimental observations suggest a set-point error such that a lower than normal serum calcium level is needed to suppress parathyroid hormone release in the presence of hypomagnesemia. Magnesium deficiency is associated with renal potassium wasting. The exact mechanism is unknown but may be related to the fact that magnesium is an important cofactor in activating Na^+,K^+-ATPase, the enzyme that normally maintains a high concentration of potassium within cells.

6. What are the principles of treating hypomagnesemia?

Magnesium deficiency is treated by replacement with magnesium salts. The tempo and route of replacement are dictated by the presence or absence of symptoms and by assessment of ongoing losses. In the asymptomatic patient with mild hypomagnesemia, oral supplementation with subcathartic doses of a magnesium salt (e.g., magnesium oxide, 400 mg t.i.d.) is usually sufficient. Parenteral magnesium is preferred for the treatment of severe hypomagnesemia (serum level < 1.0 mEq/L) or in any symptomatic patient. Because magnesium equilibrates slowly with the intracellular compartment, therapy should generally be continued for at least 5 days.

7. What parenteral regimens are used for treating severe hypomagnesemia?

	Day 1	Days 2–5
Intramuscular route (50% $MgSO_4$ solution)	2 gm (16.3 mEq) every 4 hours	1 gm (8.1 mEq) every 6 hours
Intravenous route (50% $MgSO_4$ solution)	6 gm (49 mEq) in 1 L of 5% dextrose-water during the first 4 hours; then 6 gm every 8 hours	6 gm daily in divided doses

8. What are the causes of hypermagnesemia?

- Common
    - Acute renal failure
    - Chronic renal failure with excessive magnesium intake
    - Therapy of eclampsia
- Less common
    - Chronic renal failure without exogenous magnesium excess
    - Rectal administration of magnesium salts
- Uncommon or producing only mild hypermagnesemia
    - Addison's disease
    - Acute diabetic ketoacidosis
    - Hypothyroidism
    - Pituitary dwarfism
    - Lithium therapy
    - Milk-alkali syndrome

9. What are the consequences of hypermagnesemia?

Hypermagnesemia decreases impulse transmission across neuromuscular junctions and, when severe, can result in a curare-like effect leading to lethargy, somnolence, depression of deep tendon reflexes, and coma. Magnesium levels above 4–5 mEq/L have been associated with ECG changes (prolonged PR and QT intervals, broadened QRS complexes) and conduction disturbances such as complete heart block. The inhibition of neuromuscular transmission can also result in vasodilatation and severe hypotension.

10. What is the treatment for hypermagnesemia?

Because severe hypermagnesemia most often occurs in patients receiving magnesium salts, prevention can be accomplished by judicious use of these agents. Calcium acts as a direct antagonist to magnesium. Intravenous administration of 1 or 2 gm of calcium chloride or calcium gluconate over 5–10 minutes can transiently reverse potentially lethal depressions of cardiac conduction or neuromuscular function. As in the treatment of hyperkalemia, infusions of hypertonic glucose and insulin may produce a transient influx of magnesium into cells. If renal function is adequate, volume expansion with saline and simultaneous administration of a loop diuretic will promote urinary excretion of magnesium. Dialysis is very effective and is especially suitable in patients with severe hypermagnesemia and renal failure.

BIBLIOGRAPHY

1. Abbot LG, Rude RK: Clinical manifestations of magnesium deficiency. Miner Electrolyte Metab 19:314–322, 1993.
2. Al-Ghamdi SM, Cameron EC, Sutton RA: Magnesium deficiency: Pathophysiological and clinical overview. Am J Kidney Dis 24:737–752, 1994.
3. Ellison DH: Diuretics drugs and the treatment of edema: From clinic to bench and back again. Am J Kidney Dis 23:623–643, 1994.
4. Hricik DE: Magnesium: In Kassirer JP, Hricik DE, Cohen JJ (eds): Repairing Body Fluids: Principles and Practice. Philadelphia, W.B. Saunders, 1989, pp 118–129.
5. Quame GA: Renal magnesium handling: New insights into understanding old problems. Kidney Int 52:1180–1195, 1997.
6. Sutton RA, Sakhaee K: Magnesium balance and metabolism. In Jacobson HR, Striker GE, Klahr S (eds): The Principle and Practice of Nephrology, 2nd ed. St. Louis, Mosby, 1995, pp 1005–1008.

INDEX

Page numbers in **boldface type** indicate complete chapters.